Responding to Men in Crisis

Increasing rates of male suicide have been well documented, as have the problems of mental health provision for some minority male groups. However, the complex and often problematic position of men within the psychiatric system has seldom been discussed in a context informed by both feminism and the psychiatric survivor movement. Furthermore these issues appear to have been overlooked within the critical literature on men and masculinities. *Responding to Men in Crisis* addresses this difficulty by reviewing the relationship between postmodernity and madness and proposing a pluralist politics of complexity.

Key features include:

- postmodern and feminist critiques of Enlightenment rationality
- biographical studies of Nietzsche, Foucault, Antonin Artaud and Daniel Schreber tracing connections between masculinity, distress and madness, the formation of philosophy, and the construction of case history.
- an exploration of the political uses of experience
- various perspectives on the key issues of risk, 'dangerousness' and suicide
- a discussion of the tension between profeminist injunctions for men to explore personal issues, and critiques of therapeutic normalisation
- autobiographical fragments locating the writer's speaking position and illustrating issues around masculinity, distress, and bereavement.

This book is based on new work relating gendered assumptions about rationality to men's mental health. It offers the reader a theoretical exploration of a topically and politically sensitive issue and provides a valuable critique of postmodern theory and theorists. It is relevant to practitioners and activists in the mental health field, will be of interest to profeminist theorists, and is essential reading for academics and students of sociology and allied disciplines.

Brian Taylor worked as a community development worker between 1984 and 1993, mostly for one of the first user/survivor led MIND groups in England. He draws on a range of personal experience including involvements in informal crisis support, self-help therapy and anti-sexist men's groups, and has recently completed a PhD with the Department of Social Sciences and Humanities at the University of Bradford.

Responding to Men in Crisis

Masculinities, distress and the postmodern political landscape

Brian Taylor

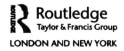

Routledge
Taylor & Francis Group

LONDON AND NEW YORK

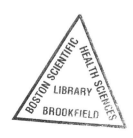

First published 2006
by Routledge
2 Park Square, Milton Park, Abingdon, Oxon, OX14 4RN

Simultaneously published in the USA and Canada
by Routledge
270 Madison Ave, New York NY 10016

Routledge is an imprint of the Taylor & Francis Group

Transferred to Digital Printing 2008

© 2006 Brian Taylor

Typeset in Goudy and Gill by BC Typesetting Ltd, Bristol

British Library Cataloguing in Publication Data
A catalogue record for this book is available from the British Library

Library of Congress Cataloging in Publication Data
A catalog record for this book has been requested

ISBN 0–415–34650–9

Publisher's Note
The publisher has gone to great lengths to ensure the quality of this
reprint but points out that some imperfections in the original
may be apparent

I have seen a world from which
my own reflection has been erased,
and have understood that all clouds
and symphonies are fragments of myself.

Rod Hartle

Contents

Preface

This book has emerged from an enjoyable eight-year period of part-time post-graduate study at the University of Bradford, which I embarked upon, in part, as an antidote to the daily reality of long-term health difficulties. My original intention was to undertake a research project that would identify distinctive issues arising in relation to men within the 'mental health' system, and responses to men's distress or madness. An exploratory study using discourse analytic methods looking at how four consultant psychiatrists talked about issues around masculinity, gender and the boundary between the personal and professional in their lives, exists as an MA dissertation, but deteriorating health levels meant that I was unable to contemplate doing any more 'fieldwork'. I therefore changed direction, and set off along a route signposted 'theory'. The resulting piece of work has been adapted from a PhD thesis, and is theoretical primarily in the sense of being about how we understand and talk about social and political realities. During the writing process I became increasingly convinced of the value and necessity of such reflection. In a field where assertions of scientific truth, political convenience and rigid moral certainty arguably do much harm, my priority has been to open up avenues of enquiry rather than to achieve analytical or conversational closure.

During what now feels like a rather distant 'past life', I had the great good fortune to work for the Rochdale MIND of the mid to late 1980s. As one of the first user/survivor-led voluntary organisations in England, the group advertised for, and employed, psychiatric survivor workers, and hosted some independent psychiatric survivor initiatives. As well as facilitating self-advocacy groups (including an enthusiastic user/survivor group that produced a video on employment issues) and supporting user-representatives in service planning, I helped set up an employment service, and an advocacy project that began to address the needs of Asian communities in a metropolitan district. I remain indebted to former colleagues there, and learned much from them. Regrettably circumstances have prevented me from keeping in touch as much as I'd have liked in recent years. Part III of the book, reviewing contemporary debates, revisits some of the questions we faced at that time.

I've also drawn upon several strands of experience in the private realm, some of which are referred to in the book. As a participant in, and beneficiary of, informal crisis support, initially in the context of community action in the early 1970s, I soon discovered that making meals and cups of tea, and 'being there' for someone, are not always enough to assuage extreme anguish. But psychiatry is no panacea either: we helped one friend recover after a very difficult stay in one of the large psychiatric hospitals. This kind of quite intensive human support – before, after or instead of spells in hospital – has often proved valuable, and may soon be needed more than ever. In another 'past life' I was involved in various more or less successful anti-sexist men's groups and self-help therapy networks, and have learned much from two very different life crises. Although any book like this is bound to have a lively subtext of stories, I have not wanted to recount other people's experiences, and have felt protective about several ongoing aspects of my own life that crucially inform my viewpoint. One of these has been so important that I feel it would justify my attempt to address these issues, even if I'd had no public involvement in the field.

A conversation with one of my former colleagues, who is a philosopher by training, revealed that we had opposite prejudices about language. He was prejudiced against 'common sense' for its tendency to exacerbate internalised oppression, while I was prejudiced against those who write about emancipation in terms that hardly anyone can understand. I was impressed by the strength of his conviction that there were no easy answers – that it may even be healthy to avoid rushing to resolve such differences – and decided to investigate the postmodern social theory he had become immersed in. I already had a strong interest in issues surrounding the telling of personal stories, and had begun to read some of the poststructuralist work on auto/biography. The whole question of stories, and who gets to tell them, is of course central to postmodernism, and not surprisingly has become a central theme in this book. If I appear to have become one of the people I used to be prejudiced against, this may be because I haven't had sufficient time or energy to undertake a radical revision of the thesis upon which the book is based. I hope the result is not too obscure. My intention, still, is to facilitate careful thought and discussion with practical and political consequences.

Brian Taylor
30 April 2005

Acknowledgements

No piece of work like this could be completed without the direct and indirect help of many people. I am particularly indebted to my PhD supervisors, two of whom found the whole thing so stressful that they left the country! Dr Barbara Fawcett (formerly Head of the Department of Social Sciences and Humanities at the University of Bradford, and now Professor of Social Work and Policy Studies at the University of Sydney) gave the project her enthusiastic support from its inception, and throughout its various twists and turns. Dr Pat Bracken (Clinical Director, West Cork Mental Health Service, Bantry, Co. Cork) contributed his philosophical/post-psychiatric perspective, and interest in Artaud. Dr Phil Thomas (Senior Research Fellow, Centre for Citizenship and Community Mental Health, at the School of Health Studies, University of Bradford) took over and nurtured the later stages of the writing process. Professor Jeff Hearn (University of Huddersfield and Swedish School of Economics, Helsinki) and Dr Ian Burkitt (Department of Social Sciences and Humanities, University of Bradford), who examined the thesis, also made helpful suggestions. Needless to say, all misunderstandings, errors, omissions and mysteries are entirely original. I am indebted to various friends who have taken a supportive interest, especially Peter Goode for sharing the journey and for being there when needed, and Chris Drinkwater for suggesting the possibility of embarkation, and commenting on the Nietzsche chapter. The poem that is the epigraph at the beginning of the book comes from an unpublished series entitled 'Fragments', written by Rod Hartle not long before his untimely death from a heart attack. Amanda Ravetz and the late Jill Fincham asked some helpful questions during the early stages. Lastly, I am indebted to Portia Fincham, advocate for the Marsh Marigold, Red Bartsia and Common Toad, with whom I've shared twenty-five years of life, love and laughter, for doing her own thing while I've been doing mine.

Part 1

Introduction

My present moment

As a thirty-something community worker, I seemed to be able to bring energy and optimism to bear upon difficult circumstances, and remember some very generous comments, such as 'There'd have to be something wrong with anyone who didn't like you, Brian' – this from a woman, of course. Twenty years on, I'm still optimistic at heart, and perhaps more contented than I was, but I have elicited some strikingly negative responses, from people ranging from pensioners in my local post office apparently afraid that I might be the next armed robber, to market traders suspecting me of shoplifting. Someone even thought I was 'shy'. So what has changed?

For more than ten years now, I've been sidelined by long-term health difficulties following a fairly devastating bereavement that was compounded by concurrent exposure to unavoidable and protracted conflict in two important non-domestic areas of my life. As emotional exhaustion gave way to a variety of physical symptoms I found myself living in a world of prematurely diminishing horizons, but hope of recovery made it difficult to acknowledge these as impairments, even fluctuating and invisible ones. I won't rehearse the boring detail, but thinking and writing happen in a space defended against encroaching tiredness. Physical discomfort, mixed with exhaustion, anger or despair, sometimes makes it difficult to appear friendly, or respond generously towards an uncomprehending, and increasingly fearful, world. When that happens, close friendship, with people who don't need explanations and aren't going to make snap 'essentialist' judgements about me, becomes a vital lifeline. Fortunately, however, I'm resilient and have much to celebrate.

Chapter 1

Approaching the politics of complexity

The historical analysis of this rancorous will to knowledge reveals that all knowledge rests upon injustice (that there is no right, not even in the act of knowing, to truth or a foundation for truth) and that the instinct for knowledge is malicious (something murderous, opposed to the happiness of mankind). . . . Where religions once demanded the sacrifice of bodies, knowledge now calls for experimentation on ourselves, calls us to the sacrifice of the subject of knowledge.

(Michel Foucault (1971/1984) endorsing Nietzsche)

The masculinity or maleness of knowledge remains unrecognised as such because there is no other knowledge with which it can be contrasted. Men take on the roles of neutral knowers, thinkers, and producers of thoughts, concepts, or ideas only because they have evacuated their own specific forms of corporeality and repressed all traces of their sexual specificity from the knowledges they produce.

(Grosz, 1993)

Orientation

Perhaps the best place for me to start is at the beginning. This project emerged during, and as part of, a long and difficult process of coming to terms with a sequence of transformative life experiences, a process, moreover, that left me with a strong impulse to write something of myself into its pages. I was not surprised, therefore, to find that experiences of ill-health and loss frequently inspire autobiographical writings, not only because they radically disrupt the life-course, destroying and reconstituting familiar worlds and cherished assumptions, but also, no doubt, because they simultaneously expose us to the disciplinary demands of a medicalising gaze that incites us to redescribe and regulate ourselves as objects of scientific and administrative knowledge. From the outset I have grappled with this impulse, not least because of an uncomfortable and apparently ineradicable tension between a postmodern and pro-feminist sense of the importance of speaking personally, of locating the position from which

I am writing, and of working, perhaps even therapeutically, to understand and change the 'selves' or subjectivities behind my various voices, and, on the other hand, a conflicting resistance against disclosure, motivated in part by a need to protect the scar-tissue at the site of some slowly healing wounds; but mainly because I am currently living a described life, and have also wanted to protect my personal story by forestalling uninvited diagnostic curiosity, whether lay or professional. Because a parallel tension, reflected in the paired epigraphs above, arguably underscores political understandings of men's 'distress' or 'madness', particularly where the quite postmodern process of self-advocacy is involved, there is an intimate connection between my recurrent personal dilemma and the primary project of the book – an exploration of the politics of male subjectivity in this most sensitive and particular context.[1] The tension between reconstructive self-disclosure and strategic self-protection forms an animating thread amongst and between the book's two major substantive sections, which focus respectively on a series of critical biographical studies, and on contemporary debates.

While grappling with the labyrinthine complexity of certain strands of personal experience, and the contradiction between different selves and voices competing to reinterpret them, I was impressed by some work that has been done within the diverse traditions of critical autobiography. Jackson's critical deconstructive enquiry into his own life story, read as a series of engagements with institutions shaped by hegemonic masculinity, in which he draws on post-structuralism and feminist life-history work in order to challenge conventional assumptions about the linear progress of a unified male subject, was particularly influential (Jackson, 1990). I also felt considerable affinity with Church's account of her involvements with 'consumer participation' and then with the Canadian psychiatric survivor movement, between the mid-1980s and early 1990s. During this same period I was doing similar work, and despite some significant differences between our speaking positions, found quite close parallels between our respective preoccupations and experiences (Church, 1995).[2]

Another, more theoretically orientated piece of writing that was resonant for me at a personal level was Price and Shildrick's 'Uncertain Thoughts on the Dis/abled Body' (1998). Despite the inclusion of a postmodern caution about standpoint epistemology and appeals to experience, here was a discussion con-testing the notion of the disabled body as a 'fixed object of concern', that clearly reflected the personal history of one of its authors, who had been living with the 'material instability' induced by the 'twists and turns' of ME for eight years.[3] They argue that instabilities and ambiguities necessarily constrain even our own 'fantasy of intimate knowledge', and limit the normative capacity of dis-ciplinary regimes – including those implicit in the terms of any emancipatory politics which preserves the modernist binary framework of unequal couplets such as disabled/able-bodied or mad/sane. Although deconstructive approaches are not without risk, they can move us towards 'an ethical openness to . . . dis-ruptive otherness both without and within', based on abandoning fantasies of control, accepting irreducible difference, and acknowledging that vulnerability is intrinsic to the condition of all of us, and not just to marginalised groups (Price and Shildrick, 1998 pp. 233, 243, 246). Clearly the challenges inherent in this proposition apply with particular force to men, and in Chapter 10 I discuss some theorisations of, and ways of working with, men's distress, that are consistent with this kind of thinking. Price and Shildrick's exploratory review had suggested further elements for the conceptual map I needed, and a sense of the direction from which I might approach some key issues that seemed to need clarification, such as how to understand and negotiate relationships between personal experience, political knowledge and entitlement to speak, and between adjacent political interests and arenas.

Encouraged by the work of Jackson and Church, whose far-reaching political analyses had been wrought from the experiential crucible of health crises, an insistent inner voice urged me to follow suit. Against this, however, a more editorially cautious voice reminded me that although my speaking position was perhaps more complex than either of theirs, my need to protect myself and others whose life-paths have crossed my own over the years meant that I would be unable to demonstrate this complexity adequately. Unlike Jackson, who as a high-flying male professional (albeit from working-class origins) had eventually encountered feminism, or Church, who as a (feminist) mental health professional had encountered the survivor movement, I was not sure that I'd ever succeeded in assembling a sufficiently monolithic primary identity around whose deconstruction I could develop a comparable narrative of painful disengagement, culminating in the gradual emergence of countervailing subjectivities. Although I don't believe it's possible for us to understand ourselves, or the positions we are called/or have chosen to occupy, with anything like complete clarity or finality, or that it's possible to circumvent all complicity in the effects of social inheritance, even the briefest review of my early life reminds me that it was characterised by a profound discomfort with an evolving sense of the implications of privilege. After reading Jackson, I was able to look more systematically at how my young life, not atypically I suspect, became an endless sequence of negotiations, compromises and evasions – survival manoeuvres within and against a harsh masculinist world that lured and coerced its recruits into adopting postures, wearing uniforms, and learning to think and speak in ways that seemed to signify a radical constriction of sensitivity and ethical concern. Like many young men, I felt such a strong sense of 'powerlessness within power' that it would be relatively easy for me now to emerge from autobiographical reflection with a sense that 'we' too are simply victims in all of this (Kaufman, 1994). For men who are users/survivors of psychiatry, most of whom have also experienced other forms of marginalisation, the appeal of constructing politicised identities based solely on victimhood should not be difficult to understand. The need for such men to negotiate a contradictory positioning in relation to hegemonic masculinity is a second core theme throughout.

In terms of the politics of 'mental health', I was mindful that, although my main purpose in writing an autobiographical strand would not be to attempt to legitimate my speaking position – I shall be arguing against uncritical assumptions about the authenticity of voices speaking from raw experience, and citing postmodern feminist arguments against a paradigm of victimhood – devoting too much space to my own experiences would distract attention from the systemic oppressions and intense personal challenges faced by most users and survivors of psychiatry.[4] I had been excited by the emergence of the survivor movement in the UK from the mid-1980s, and was involved in facilitating the development of self-advocacy initiatives, but, because I had managed to avoid hospitalisation when in crisis some years previously, was regarded as an 'ally' whose personal story was inadmissible in survivor circles. Perhaps one of my motivations for wanting to speak personally here, then, was to compensate for the ambivalence and discomfort I had felt about that experience of censorship? More recently, the difficulty of negotiating wildly fluctuating physical symptoms associated with emotional exhaustion and 'overwhelm',[5] has confirmed the relevance for me of Price and Shildrick's critique of the way in which the boundaries of politicised identity come to be policed within discourses of liberation (Price and Shildrick, 1998). I now feel much less apologetic about being something of an 'undecideable stranger' in worlds administered according to categories and counter-categories, which in terms of local political sensitivities means that I might want to declare myself to be neither 'mental health' professional nor psychiatric survivor.[6] My hope is that my work will be received on the basis of what I have to say, and perhaps what I have done, rather than how I might be politically labelled.

Considering the same editorial dilemma from a pro-feminist viewpoint, my somewhat different conclusion was that sharing accounts of men's experiences of bereavement, and of other kinds of distress that fall somewhere near the middle of a long and complex continuum, might help undermine the far-reaching discursive power of a historically prevalent binary distinction between presumed masculine rationality, long privileged as the engine of modernity, science and progress, and devalued 'feminine' unreason (Foucault, 1961/1971; Seidler, 1994).[7] Although much has been written either dismissing or defending 'soft men', whose identities appear, often perhaps somewhat unconsciously and chaotically, to subvert this divide, there seemed to be a dearth of first-hand accounts of the lives of men so described.[8] Since my younger self had memorably attracted such an attribution, both from his father and from feminist friends, I decided to flesh out some connections between this kind of orientation towards masculinity and experiences of distress, using a series of brief autobiographical sketches. Although these selective reconstructions would enable me to give a strategically partial picture of the tensions within my speaking position, their main purpose would be to suggest the possible value for men of taking a more detailed look at our individual – but historically contingent and socially formed – 'paths towards (and/or away from) masculinisation' as a way of illuminating the social construction of 'our' diverse selves, 'our' equally diverse experiences of distress or madness, the impact of our experiences on those around us, and possible routes to recovery.[9]

But the most significant outcome of my foray into the critical autobiographical literature was that it also led me away from myself in a quite unexpected direction. Initially prompted by the political difficulty of representing other men's experiences of crisis, I decided to turn to some history, and became so interested in the material that Part II of this book (Chapters 3 to 7) has been devoted to the lives and work of four prominent male figures. Since madness, and its exclusion, have arguably been an important theme in postmodern writings, two chapters are devoted to critical biographical studies of highly influential theorists, based on a rereading of secondary sources in the light of critical commentaries on masculinity. Foucault, who still exerts a profound influence on critiques of psychiatry and on the contemporary debates discussed in Part III of this book (Chapters 8 to 10), privileged Nietzsche among a pantheon of philosophers in whom madness appeared to accompany exalted lucidity (Bouchard, 1977). Prompted by feminist responses to postmodern social theory, I wanted to look at the lives of these men in order to evaluate both hegemonic masculinity and experiences of distress or madness as formative influences on the genealogy of postmodern thought – to undertake a biographical reading of theory (Warner, 1986). But my main concern was to explore the inter-relationships between masculinities, men's distress and the normalising function of psychiatry – to use biography to read social forces and patterns of oppression.

Chapters 3–7 point forwards towards a subsequent discussion (in Chapter 10) of social readings of biographical experience in the practices of self-advocacy and life-history research, where these apparently opposing directions of enquiry occur simultaneously. In Part II the tension between various contradictory imperatives towards disclosure and self-protection, which becomes particularly apparent in relation to masculinity and madness – informing valid resistance against therapeutic normalisation and more recently against a trend towards therapeutisation in Western culture, but also foreclosing transformative possibilities – remains an implicit theme (Rose, 1999). The dual positioning of men who experience distress is more explicitly discussed. Chapter 5 considers the life and work of Antonin Artaud, another figure exalted at the close of *Madness and Civilisation* (Foucault, 1961/1971), whose encounter with, and resistance against, psychiatry has informed postmodern commentaries. A fourth biographical chapter deals with the appropriation of biographical experience in the extensive body of case history constructed around the life of Daniel Schreber. The published material surrounding the lives of these two men effectively dramatises the interface between the politics of 'mental health' – what Coleman has called 'the politics of the madhouse' – and the politics of masculinity (Coleman, 1998). Not least since lived context has long been excluded from serious consideration as an aspect of the origins of social thought, genealogical approaches to biography are discussed further in Chapter 3 (Gane, 1993 pp. 14–16, citing Warner, 1986).

An introductory overview

Because I needed to rethink this political interface for personal reasons, I was already aware that it was a potentially sensitive area, but as I embarked upon writing, I began to wonder whether I was entering something of a Bermuda Triangle between adjoining literatures. Pro-feminist writers did not appear to be conversant with contemporary critiques of psychiatry, while few commentaries on men's 'mental health' seemed to engage meaningfully with feminism.[10] On either side there seemed to be a marked reluctance to enter a liminal zone characterised by complexity and contradiction. Pro-feminist commentators, necessarily focusing on violence and other practices of domination, may have felt wary about attending to male vulnerability, and appearing to recentre men as subjects and objects of discourse. Commentaries about men and 'mental health', on the other hand, have frequently conceptualised men's distress in terms of gender role theory, an approach which problematically implies a historical reciprocity between two complementary and unitary categories, men and women. Although some studies link 'mental disorder' in men with the erosion of patriarchal privilege in employment and marriage, gender role discourse effectively precludes constructive engagement with masculinity and has often been associated with the adoption of a petitioning stance, sometimes to the extent of constructing men as the new victims of women's political advances (Jorm, 1995; Morgan, 1987; Coyle and Morgan-Sykes, 1998).[11] Critics of this approach memorably point out that no one talks about 'race roles' (Messner, 1997; see also Whitehead, 2002). I shall be suggesting that postmodern social theory is potentially helpful in the work of facilitating dialogue between adjacent political interests.

The lack of interchange between critiques of hegemonic masculinity and of the dominant stories of masculinist psychiatry looked particularly surprising, given that the historical privileging of 'male' reason over 'female' emotion in Western culture has both shaped and been shaped by psychiatry and been identified as a defining characteristic of hegemonic masculinity – and given the close similarity of appeals to biological essentialism in relation to both masculinity and madness (Foucault, 1961/1971; Seidler, 1994). Unless such exchange takes place, hegemonic masculinist discourse about men will go unchallenged within developing discussions of men and 'mental health'. Claims that masculinity is innate, that men are biologically predisposed (by evolutionary inheritance, genetic constitution or hormones) towards aggression and dominance, have been countered, for instance, by highlighting the contradictory nature of findings about, and the complexity of linkages between, the presence of testosterone and aggressive or violent behaviour, and stressing that talk about 'man the hunter', a 'male sex drive' or 'female passivity' is just that – influential discourse in which cultural assumptions are presented as timeless truths.[12] Interestingly, the case for essential masculinity has been made in relation to a striking male majority among people given a diagnosis of high-functioning autism, and has been linked to claims that such men face discrimination in a world that 'stigmatises the extreme male brain' because of their inability to empathise (Baron-Cohen, 2003). A second pervasive discourse claims that men and masculinity are 'in crisis', not least because of advances made by women and the challenge of feminism. Far from being a unique response to contemporary social conditions, fears of feminisation and 'masculine retreat' have been shown to be a recurrent theme over the last two hundred years (Kimmel, 1987).[13]

Questions around what happens when 'we' men, who are not meant to cry or show vulnerability, and may well have had difficulty with intimacy of any kind, really do find ourselves 'in crisis' have mattered a great deal to me on a personal level – as a participant on both sides of informal crisis support – but they also matter, I believe, in terms of the kinds of communities we construct, and the kinds of support networks and crisis services we create. Relations between public and private worlds have long been a central concern within feminism, and are also, arguably, pivotal to the intrinsically personal politics of 'mental health'. Any attempt to understand the workings of psychiatry involves attending to this interface, which several decades of feminist scrutiny has rendered amenable to renegotiation and change. At times of crisis, innermost private worlds come into collision with the all too often uncomprehending faces of the public domain, and when the person in crisis is a man, a distinct set of issues and difficulties arise which have seldom been addressed without recourse to a modernist paradigm of medicalising knowledge. My reason for choosing to use the term 'in crisis' in the book title, rather than 'madness' or 'distress', was firstly that it created a non-medicalising space within which experiences like my own could be located on a continuum, while still sufficiently evoking an arena where key issues such as risk and fears of 'dangerousness' arise. It also enabled me to avoid headlining the discomfort many people feel with other people's use of language, and to flag up the tension between discussions about 'mental health' crises and discourses claiming that masculinity, or men in general, are in a state of crisis (e.g. Clare, 2001).

Over recent decades a considerable feminist literature has debated the impact of patriarchal culture and psychiatry on women. Issues particular to women in the 'mental health' system, such as concerns about violence and harassment, have recently been written into policy, but remain far from resolved on the ground (Department of Health, 2003b). Despite cautioning against an essentialist identification of insanity as feminine, some feminist commentators may have inadvertently encouraged a belief that women are intrinsically psychologically vulnerable and that madness is a 'female malady' (Showalter, 1987; Pilgrim and Rogers, 1993/1999). While acknowledging the strategic importance of second-wave feminist analyses of gender and 'mental disorder', Busfield criticises their almost exclusive focus on what happens to women. In a book entitled *Men, Women and Madness*, she argues that although this focus may have been strategically necessary given an over-representation of women in the system, and a long-standing silence in relation to their needs, men's experiences and treatment also need to be 'kept in the frame'. Acknowledging that men are prominent among some psychiatric populations, and that some groups of men have been subject to as much if not more coercion than women, she advocates moving towards 'more subtle and complex forms of analysis that fully allow for the presence of male . . . patients' (Busfield, 1996 pp. 6, 231–2).[14]

Prior also concludes that the assumption that women are universally over-represented in psychiatric statistics has been based on over-generalisation, and finds evidence for an increasing visibility of men (Prior, 1999). Boys are over-represented by between two and ten to one in apparently bio-medical disorders such as attention deficit hyperactivity disorder (ADHD) (Timimi, 2005 p. 149). Rising male suicide rates also indicate serious systemic problems that need to be carefully contextualised (see Chapter 9 below). There can, however, be little doubt that many of the most vulnerable users and survivors of psychiatry have been and continue to be women. Moreover, given that some diagnostic categories in which men predominate (notably substance abuse and antisocial personality disorder, neither of which are classified as 'mental illnesses' per se) have been linked, for various reasons, with violence, any shift in the overall gender balance of the psychiatric patient population is unlikely to favour claims about a new parity of victimhood for men. Clearly such statistics depend upon how distress is theorised, on the contingencies of social and diagnostic processes, and on how evidence is evaluated and presented within various discourses. Empirical evidence about changing patterns in the relationship between gender and distress or madness are summarised and evaluated elsewhere (Pilgrim and Rogers, 1993/1999; Rogers and Pilgrim, 2003; Prior, 1999; Archer and Lloyd, 2002). Given a tendency within non-feminist 'mental health' discourse to mask the gendered nature of 'dangerousness', and under-theorise the relationship between masculinity and suicide, there would, I believe, still be a pro-feminist case for looking carefully at these concerns even if men were under-represented as service-users.[15]

Despite the apparent reluctance of many writers to discuss men's distress and/ or madness, a variety of personal experiences had left me with a strong sense that some difficult issues needed to be addressed in a context informed by both feminism and the psychiatric survivor movement. Within academic discourse 'mental health' issues have tended to be consigned to a specialist literature, an isolated conceptual asylum among the bookshelves. Even in disciplines where silenced voices are routinely championed, survivor politics has either been subsumed within the category of disability and/or overlooked.[16] One of the clearest messages emanating from the survivor movement over the years, ironically, has been that users and survivors of psychiatry have not been listened to, either individually or collectively. There have been repeated claims that the needs of women, people from ethnic minorities, gay men and lesbians and disabled people have at best been poorly served by a psychiatric system dominated by men from a privileged social background.[17] The histories of mistreatment of gay men and African-Caribbean men, and increasing rates of male suicide, are well documented, but the position of men within the psychiatric system remains complex. There is arguably, therefore, a clear need to theorise and respond adequately to men's experiences of extreme distress, and not least to a small minority of male service users who may be threatening as well as vulnerable, while also challenging the pervasive and damaging stereotyping of psychiatric patients, especially those who happen to be young black men, as dangerous. A recent review of the mental health system in the UK referred explicitly to the social exclusion faced by service users, but has been dominated by a vigorously contested mental health bill apparently based upon a conflation between 'mental illness' and dangerousness.[18] Campaigners opposing potentially draconian proposals for increased coercion have called this the 'Dangerous Men Bill', thereby highlighting the need for good understandings of the kinds of contradictions that can arise at the interface between gender, 'mental health' and other oppressions.

Psychiatric ward environments are frequently experienced as depressing and unsafe places. A consultant has even admitted that under the impact of NHS reforms 'everyone in the community team, including himself, was at times sobbing' (Bruggen, 1997 pp. 167–8).[19] In response to demands for holistic and democratic alternatives to the hospital-centred biomedical model, an exploratory programme of user/survivor-led crisis houses has recently been established. Although some critics claim that such services only provide 'respite' and prevention, it has been argued that a prompt and flexible response can often avert a full-blown emergency and hospitalisation (Faulkner et al., 2000). Issues around working with men in such settings have still not been widely aired in the associated literature, but some years ago an article entitled 'So You're Thinking of Setting up a Crisis Service?' (Strickland, 1993) drew attention to the need for women-only space for women who have been abused by men. The text of the article was arranged around a photograph of a man, holding a large suitcase and a carrier bag of belongings, arriving at the front door of a house. There was no direct discussion of the significance of this figure, but his inscrutable and presumably potentially threatening presence effectively raised necessary questions in the minds of groups hoping to set up a crisis house.[20]

Rather than commenting on familiar debates about how changing political, cultural and material environments shape institutional responses to distress and madness, or on the development of crisis resolution services, my intention here is to step back from the moment of crisis and open up an area of discussion – around the significance of reimagining masculinities so as to revalue and reconstruct men's sense of selfhood and identity – that has been relatively neglected within critical 'mental health' circles. I make this move in the hope that pro-feminist political change, and cultural renewal involving the promotion of more egalitarian and supportive social practices among men, will prove relevant to crisis prevention of any kind.

Part III of the book looks at contemporary debates from a critical postmodern perspective in order to explore points of convergence and tension between discourses, taking account of the respective investments and sensibilities of various stakeholders. A discussion of politics and experience (Chapter 8) reviews postmodern appropriations of the imagery of 'schizophrenia' as a metaphor for cultural fragmentation, before discussing self-advocacy and political uses of experience, and the relationship between postmodernity, masculinities and distress. This is followed (in Chapter 9) by a consideration of issues around risk, 'dangerousness' and suicide. Chapter 10 looks at the tendency within critical discourse to pathologise masculinity, and explores the apparent contradiction between pro-feminist recommendations that 'we' men should turn to therapy in order to refashion ourselves, and Foucauldian critiques of normalisation and therapeutisation (Seidler, 1994; Rose, 1999). Rather than attempting a comprehensive overview of empirical material, these discussions explore postmodern philosophical perspectives that are potentially applicable across a wide range of local debates about ongoing attempts to secure genuinely anti-oppressive practice and establish environments that are safe and healing places for all who need them.

Descent and return?

> through suffering, Dumuzi awakens fully to the reverence of fear and to his mortality. He is wrenched from his regal, godlike state and made suddenly aware of time's limit and of human insecurity and death.
>
> (Perera, 1981)

During the long aftermath of a difficult bereavement I became fascinated by mythical stories of descent and return, and began to think about how contemporary retellings of these stories have reflected the cultural context within which we approach questions of gender and distress. The links between mythological underworlds and the notion of descent into 'madness' will hopefully soon become clear, but an interesting historical reference illustrating the archaeology of this metaphor came to hand at the time of writing. When a Roman town was founded, a round hole would be dug, and a stone, representing a gate to the underworld, would be placed at the bottom of it. At festivals held during the Romans' month of the dead, the stone would be removed so that angry infernal deities, known as Manes, could pass through. A cult was devoted to appeasing their anger, and like Dis, the Roman god of the underworld, whose name meant 'rich', they were also paradoxically named. 'Manes', apparently, was derived from an archaic word meaning 'good', and the connection with madness was through their mother, the fearsome female divinity, Mania (Guirand and

Pierre, 1953). Many centuries later, we find Mania transformed into a male figure adorning the gates of Bedlam (Porter, 1987). Stories of descent and return certainly seemed to resonate with the experiences of various men with whom I have shared travellers' tales of recovery from periods of distress following significant loss or emotional injury.

Because critics of the work of Robert Bly often characterise mythopoetic approaches as inherently anti-feminist – a view arguably rooted in the same masculinist prejudice against the imaginal realm that fuels discrimination against psychiatric patients – it is perhaps worth emphasising that many feminist psychotherapists and psychologists have deployed the mythological motif of descent into an underworld and subsequent renewal, and that Bly's particular orientation is not the inevitable product of his narrative method. Hillman's *The Myth of Analysis* (1972), for instance, which is in some ways comparable with the almost contemporaneous English version of Foucault's *Madness and Civilisation* (1961/1971), developed a mythopoetic critique of the misogyny of both late nineteenth-century classical scholarship and psychiatry, and inspired Rowan's anti-patriarchal therapeutic work (Rowan, 1987, 1997).[21] I shall not be proposing an uncritical endorsement (or totalising rejection) of psychotherapeutic responses to distress or 'madness', however, and I approach recent therapeutically orientated appropriations of this remarkably archaic narrative tradition in a deconstructive spirit.

Although I'm still not sure why the mythology spoke to me so powerfully, the process of carefully locating individual loss within a panoramic framework of continuous cosmic renewal can provide a comforting sense that return, however circuitous, is ultimately inevitable. There is also a sense in which poetic and elliptical language protects profound injury from the emotionally clumsy scrutiny of reason, and can evoke that mysterious moving ground of existence, which many of us feel we glimpsed, for the first time, amidst the chaos of crisis (Barker *et al.*, 1999). I soon became aware, however, that something was missing from the stories to hand. I searched in vain for a male figure who negotiated a journey of grieving similar to my own, a counter-hero who was able to transmute the visceral and venomous intensity of its rages. Was there no male traveller who, after immersion in tears, entered a calm space of tender vulnerability, before returning with renewed awareness to the everyday world? Was there no male figure, torn apart by madness, who eventually found his way back to the embrace of a nurturing community? If cyclic experiences of descent, transformation, survival and return were represented as enacted by female characters, did this not reflect assumptions about gender and madness in Western culture?

Probably the most notable deployment of an underworld story in this context has been Phyllis Chesler's retelling of the myth of Demeter and Persephone in the introduction to *Women and Madness* (1972). This torrential radical feminist/anarchist indictment of patriarchal culture and psychiatry awakened feminist concerns about gender and 'mental health' some thirty years ago, and remains a landmark text. Finding the mythology of descent and return here is significant, therefore, and establishes its presence at a decisive moment in the literature (Chesler, 1972). Chesler presented the myth as a starkly drawn drama of gender oppression, in order to place women's 'madness' firmly in the context of women's subordination, and directed it with considerable rhetorical force against the political silences of its time.[22] The story, as she tells it, begins with a period of primordial bliss in which Demeter, the goddess of life, and her four daughters, live happily together, until one day their celebration of Persephone's first menstruation is interrupted by Hades. The 'middle-aged god of death' appears in his chariot, carries the young woman away, rapes her, and makes her his queen 'in the realm of non-being below the earth', thus committing 'the first act of violence earth's children had ever known'. Demeter's remaining daughters observe that the intruder is old enough to be Persephone's father, and Chesler comments 'perhaps he was: who else could he be?' Demeter rages and cries with grief, threatening to render the earth barren, until a deal is struck whereby her daughter is allowed to return for half the year, but has to stay in the underworld with Hades during the winter months.

For Chesler, both Demeter and Persephone embody earth-mother passivity, the sacrifice of women's selves to biology. They react rather than act, and demonstrate the denial of 'uniqueness, individuality, and cultural potency', which results when individual women are 'broken on the wheel of biological reproduction'. Her project was to show how modernist psychiatry reinforced their descendants' socially constructed passivity. Like Persephone, 'most women today are not bold, forceful, knowledgeable, physically strong, active, or sexually potent'. Such women's madness incorporates the meaning of the mythical sacrifice of the maiden for purposes of male renewal (Chesler, 1972 pp. xiv–xxiii, 22–30, 264). Chesler's analysis of a system in which most clinicians were men, and most of their patients women, used the then recently published work of the Brovermans, and developed the case for a gendered double standard of mental health (Broverman et al., 1970). The abduction of Persephone symbolised a prevalent structural dynamic, a dimension that had to be foregrounded if women's madness, and social and psychiatric responses to it, were to be understood.

By contrast, Chesler argued that Persephone's male counterparts, the divine male child and male adult hero, were defined in terms of their uniqueness and heroism.[23] What is immediately striking about the myth she uses, however, is the one-dimensional nature of the figure of Pluto, a menacing perpetrator, interested only in the pursuit of self-gratification and undiluted power, said to represent 'men in general', positioned as unambiguous oppressors in relation to a 'rape-incest model' of sexuality (Chesler, 1972 p. 30). Whereas this late Greek myth depicts the underworld as a place of utter negation where Persephone is held hostage, Goodison, for example, points out that equivalent female figures from the earlier Bronze Age went there of their own accord (Goodison, 1990). She invites readers to look at myths as specific products of their time in order to understand their constructed nature, and grasp the creative potential of contemporary remythologising. Thus the story of Demeter and Persephone might be adapted, and consulted for insights into a broader range of issues (Goodison, 1990).[24] Older versions of the underworld mythos, interweaving seasonal imagery from nature with allegories about human life, have circulated widely since *Women and Madness* was written, and like Chesler, various post-Jungian feminists have used them to elaborate on the progressive dilution of female cultural and religious imagery across the millennia. Seeing the underworld as a repository of long-dormant female power, they have introduced vivid and powerful goddess figures into the cultural debates of late modernity (Perera, 1981; Baring and Cashford, 1991; also Lloyd, 1984).

Perera's influential psychotherapeutic reading of 'The Descent of Inanna' also touches directly upon questions of 'mental health'. Here, the Queen of Heaven, who is less concerned with a fixed domain above the earth than with liminal and intermediate realms, with transitions and border crossings, decides to enter the underworld in order to attend the funeral of her sister's husband. But her sister, who happens to be Ereshkigal, Lady of the Great Place Below, becomes furious at her approach, and orders that the Queen of Heaven be judged, and progressively stripped of her regalia, at each of seven gates. When Inanna finally arrives, the grieving Ereshkigal kills her and hangs her corpse on a peg, where it turns into rotting meat. But after three days, a period familiar to us from the story of Christ, a prearranged rescue plan is set in motion. Enki, male god of waters and wisdom, creates two little mourners from the dirt under his fingernails. They slip unnoticed into the underworld and commiserate patiently with the raging, groaning Ereshkigal, who eventually hands back her sister's body. Once revived, Inanna can return, but must select a substitute to go down in her place. Seeing her consort, Dumuzi, enjoying himself on his throne, and oblivious to her suffering, she immediately nominates him. Thus the year-god is challenged to make the journey she has had to make, and to undergo the torments and humiliations she has undergone. Abducted by her demons, he must die so that creation can renew itself. Terrified by this ordeal, Dumuzi offers his tears and appeals to the solar god Utu to be transformed into a snake, in which guise he discovers that although life's forms are continually lost and renewed, nothing ultimately dies (Perera, 1981 pp. 81–6).

For Perera, this story of life-enhancing descent and return encodes an image of the rhythmic order of nature, and presents a paradigm for a form of psychological healing demanding active receptivity, a process of controlled regression to dark repressed levels and subsequent rebirth, understood in Jungian terms as engaging with 'the feminine' in men as well as women. The story also works as an allegory for initiation into magically archaic and transformative pre-verbal realms, modes of consciousness radically different from the intellectual secondary process levels privileged in Western culture, realms where we might be 'shaken to the core' by an experience of unity with nature and the cosmos. Finally, it is claimed that the relational dynamic symbolised by the dialogue between the returning goddess and her consort might engender 'a new model of equal and comradely relationship between woman and man'. Perera hopes that therapists will '"manage" or companion' such descents, but cautions that, like shamanic journeys, deeper forms of descent entail real peril, and that some will 'fall beyond the therapist's capacity . . . into the unseen crevasses of psychotic episodes'. This, of course, raises questions about the intrusion of professional discourse into lifeworlds, about the medicalisation of distress, and about the boundaries between psychotherapy and psychiatry (Perera, 1981 pp. 13–15, 50).[25]

Despite these reservations, I found this five thousand-year-old story powerfully evocative of what can happen during intense bereavement, and I could readily identify with the dark fury of Ereshkigal. I was also pleased to find a much less bleak positioning of male characters. Indeed, the figure of Enki, Lord of the Earth, a bisexual god of water and wisdom who lives in the abyss and rules the flow of rivers and seas, is so helpful that Perera proposes him as patron of therapists.[26] In this telling of the myth, however, it is still a female figure who demonstrates exposure to vulnerability, and who by default symbolises the client. Much depends, then, on the reluctant Dumuzi, who according to Perera's case notes has 'a very poor relationship to his own vulnerable sensitivity and depths'. His initial unwillingness to accept an arrangement whereby he is contracted to spend half the year in the shades emphasises that willing descent, involving self-sacrifice and the painful renegotiation of identity, was already regarded as the domain and perhaps the duty of women.[27] Perera argues that until recently most men have simply not needed to face their own repressed depths. Once freed from childhood, their identification with the ideals of the culture has been supported, and they have felt no dissonance with the world. As the heroic ego ideal has been found inadequate, however, men are increasingly being forced to confront 'repressed instinct and image patterns'. Male flight into passivity or aloofness betrays an increasing need to descend, and relate to the 'inner feminine' (Perera, 1981 pp. 84, 102).

Whereas early goddess mythology symbolises the organic unity of life, and shows a young goddess undertaking an initiatory journey in which she 'opens her ear' to the hidden dimension of the underworld, feminist historians of a present and pervasive desacralisation of nature argue that patriarchal mythology increasingly split life into 'light' and 'dark' aspects, portraying the latter as fearful, absolute and geographically remote. No longer could death, or loss of any kind, be seen as a transformative passage into a new cycle of existence (Baring and Cashford, 1991 p. 282). Unlike Ereshkigal, the clenched and rigid figure of Pluto, constructed out of this long-standing masculinist fear of all that darkness signifies, is neither offered, nor presumably seen as deserving, unconditional sympathy. Even if it were offered, he seems singularly ill equipped to respond. Given that 'men's violences to known women', towards children, and against other men have been endemic within patriarchal cultures, and that few women actually murder their sisters, the implications of portraying a male figure such as Pluto as a rapist, and a female figure such as Ereshkigal as a murderess, are quite different.[28] Ereshkigal's actions seem safely symbolic. Given sufficient sympathy she is shown to be capable of relenting, whereupon her victim not only recovers, but turns out to have benefited from the indignity of her temporary death. Pluto's actions, by contrast, might well seem disturbingly real. He is represented as beyond reach or redemption, and although Persephone's abduction has been used as a metaphor for states of depression in which latent psychic growth depends upon a loss of innocence and exposure to overwhelming experience, such interpretations surely remain problematical.

Rather than serving as a constructive repository for material censored by masculinist reason, or as a cautionary tale, Pluto's story seems likely to reinforce the notion of male violence as an innate, anatomically 'hard wired', and thus irrevocable, instinctual legacy. Whitmer has described this kind of perspective as the 'violence mythos', and identified it as a key metanarrative of Western culture (Whitmer, 1997). Although for Chesler, Pluto, as perpetrator, may have usefully dramatised a major route by which women are driven towards distress or madness, his incorporation into discussions about 'mental health' inevitably summons up the spectre of the male monster who is not only menacing but 'mad'. Such a spectre, of course, periodically haunts public discourse where it crystallises into a damaging and unrepresentative stereotype of the psychiatric patient. Thus the mythology draws us towards a vortex of unspoken tensions reverberating beneath debates about men's distress or madness, but leaves the journey of men who are injured by male-on-male oppression and violence unportrayed.

Unfortunately Pluto is not alone among male mythological figures for whom the underworld becomes a site of material power. During his sojourn there, Aeneas meets the shade of his long-dead father, is instructed in the inevitability of the rise of Rome, and witnesses a parade of its future heroes. The story of Hercules, by contrast, is self-evidently satirical. Jungian analyst James Hillman describes him holding on to his muscular upper-worldly manner, wounding Hades in the shoulder, slaughtering cattle, wrestling the herdsman, choking and chaining Cerberus, and insisting on testing the reality of every phantom. Intent on plunder, his conspicuously bungled, almost slapstick descent, epitomises a masculine refusal to concede the necessity of death, even to 'die to metaphor'. Hillman cites Freud's identification of the origin of aggression in such a refusal, and draws attention to the proliferation of monuments to a heroic Herculean ego, which is unfamiliar with the language of dreams and 'does not know how to behave' in the underworld. The solution for Hercules, it seems, was 'to go mad, literally, in order to understand the underside of things' (Hillman, 1979 p. 110). As we shall see, Hillman is not alone in this description of 'madness' as a remedy for the excesses of masculinity. I therefore want to conclude this introductory chapter by looking at some apparently transformative male imagery, and at how such imagery might relate to men's experiences of crisis and recovery.

The mad god

> To evoke Dionysos scares up a flight of shadows.
>
> (Hillman, 1972)

> In the remotest depth of the European unconscious an inordinately black hollow has been made in which the most immoral impulses, the most shameful desires lie dormant. And as every man tries to climb up towards whiteness and light, the European has tried to repudiate this uncivilised self. . . . When European civilisation came into contact with the black world, with those savage peoples, everyone agreed: Those Negroes were the principle of evil.
>
> (Fanon, 1952/1986)

Bly talks about men's need for Katabasis, a consciously or unconsciously arranged process of descent into, and passage through, states of 'lowliness'. As well as historically failing to notice women's suffering or 'madness', men in Western culture fail to notice their own, and are only supposed to express grief at funerals. We don't have to concur with Bly's problematic model of deep masculinity, depicted in the hairy figure of the wild man, or share his perspective on gender issues, to sympathise with the direction of his claim that this has some implications for understanding men's experiences of depression. But this is a relentlessly individualising account, in which the social dimensions of forms of 'descent' such as addiction, depression and deprivation are eclipsed by a seductively psychologising rhetoric that comes close to justifying oppression for its healing potential.[29] In keeping with Bly's emphasis on young men's relations with their fathers and with older men, rather than with women, he proposes male descent as 'a way to move to the father's house'. Rowan has pointed out that for unreconstructed chauvinists, the notion of a wild man could appear to legitimise further aggression, and that Bly has little to say about how his allegorical figure relates to women (Bly, 1991 pp. 75, 88–90; Rowan, 1987). Given that Rowan was proposing the horned god as another model of masculinity, however, it is perhaps not surprising that he shares with Bly an interest in the Greek god Dionysos as a potentially transformative symbolic figure.

Stories about this god and the observances of his followers are often extravagant and vary considerably over time and between different cultures, but some of the material relates closely to the present discussion for at least two reasons (Allison, 2001 p. 21). According to the Cretans, Dionysos was the son of either Demeter or Persephone, and thus intimately related to the mythical genealogy of underworld deities. Even more intriguingly, he was known as the 'mad god'. In one version, subterranean Zeus (who in this guise was interchangeable with Pluto) came to his daughter Persephone in the form of a snake.[30] Persephone, who had been sitting in her cave weaving the threads of destiny, gave birth to the horned infant Dionysos, a mystic child who would come to share his father's divinity. This account draws upon an earlier symbolism of a creative and regenerative underworld reflecting the seasonal cycle of nature. Zeus, who refers back to the year-gods who as son-lovers of the goddess had to die to ensure the renewal of life, and Ploutos, whose name evokes the wealth of nature, were subsequently refashioned into the great father and his chthonic counterpart: the rigidly polarised icons of light and darkness characteristic of patriarchal culture. Interpretations of the madness of Dionysos are therefore doubly enmeshed in social construction, and need to be read in terms of changing contemporary perspectives on what was always a fluid and contested symbolic iconography (Kerenyi, 1976; Baring and Cashford, 1991 pp. 139–41, 317–18).

Bly introduces Dionysos at a point where he talks about men and grieving, and clearly regards the image of this god as potentially pivotal in processes of emotional healing. Once young boys enter 'the domination system', they lose their ability to cry easily, and some learn to become cruel. Rape and brutality are the work of 'unfinished men, dangerous in their inability to shudder'. For Bly, Dionysos is 'the shudderer, the one who could feel grief', and presides over processes in which young men reopen their hearts (Bly, 1991 pp. 84–5). Psychotherapeutically inclined commentators such as Bly and Rowan focus on processes of cathartic initiation and shamanic wounding in which 'the ecstasy that can come from tearing and being torn' distils new vision (Bly, 1991; Rowan, 1987). In doing so they invoke the reconstituted and redemptive Dionysos, who symbolised infinite life in the Orphic mysteries as 'the god who is destroyed, who disappears, who relinquishes life, and then is born again' (Guirand and Pierre, 1953 p. 160). Indeed Dionysos was sometimes known as Megapenthes, he of great suffering, in order to emphasise his capacity to survive ordeals. But the mythology also reflects a sense that grief and catharsis are unmasculine. We learn that as a child Dionysos changed his appearance and was raised as a girl, and Rowan argues that although he is phallic, 'there is no misogyny in his structure of consciousness because it is not divided from its own femininity' (Rowan, 1997 p. 259; Allison, 2001 p. 23).[31]

When proposing the horned god as a positive image of essential maleness in the service of a goddess, Rowan cites Starhawk's vision of a god who is gentle and tender yet also a hunter, a god whose dying represents a willingness to work with the pain of loss, and who embodies sexuality as a 'deep, holy, connecting power'. Starhawk argues that dramatic tragedy, which first arose out of the rites of Dionysos, was originally intended to facilitate the removal of emotional toxins, and constructs the god as representative of 'the undivided self', in which mind is not divided from body, nor spirit from flesh' (Rowan, 1987 pp. 85–7; Starhawk, 1979). In the context of men and 'mental health' this image inevitably recalls Laing's The Divided Self (1959/1965), which Connell visits for its 'vivid pictures of men's activities in the emotional interior of families' (Connell, 1995 p. 19). Rowan's recommendation of the 'mad' dancing god as an exemplar for men also draws on Hillman's Jungian reading, and calls for an embodied resolution of apparent contradictions, an ability to transcend hierarchy and move between worlds. Like Inanna, Dionysos dissolves dualisms, and because he is concerned with 'borderline' phenomena, with joining rather than separation, 'we cannot tell whether he is mad or sane, wild or sombre, sexual or psychic, male or female, conscious or unconscious' (Rowan, 1987, 1997 pp. 259–60; Hillman, 1972 pp. 258, 275). Rowan juxtaposes these fluid qualities against a generalised and universalised 'male ego', which he characterises as completely unable to admit vulnerability, and controversially, I hope, declares 'actually sick'. Thus worship of the 'mad god' becomes a remedy for a pandemic pathology of masculinity. Although Rowan is among those who feel that homophobia is not a good term for heterosexist prejudice, his uncritical use of terms such as 'neurotic and borderline *client*' and 'psychotic *patient*' (italics added) overlooks survivor critiques of medicalisation, and disappointingly contradicts both his own anti-sexist identification with Dionysian liminality and Hillman's deployment of the story of the 'mad' god in the context of a critique of Apollonian scientific psychology (Rowan, 1997 p. 173; Hillman, 1972).

Whatever conclusions we reach about the mythology, there can be no doubt about the extensive influence of Nietzsche, who decisively conjured the return of Dionysos into the Western psyche and whose personal tragedy makes this invocation poignant, upon subsequent interpreters of Dionysos, and upon the formative philosophers of postmodernism. For him Dionysos was 'the frenzy which circles round wherever there is conception and birth, and which in its wildness is always ready to thrust forward into destruction and death. It is life.' Dionysian enchantment led to exuberantly altered states during which an ecstatic reconciliation between people, and with nature, became possible 'as though the veil of *Maya* had been torn apart and there remained only shreds floating before the vision of mystical oneness'. At such times 'man [sic] . . . feels himself to be godlike' (Kerenyi, 1976 pp. 134–5). 'No longer the *artist*, he has himself become *a work of art*' (Nietzsche, 1871/1956 pp. 23–4).

Male commentaries on the creative madness associated with Dionysos often seem to be identifying an alien condition, perilously balanced between descent, with implicit references to the wildness and trauma of childbirth, and ecstatic flight. It may be significant that the first use of the designation *mainomenos Dionysos*, 'mad Dionysos', is attributed to Homer, a shadowy figure who was interpreting older traditions for an aristocratic audience at a time when patriarchal power was becoming entrenched, and the symbolic demarcation between male deities controlling the heavens, and female deities banished to the earth, reflected a growing split between mind and body, spirituality and sexuality (Goodison, 1990). What drove Homer to reach for the label *mainomenos* was the god's apparent propensity to inspire madness in women, to turn them into *mainas*, raving women prone to violent rage. It was said that followers of Dionysos sacrificed animals by tearing them to pieces and eating them raw, in rites recalling the identification of archaic hunters with their prey. Dionysos was known as 'eater of raw flesh', and 'no single Greek god even approached

[him] in the horror of his epithets, which bear witness to a savagery that is absolutely without mercy' (Kerenyi, 1976 p. 85). Clearly, in view of concerns about the stereotype of the mad axeman, this aspect of the mad god's mythology is far from reassuring, but like those deemed mad today, he may well have been subject to gross misrepresentation.

We should perhaps ask why a cult emphasising sensuality should be assumed to have such an affinity with 'the emotional nature of woman' (Kerenyi, 1976 p. 130). Goodison finds a monstrous mythical figure in Hesiod, who (like Dionysos) was born in a cave, was half nymph and half snake, and ate raw flesh. Interpreting this in terms of the equation 'earth-cave-woman-snake-raw meat equals horror', she locates it in a context of mounting patriarchal distaste for the body, and anxieties about death and personal survival. Thus this most disturbing element in the portrayal of Dionysian madness, to which 'irrational' women were most susceptible, seems consistent with a particular set of historically identifiable masculine existential fears (Goodison, 1990 pp. 160–1).[32] Kerenyi was quick to medicalise the mythology, grouping the symbolism of wine and bull, woman and snake, into 'syndromes' of 'an acute Dionysian state', and criticising Otto for his failure to 'recognise the symptoms' of Nietzsche's pathology (Kerenyi, 1976 pp. 52, 132, xxv; Otto, 1933). Hillman, on the other hand, warns against literal readings of myth or ritual, and talks about the need to 'unbind' the story of Dionysos from fixed and frightening interpretations. Apparently horrible aspects of the mythology may even be especially effective in evoking 'the emotional, instinctual level of the psyche' (Hillman, 1972 pp. 277–81). Our most savage feelings might be the very ones we need to address in order to heal the emotional injuries associated with distress or madness, and forestall the eruption of violence.[33]

According to Allison, Dionysos was also known as 'the gentle one'. Since his adherents were mainly peasants or serfs, and women, for whom the cult's transgressive festivals offered an escape from poverty and tedium, he was clearly a danger to the patriarchal social order (Allison, 2001 p. 23). If Allison is right, there is a pleasing irony in the prospect of turning the imagery of a god once demonised by the ideologues of this order – presumably during an early 'crisis of masculinity' – towards subversive ends. This said, there are clear difficulties with mythopoetic approaches. Nietzsche cautioned against reducing the mythopoetic element in tragedy to a vehicle for rational strategy and characterisation (Allison, 2000 p. 75; Nietzsche, 1871/1956 p. 104). Mapping experience against mythology can become a reductively individualising and universalising exercise that gives simplistic ideas a spurious patina of authority, and can work to naturalise oppression by reinforcing the very dualism that many hope it will heal. Recent critiques of masculinity, for instance, alert us to the danger of over-emphasising male psychology at the expense of material practices (Petersen, 1998). As well as conflating woman, madness and nature, the European imagination has constructed a seething repository of racist associations between blackness, evil and the 'baser inclinations' (Fanon, 1952/1986 p. 190). Given a critical appreciation of the genealogy of hegemonic patriarchal thought, how-ever, this archive might continue to inform an open-ended restorying that challenges the major exclusionary processes of Western culture. Some interest-ing questions certainly arise, such as: To what extent can men's distress be regarded as counter-cultural, or even as a possible remedy for Herculean harm?

I shall be arguing that the compression of difficult experiences and convo-luted issues into simple public narratives is both a key feature of 'mental health' environments and debates, and a characteristic problem in postmodern politics, where different political dimensions and discourses continually inter-sect. Perhaps because contradiction can feel uncomfortable, and ambivalence irresponsible, there is a marked tendency to resort to generic terms, such as 'men', 'men in general', 'the masculine', 'wild man' or 'the male ego', which encourage essentialist understandings and over-generalisation. Once we turn away from contradiction, ambivalence, reflection and curiosity, we find our-selves entering a closed conceptual world of polarised qualities and rigidly opposing blocs, and facing the considerable perils of othering. In the next chapter I make the case for a critical postmodern framework – a politics of complexity capable of engaging with a variety of voices, understandings and interests, as well as with overarching patterns of oppression, and with the need to temporarily 'fix' and articulate collective positions while still addressing the sensitivity of emotional process, and fostering an open and flowing awareness not unlike that suggested in the liminal imagery of figures such as Inanna and Dionysos.

Disturbing normalities

On her 101st birthday my grandmother addressed a throng of about seventy people. Because I was very close to her, I identified intensely with her stories of hardship from another era. She'd seen Queen Victoria, and had been in service from the age of eleven. As a young woman she'd had all her teeth removed, with only whisky as an anaesthetic (this would have been in order to make some money), and then had to 'go back and cook a full course meal'. When her husband was ill she'd done night nursing as well as her daytime job, for four years, but when my mother was born had been unable to afford a doctor. From her I acquired a strong sense of social justice. At the age of ten, for example, I thought it outrageous that almost all of my primary school class were destined for grammar schools, while almost all of the 'B stream' in the adjoining room would be sent to the local 'secondary modern'. Nan's renunciation of the violence she'd experienced in childhood also made a deep impression on me.

With hindsight I'm impressed by my dad's resolute gentleness. Robins would come and perch on his hand. As a boy, he'd cried himself to sleep from the age of seven, in an orphanage where sadistic physical punishment was routine. One of his favourite sayings was 'it never did me any harm'. He'd wanted to work on the land but his family found him a job for life in the sunless basement of a Lombard Street bank, which in the 1930s counted as good fortune. During the war he survived the sinking of the *Lancastria*, having spent twelve hours in the water, surrounded by bodies. Although he rarely talked about the war, a facial expression would occasionally suggest the magnitude of its horror. As a young boy, I remember proudly showing him an Airfix model of a 'Stuka' bomber I'd assembled. He became visibly upset, and mum ushered him away.

Eventually I learned that these were the planes that had bombed the *Lancastria*, and then returned, dropping flares into the oily sea and strafing survivors with machine gun fire. He was sent back to France, and when hostilities ceased, took turns guarding 10,000 Waffen-S.S. prisoners-of-war, four miles from Belsen, where he saw huge piles of discarded clothing and number discs, and was told that the parade ground they were using was a mass grave.

I loved it when my mother played Chopin. She'd been one of the first small intake of women employed by Lloyd's Bank beyond the typing pool. Commuting to work during the blitz, and assessing bomb-damaged branches to see what could be salvaged, she'd also seen the human effects of bombing at close hand. When the war ended, she taught my father the job he returned to. Within two years, they were married, and she became a housewife. Within three, I was born.

Rereading some notes of a conversation I had with my grandmother when she was ninety-eight reminded me that I'd been investing in a somewhat nostalgic view of my family's past. On that occasion she told me about difficulties and conflicts in the early stages of both generations' married lives, described dad's condition after the war as 'shell-shock', and mum's quite protracted periods of illness around childbirth as 'more than her ordinary worries'. Although distress was not generally talked about, and any setback would be greeted with the wartime catchphrase 'carry on London', it had clearly been the women's job to conjure comfort out of chaos, keep the peace domestically, and 'cure' or rescue damaged men.

Chapter 2

Why postmodernism? Conceptualising the politics of complexity

> Genealogy turns the problem of knowledge into a problem about power and freedom: truth becomes a 'thing of this world . . . [that] induces regular effects of power'. . . . Genealogy thus introduces the problem of how, by becoming constituted as subjects, we come to be subjected within a configuration of practice. And therefore at the same time it introduces the politics of the *freedom* we also have to criticise those very practices.
>
> (Rajchman, 1985)

> During the past twenty years, the self-advocacy discourse has begun to generate its own discursive practices through survivor-led services. It is now possible to discern a clear alternative discourse relating to the phenomena of severe distress, non-rational behaviour and beliefs.
>
> (Wallcraft and Michaelson, 2001)

Poststructuralist and postmodern social theorists have had much to say about madness and its exclusion, and although their contributions have often included a problematic appropriation or romanticisation of 'schizophrenic' experience, some of their central concerns have been profoundly consistent with the politics of the madhouse. An intense interest in critiquing the influence of Enlightenment science, for instance, effectively extended analysis of the operations of power beyond the state and the economy, across domains such as 'mental health' (Nicholson, 1990). The work of Michel Foucault, in particular, which was informed by direct experience of distress, placed debate about the social origins of madness close to the heart of contemporary critical thought, developed a vocabulary of resistance against regulatory power, helped galvanise the anti-psychiatry movement, and continues to inspire critics of psychopathology. This chapter opens an exploration of the relevance of debates about the 'postmodern condition' for understandings of gender and 'mental health', and draws attention to the overlap between feminist and postmodern challenges to rationalist assumptions about who we are, and what we can know, noting the indebtedness of the latter to the former.[1] Because of a continuing need to theorise enduring formations of power, I shall be making the case for an explicitly social and critical postmodernism, and a corresponding politics of complexity, and have sought theoretical refuge among those variants of postmodern social theory that are being reconstructed in relation to challenges from feminism and other contemporary social movements (Nicholson and Seidman, 1995).

Given that diversity and instability are such defining features of post-modernity, it should come as no surprise to find that 'there is no one postmodern paradigm of social knowledge' (Seidman, 1994 p. 21). In order to avoid repetition of lumbering formulas such as 'poststructuralism and postmodernism', I will sometimes use the term postmodern inclusively as a generic term for post-Enlightenment cultural criticism and social theory. Such is the plurality of theoretical contributions subsumed within both poststructuralism and post-modernism, and the continual need for clarification and qualification of both terms, that the danger of conflation between them can perhaps be over-stated.[2] Although there is a potential danger of appropriation in such an approach, I suspect that this mainly arises in relation to the tendency of an unbounded post-modernism to lapse into hegemonic generalisation as a way of 'incorporating others through the language of crisis' (Ahmed, 1998 p. 6). Both Lyotard, who identifies the pretence of speaking for others as a key injustice, and Foucault, who once remarked that there is something shameful about speaking on behalf of others, seem fairly clear on this, and Seidman has argued that if the term 'postmodern' is to become a meaningful way of 'mobilising discontents . . . in the Western organisation of knowledge and culture', social postmodernism needs to ground its conceptual strategies in an inclusive politics of diversity (Seidler, 2001; Macey, 1995; Seidman, 1994 pp. 21, 121).

Within the 'mental health' field, the willingness of postmodern social theory to address complexity, uncertainty, ambiguity and contradiction makes it relevant for the development of democratising and pluralistic perspectives, and in particular for facilitating exchange across the boundaries between adjacent political interests and concerns, such as that between survivor critiques of psychiatric hegemony and pro-feminist critiques of patriarchal power. In particular, postmodernism invites us to look at truth claims as socially situated and legitimated stories. Bracken and Thomas draw an analogy between the position of anthropologists, who have had to come to terms with post-colonial challenges to the authority of Western academics writing about non-Western peoples, and the position of psychiatrists expecting to write about the lives of people experiencing distress and madness from an ostensibly value-free vantage point. Psychiatry must now take responsibility for the effects of its objectifying constructions of others as cases (Bracken and Thomas, forthcoming). Writing about a crisis of representation in ethnography, Clifford talks about indigenous discourse 'interrupting the privileged monotone of "scientific" representation'. What once seemed to be empirical interpretation now appears as just another level of allegory, 'no longer *the* story, but a story amongst other stories' (Clifford, 1986 pp. 103, 109). Likewise Plummer, writing about sexuality, observes 'stories of authority (given to us from on high by men in black frocks and white coats) . . .

fracturing in the face of *participant stories*', stories of essence . . . fracturing into '*stories of difference*, multiplicity and a plural universe', and 'stories of the categorically clear' displaced by '*stories of deconstruction*'. Late modernity is characterised by a proliferation of new kinds of stories (Plummer, 1995 pp. 133–4).

The tradition of self-advocacy, developed within the survivor movement, has emphasised the validity of accounts and understandings that have been comprehensively undermined, historically, by stereotypes fostered by the medical model of distress, and its pervasive labels such as 'psychotic', 'neurotic', 'schizophrenic' or 'manic' (Plumb, 1993 p. 177; also Campbell, 1989). Because of this legacy of devaluation and exclusion, self-advocacy has attended to the quality of the political process itself, in an attempt to ensure that individuals have the opportunity to develop informed understandings and self-definitions, and that groups can construct collective positions with great care. At least in respect of this painstaking acknowledgement of diverse views, and of contradictions between respective explanatory models – even sometimes at the expense of political focus – self-advocacy can be regarded as quintessentially postmodern. At this point, however, it is important to note that adopting a postmodern perspective by no means guarantees either democratic intent or democratic outcome. One of the key issues facing anyone wishing to put postmodern social theory into practice is the notoriously opaque style of much of the writing. In a field where many people experience difficulties with the processes of thinking and communicating – often because of the intrinsic difficulty of coming to terms with traumatic experience – and may also have difficulties with reading and writing for various reasons, this constitutes a formidable barrier against access to some potentially empowering and relevant ideas. Although this is a problem shared by other strands of social theory, postmodernism professes a particular concern for issues of power, difference and marginalisation, and would surely benefit from creative exchange with a wider constituency.[3] The intellectual momentum of postmodern debates seems to exacerbate a historical reluctance on the part of academics and professionals to engage with the discourse of service-users' movements (Beresford and Croft, 1998). Some contributions to the field even contrive to use Foucault while overlooking survivor writers and theorists.

My sense, though, is that such difficulties can be overcome. Seidman, for instance, repudiates the giddy obscurity of much postmodern writing and proposes that postmodern social critique should be socially relevant, pragmatic, specific and accountable (Seidman, 1994). Postmodernism, after all, fundamentally challenges a traditional masculinist view of the 'expert' as the remote and disembodied voice of objectivity, uniquely authorised to reveal underlying truths. Unless we clarify theoretical understandings it will be difficult to generate insights into emancipatory processes and facilitate engagement with some quite thorny issues (Parton, 2000; Bracken, 2002). Yet under some circumstances, such as when evoking experiences of 'madness' in ways that challenge the hegemony of reason and science, there may be a case for resorting to poetic forms of language that unsettle taken-for-granted processes of reading and writing (Rajchman, 1985 pp. 17–18). Obscurity may be an inevitable, even 'precious ingredient' of occulted histories awaiting reclamation (Lionnet, 1989 p. 4). We might also conclude that ceding the terrain of philosophical discourse to those in positions of relative power reinforces internalised oppression. Because there is no single postmodern paradigm of social knowledge, there can be no single solution to the question of how to write postmodern theory, but following Nietzsche's deconstruction of authority within texts, the prevailing tone tends to be pluralistic, dialogical, reflexive and provisional (Schrift, 1995). I have wanted to avoid imposing theoretical closure that might forestall participation in the construction of meaning, talk across others' theorisations, or short-circuit the dramatic tension between various kinds of stories, and have chosen to include something of myself in the text, partly to show something of its production. My intention has been to write in a way that facilitates dialogue between discourses, invites readers to reconsider familiar worlds, and creates a resource for thoughtful action.

Cultural prejudice against the imaginal realm appears to have ancient taproots, but was significantly invigorated during the Enlightenment period when the conceptual ground was being prepared for the advent of modernist psychology and psychiatry. Unconscious processes came to be seen as a 'waste bin of undigested sensations', and although Kant specifically described his 'field of dark ideas in man' as 'immeasurable', Bentham was suggesting a 'felicific calculus', and measurement began to take precedence (Hillman, 1972 pp. 175–6). This gendered marginalisation of emotion, poetry, metaphor, fantasy and vision has been widely regarded as integral to the social and material marginalisation of women, black people, lesbians and gay men, disabled people, and not least people deemed mad (Seidler, 1994). Haraway opens her feminist critique of technoscience with a reproduction of an oil painting based on an advertisement for a Hitachi Magnetic Resonance Imaging device. 'Immeasurable Results' by Lynn Randolph shows the draped body of the artist with her head inserted into this apparatus, while above her a picture-within-a-picture illustrates 'projected dreams and nightmares that remain immeasurable within the machine's information calculus'. Among these a red demon hammering on a skull echoes the pounding heard by the woman inside the MRI machine. The 'material grammar' of such machines is designed to exclude not only non-rational imaginings, but also any information about the social worlds in which its 'gender-and-race marked patients' live, feel and dream (Haraway, 1997). Positioned inside a huge machine, the service user's voice seems particularly unlikely to be heard.

Randolph's powerful symbolic image highlights, and works to undermine, the markedly gendered sociotechnical production processes of psychiatric research, and prompted me to think about the distinctive issues that might arise when the body of a male figure enters one of these gleaming machines. What kinds of projected dreams and nightmares, what field of dark ideas, what social realities,

might then haunt its instrument panels and monitor screens? At the most basic
level, we might expect this to depend upon who the male figure was. Magnetic
resonance imaging is one of the technologies currently being deployed in the
investigation of 'psychopathy'. In a documentary broadcast in December 2000,
Adrian Raine, a British neuroscientist working in California, announced that
we would see the first microchip brain implant within a decade. Warning us
that this would raise important moral and ethical questions about the treatment
of people diagnosed as having a 'severe personality disorder', and hitherto
regarded as 'untreatable', he posed the question 'Do we reshape them entirely,
make them a new person? Is it really right of society to go into that holy of
holies, go into a person's brain, their essence, and change the neural wiring
and structure?'[4] The programme opened with an authoritative-sounding male
voice-over intoning the following words accompanied by sinister music.

> They are dangerous, without conscience, and all around us. In Britain it is
> estimated that one in every two hundred of the population is psychopathic.
> The kind of harm that psychopaths can cause at home and in the work-
> place is deeply damaging and costly in every sense.
> (Adrian Raine, The Science of Crime, Channel 4, 17 December 2000)

The script was laced with terms such as 'public enemy number one' and
'monsters', and invited speculation about those who are 'still out there'. Raine
left little doubt that he would favour drastic intervention, and the concluding
commentary urged that unless psychopathy was eradicated 'one of the most
dangerous forces of our time will continue to plague society, and the answer
must lie in treatment'. Surgical intervention in the brain might polarise opinion,
but the cost of evasion would be too high.

Although the broadcast coincided with mounting concern over proposals to
incarcerate people in the UK on the basis of a diagnosis of personality disorder
alone, no space was given for the exploration of the complex matrix of issues
that arise in this context. There was no mention of gender or of 'race', for
instance, and no exploration of the possibility that the 'recidivists' and 'paedophiles' highlighted in the programme might have little in common with most
of the men who experience madness or mental distress. All of these groups
were being subsumed within the same institutional framework and public
safety rhetoric, already familiar from media coverage of instances involving
'dangerous madmen'.[5] Given the quite high incidence of male violence in our
communities, issues around risk and 'dangerousness' will continue to reverberate
within and around discussions about men in crisis, and we must expect tensions
between different interests. In an environment of both social and technical
complexity, the sensitivity of debates about psychopathy epitomises the need
to develop clear theoretical approaches, ways of thinking about practical
issues that facilitate dialogue. Effective resistance to the kinds of dystopian
agenda invoked in programmes like The Science of Crime will depend upon the

ability of a wide range of stakeholders to exchange insights and negotiate common ground around some difficult and contentious issues. Discussion of these concerns is continued in Chapter 9 below.

Towards critical postmodernism

Although the Enlightenment project undoubtedly delivered advances, both politically and in the fields of science and technology, even the most cursory review of twentieth-century history should reveal that some considerable shadows have irrevocably disturbed its promises of progress (Flax, 1990). Responding to developments such as the human genome project and genetic modification, Haraway talks about 'the capitalist commodification of the dance of life', and argues that 'dazzling promise has always been the underside of the deceptively sober prose of scientific rationality and modern progress' (Haraway, 1997 pp. 7, 41). When neuroscience promises to deliver a dream of purity, a world cleansed of the 'plaguing' dis-order of psychopathy, 'one of the most dangerous forces of our time', we must surely be concerned. The history of modernity has also been a history of exclusion, a history of the workhouse, the prison and the asylum. Bauman, who has pursued the unnerving insight that the holocaust is consistent with rationality, rather than a failure of its civilising process, an indicator of its normality, not its pathology, condenses this into the terse epitaph: 'modernity was a long march to prison' (Bauman, 1992 p. xvii; Beilharz, 2001 p. 236). Foucault expounds upon Bentham's design for a Panopticon, a prison whose inmates were isolated and subjected to unseen surveillance from a central tower, as paradigmatic of a new disciplinary technology with widespread application (Foucault, 1975/1977; Dreyfus and Rabinow, 1982). Compounding this insight, Hillman notes that, long before Freud, Bentham described the mind as 'a dynamic system, the source of whose dynamics lay in the mind's own pathology'. Thus it appears that the designer of the Panopticon had also paved the way for psychopathology, the science of those 'unseemly parts of the human mind' which he described as normally veiled by 'a sort of fig-leaves'. This ominous theoretical advance came in 1817, the year in which Esquirol gave the first clinical psychiatric lectures, elaborating upon the concept of 'hallucination'. Psychic events were now to be tested only for their outer 'reality'. Hillman laments that 'the demon and ghost are banished, but with them go the ancestor and the angel' (Hillman, 1972 pp. 131–4, citing Bowring, 1843/1962).

One of the ironies that repeatedly surfaces, however, is the temptation to conceptualise modernism and postmodernism themselves as radically opposed but internally coherent historical periods or philosophical systems. Our Western habit of dualistic thought is deeply ingrained, and in the face of what Hall has described as 'the massive complexification of the social', the desire to return to comforting simplicity is perhaps understandable (Grossberg, 1996 p. 147). Norris argues that Derrida has been grossly misrepresented in debates about deconstruction, which far from being a species of 'last-ditch irrationalism' is actually consistent with the Kantian tradition of enlightened critique. In his later work, Derrida questions the principle of reason and confronts its paradoxes, but does not reject it (Norris, 1987 pp. 169, 236; Derrida, 1983). Modernity, arguably, has always incorporated the seeds of its own deconstruction.[6] Bauman (1991 p. 272) envisages postmodernity as a collective developmental process representing 'modernity coming of age . . . coming to terms with its own impossibility; a self-monitoring modernity, one that consciously discards what it was once unconsciously doing'. This formulation effectively refutes Kant's pronouncement, some two hundred years earlier, that the Enlightenment was 'man's emergence from his self-incurred immaturity', an immaturity defined in terms of an 'inability to use one's understanding without the guidance of another' (Kant, 1992, cited in Bracken, 2002 p. 18). From the point of view of the politics of 'mental health' it is striking that in depicting a postmodernity of healthy reflexivity and relationship, Bauman resorts to the individualising discourse of psychotherapy. Modernity will psychoanalyse itself. He is clear, however, that the co-existence of overlapping and contradictory descriptions of the world should not be taken as signifying the end, discreditation or rejection of modernity'.[7]

What we do appear to have abandoned, according to postmodern theorists, is a belief either in the possibility of disinterested arbitration between truth claims according to universal principles or in the unimpeachable standards of over-arching higher-order stories, be they about inexorable technological advance (science), the inevitability of social progress (Marxism), the intrinsic bene-ficence of wealth creation (capitalism), or liberation through the progress of ideas themselves ('spirit'). As Lyotard memorably put it, postmodernity is char-acterised by 'incredulity toward metanarratives' (Lyotard, 1984).[8] Postmodern politics, therefore, correspondingly rejects 'the quest for a totalising general theory' based on 'one dimensional notions of domination and liberation', and looks beyond universalising visions for overturning the social order, preferring instead to think in terms of resistance and transformation (Seidman, 1994 pp. 127, 131; Halperin, 1995). Following Derrida, who insisted that such moves perpetuate the inherent limitations of binary logic, a consistent theme is the need to acknowledge complexity by creating spaces beyond a simple radi-cal reversal of values and positions (Howells, 1999). Lyotard's remarks about 'grand narratives of emancipation' came in the context of an appeal to his then fellow Marxists that they should not simply 'look round for another revo-lutionary subject to fill the vacated place of the industrial proletariat' (Lyotard, 1993, cited in Seidler, 2001 p. 130).[9] As well as cautioning against the 'intellec-tual blackmail' of being either 'for or against the Enlightenment', Foucault urges us to turn away from projects making global or radical claims, since attempts to break with contemporary reality and 'produce . . . overall pro-grammes for another society, another way of thinking', have 'led only to the return of the most dangerous traditions' (Rabinow, 1984/1991 pp. 39, 45–6).

His rejection of attempts 'to articulate the consciousness or voice of a people, a class, or a society' is well described as a post-revolutionary stance (Rajchman, 1985 p. 50).

Making the case for a Nietzschean perspectivism that multiplies points of view and 'avoids fixed and rigid posturings', Schrift comments that 'to be able to see the world with more and different eyes now appears to be a political necessity' for individuals whose social subordination results from 'traditional and/or essentialist judgements as to their diminished worth' (Schrift, 2000 p. 192). A characteristically postmodern political moment has occurred across oppositional movements mobilised around signs of unitary identity such as 'black', 'woman', 'gay' or 'disabled', as internal difference has inevitably demanded expression. In response to this crisis in minoritarian politics, queer theory has reconceptualised identity as 'open to conflicting and multiple meanings, and as always interlocking with categories of gender, race, class, and so on'. thereby enabling 'newly imagined composite, hybrid, or fluid identities', that facilitate coalition building (Nicholson and Seidman, 1995 p. 17). In postcolonial theory, Hall's analysis of the 'demise of the black subject', and of essentialist discourses of 'race', 'nation' and 'culture' has been influential. In the context of 'a multi-axial performative notion of power', Brah has signalled a need to go beyond claims that 'assert the primacy of this or that axis of differentiation over all others' (Hall, 1992; Rattansi, 1995; Brah, 1996 pp. 242, 246). Likewise, postmodern feminists have addressed questions arising from differences between women, by depicting gender as one strand in a multi-hued theoretical tapestry, and developing 'plural and complexly constructed conceptions of social identity' (Nicholson and Fraser, 1999 p. 114; Flax, 1990). I shall be arguing that this kind of postmodern political theorising has significant implications where the politics of masculinities and of 'mental health' intersect.

Feminist commentators have generated a major current of critical reflection on postmodern social theory, attributing the phenomena it describes to the dynamics of gender systems rather than to the binary logic of language and, for instance, pointing out that comparable critiques of authorship can be found earlier in women's modernist fiction (Flax, 1987; Stanley, 1992; Nicholson, 1990). Postmodern feminists have developed the theory in significant ways, however, not least by asserting that large-scale but non-foundational historical narratives are still necessary in order to grasp the pervasive and multi-faceted nature of male dominance (Fraser and Nicholson, 1994). Against mainstream postmodern declarations of the death of the subject, it has been argued that some conception of a core or continuing self remains vital for women and for people from marginalised groups, whose voices have only recently begun to be celebrated (Flax, 1990). Despite its androcentrism, many feminists have found postmodern philosophy rich in possibilities, and have also brought postmodern insights to bear upon feminist theory (Nicholson, 1990). Flax argues that a tendency within feminism to see gender as 'an opposition of inherently different beings', rather than as a social relation, has constrained understanding of powers and oppressions in particular contexts, and that feminist notions of selfhood, knowledge and truth are not congruent with a whole series of trans-historic claims – particularly those about the stability and coherence of an autonomous self and about transcendental objective reason, characteristic of Enlightenment philosophy. Postmodern theory constructively questions the reliance of social movements on ahistorical modernist conceptions that naturalise and essentialise identity, and challenges the assumption that oppositional politics confers privileged access to forms of truth and knowledge which are innocent of power (Flax, 1990 p. 54, 1992 p. 460; Nicholson and Seidman, 1995).

One way of encapsulating a necessary tension between the imperative of retaining an analytical focus on enduring and interlocking patterns of social oppression, while moving beyond the totalising modernist impulse towards once-and-for-all liberation, is to employ correspondingly compound terms such as critical postmodernism and critical deconstruction. Bracken develops a Foucauldian critique of the critical theory of Habermas and the Freudo-Marxists, whose hermeneutic reformulation of psychoanalysis treats the liberation of society from ideology and oppression as analogous to the liberation of patients from madness and neurosis. Such understandings of liberation imply a belief in the possibility of 'uncontaminated' or neutral reason, and that training and theoretical knowledge can equip some people to 'determine and remedy the distortions wrought by repression'. Foucault, by contrast, focuses on the productive capacity of power to constitute reality and subjectivity through rituals of truth (Bracken, 1995 pp. 3–7). In a field in which experience is systematically colonised by such rituals, issues of political ontology, the production of subjectivity by knowledge and power, becomes a primary concern, and one that should be no less assiduously attended to within any politics of liberation. Genealogy aims to show us when our own political positions, our visions of the good, are operating in the same register of 'political rationality' as those we presume to escape (Brown, 2000 pp. 213–14, citing Foucault). From a pro-feminist vantage point, however, Hearn notes that many malestream postmodern theorists fail to address either feminism or the category of men, as though this category itself might be 'presumed to vanish into fragments'. Where deconstructive approaches risk reducing the materiality of oppression to discourse or text, and where casting men as 'other' can be misused in order to dilute 'men's power, agency, and responsibility', critical theory is invoked as a means of affirming political orientation and intent (Hearn, 1998 pp. 790, 800). My feeling is that the term 'critical postmodernism' usefully invokes and holds the creative mutual suspicion between these contrasting perspectives, across its component elements.[10]

Postmodernism and madness

In subsequent chapters I discuss the appropriation of imagery of 'schizophrenia' by postmodern writers, but deconstructive thought, including the writings of both Nietzsche and Foucault, has itself attracted attributions of madness. One proponent of critical realism, for instance, dismisses Rorty's reading of post-modernism as 'a reductio ad absurdum of the "subjectivistic madness" of post-Cartesian philosophy' that in leaving us free only to redescribe the world 'presents psychosis as our true freedom' (Collier, 1994 pp. 99, 106).[11] It is worth noting here that many writers within or sympathetic to postmodernism also dismiss unbounded expressions of postmodernism as having a fairly tenuous connection with political reality, without recourse to such analogies. Bauman, for example, writes that the idea of language games has been adapted from Wittgenstein in such a way as to 'justify the elimination of all "tougher" extra-conversational constituents of social reality' (Bauman, 1992 p. 40). Hall feels that Lyotard and Baudrillard go 'right through the sound barrier' when they move from identifying contemporary trends to an uncritical celebration of them. He regards the discursive perspective as important, and agrees that 'the social operates *like* a language', but identifies a powerful tendency among post-modern writers to 'go all the way', and reduce everything to language (Grossberg, 1996 p. 146).

Against this, however, Rajchman believes that the potency of Foucault's analysis in fields such as 'mental health' derives from his de-realisation objects, a process which demonstrates the consequences of assuming them to be real in arbitrary and contingent ways, thereby opening up new possibilities for thought and action (Rajchman, 1985 p. 58). Writing as a translator of Derrida, Spivak insists that in the wake of structuralism, Foucault, Lacan and Derrida, set out 'precisely to question the privileging of language and . . . the notion that the best way to understand everything was to reduce it to sign systems'. For Derrida, 'the category of language embraces the categories of world and consciousness even as it is determined by them', so that text becomes 'the weave of knowing and not-knowing which is what knowing is'. This kind of understanding deepens the metaphoric reach of 'text', whilst insisting upon the unavailability of simple and unified solutions, to simple and unified rational agents (Landry and MacLean, 1996 pp. 302, 55).[12] Derrida's conception of deconstruction goes further than Kantian 'critique' because it 'interferes with solid structures' (Schrift, 1995 p. 20). Observing that the genome is both database and material substance, Haraway identifies this collapse of the modernist 'epistemological barrier between representation and the real' as characteristic of postmodernity (Haraway, 1997 p. 74). Within the 'mental health' field there have been attempts to develop notions of discourse that account for the materiality of psychological practices, and conceive of technologies of regulation as 'material, relational, and discursive'. Haraway's notion of the 'material grammar' of the Magnetic Resonance Imaging machine is a case in point (Burman et al., 1996 pp. 6, 197–8; Haraway, 1997 p. 1; Burman and Parker, 1993 p. 158). If we follow Foucault's insight that all acts of representation, all stories, all truth claims, are social acts, immersed in relations of power, questions about realism and language, about interpretation, accuracy and fidelity become ethical questions about the uses and abuses of power (Rajchman, 1985; Bracken and Thomas, forthcoming).

Harvey's post-Marxist account of the cultural implications of late capitalism suggests another way of thinking about intersections between 'world, language, and consciousness' in relation to personal crisis. He uses the notion of 'time–space compression' to conceptualise the effects of capital accumulation, technological change and imploding distance upon transformations in the postmodern 'structure of feeling'.[13] For Harvey, the intensity of the experience of time–space compression distinguishes the condition of postmodernity. When whole landscapes are destroyed 'in order to make way for the new', we respond with a sense of disorientation, foreboding, collapse and even, in some circumstances, terror (Gregory, 1994 pp. 410–13, citing Harvey, 1989; Harvey, 1990 pp. 426, 433). Harvey's economic determinism should not distract us from the potential relevance for a politics of wellbeing, of perspectives linking macro-processes with micro-processes of subjectivity (Said, 1978; Hall et al., 1992; Harvey, 1989 p. 240; Gregory, 1994 p. 412). What interests me here is both the possibility and the difficulty of thinking in more postmodern terms than Harvey does about personal crisis in the context of specific configurations of power. Any overwhelming compression of our subjective space and time by social forces beyond our control is likely to precipitate a personal crisis of representation.

When 'we' are 'in crisis', the pace and intensity of events tend to overwhelm our ability to think clearly and communicate the nature of our experiences, wishes and needs to other people. Because there are insistent demands to compress what are often unbearably complex personal stories into the confined and distorting language of formalised exchanges with the public world, self-advocacy becomes an urgent priority. But postmodern theory, for all its celebration of diversity, also questions the assumption that authors can unproblematically convey a uniquely personal perspective, and the concept of crisis of representation, which signals the micropolitics of who gets to control the terms and spaces within which speaking and writing take place, also highlights the open-ended, indeterminate and constructed nature of voices, authorship and texts (Haywood and Mac an Ghaill, 2003 p. 114; and Chapter 8 below). Although the realisation that, as Lionnet puts it in her discussion of Nietzsche, 'subjectivity (and writing) is always already filled with the voices of others' does have some paradoxically positive implications for self-expression, not least in valorising a sense of the plurality and complexity of selfhood, a worrying paradox remains in the proposition argued by Derrida against Foucault, that any quality in madness that radically challenges reason also necessarily subverts its own articulation in the realm of political rationality (Lionnet, 1989 p. 68; Derrida, 1967/1978).

Some elements of postmodern theory do seem unambiguously useful to critics of psychiatry, however. Bauman's analysis of the repressive features of a managerial modernity that seeks to 'exterminate ambivalence' in an obsessive pursuit of order has obvious resonance. He writes, for instance, that 'the other of order is the miasma of the indeterminate and unpredictable', and enumerates the tropes of this 'other of order' as 'undefinability, incoherence, incongruity, incompatibility, illogicality, irrationality, ambiguity, confusion, undecideability, ambivalence' (Bauman, 1991 p. 7). As well as looking very much like a checklist of the kinds of blemish which psychiatry has sought to erase in its mission to impose order upon the chaos of 'madness' and 'distress', this inventory of intolerance looks suspiciously masculine. Postmodern theorists consistently advocate an acceptance of ambiguity, hybridity, contradiction, even fallibility and, crucially, an ability to live with 'undecideable strangers'. Bauman also identifies an important positive dimension of postmodernity when he talks about the re-enchantment of the world. The postmodern world is 'one in which a mystery is no more a barely tolerated alien awaiting a deportation order', in which there is a growing acceptance of the incommensurable. Once again, science can no longer expect to be regarded as intrinsically emancipatory, nor claim legitimacy by setting itself above 'narrative knowledge', the merely anecdotal evidence of stories from experience, yarns, folk tales or myths told by less rational mortals. Scientific knowledge can now be approached as just another, albeit impressively tenacious and culturally dominant, fiction (Bauman, 1993 p. 33; and see Kuhn, 1962/1970; Feyerabend, 1975).

Various feminist accounts portray Western science as explicitly masculinist from the outset. Plumwood argues that the problem of 'western hyper-separation from nature' considerably pre-dates Descartes and the Enlightenment, and traces a long-term colonising process involving 'multiple interlocking oppressions and sites of separation, the denial of dependency, and the formation of an alienated, hyper-separated identity' (Plumwood, 1993 p. 73). Drawing upon this archaic Western philosophical tradition, the Cartesian 'dream of power' set the subject decisively above the object of his (sic) knowledge, a 'disembodied mind', res cogitans, above 'a mindless body' and over matter, res extensa (Plumwood, 1993, pp. 114–17). The male scientist was thereby rendered invisible by the very process that constituted him as rational, objective, active and powerful in relation to a passive and feminised nature. Since Bacon, modern science has been concerned with the potential power of its knowledge to control and dominate both nature and human nature (Lloyd, 1984).[14] Roszak discusses the influence of the Athenian atomists who imagined a world composed of, and explicable in terms of, indivisible, invariant and law-abiding particles, and cites feminist psychologists who draw an analogy between the classical atom and a stereotypically 'autonomous', 'separate', 'isolated', self-determining', 'rigid' and 'insensitive' male persona (Roszak, 2000 pp. 55–6).[15] Scheman gives a Freudian account of such a masculine self, establishing its authority in terms of disembodiment, and maintaining its unity by splitting off and 'dumping out of the self' various qualities defined as incompatible. These rejected elements are defined as wholly negative, and attributed to 'others' who can be stigmatised as different. The resulting 'paranoia' has been expressed both through oppression and through philosophical preoccupations reflecting the subject's inability to connect with its disowned physicality and sociability.[16] 'Madness', in this sense, is therefore inherent in Cartesian method (Scheman, 1996 pp. 210–11). Qualities thus erased from the realm of reason and science have often been constructed as explicitly female.

Plumwood argues that Platonic philosophy is organised around a hierarchical splitting between reason and nature, and that this division creates a defining fault-line that colours virtually every other topic, and has profound implications for the way in which gendered identity was understood.[17] The implications of this division of consciousness for attitudes towards men's 'mental health' are memorably illustrated by a passage from Plato's dialogues, in which Socrates, on his death bed, 'sends away the women' when they 'give way to undisciplined grief and fail to appreciate his reasoned approach to death'. It seems that Plato's difficulty was not so much with women as with behaviours regarded as feminine. Qualities such as disorder, emotion, amorality, gossip, incompetence and bodily desire represented a lower order of nature, set firmly below reason and excluded from the public sphere. Any softness or lack of control in men was to be eradicated by a militaristic education (Plumwood, 1993 pp. 81, 76). But while distress was inadmissible in men, certain kinds of madness were not. Plato distinguished between the 'infirmity' of emotional turmoil when passion distracted the mind, and 'divine frenzy which impels the soul through the pursuit of knowledge to an immortal joy'. This latter form of visionary madness became a gift, challenging convention and reminding the soul of its previous non-bodily contemplation of ideal forms. Such a 'growing of wings' anticipating flight into the exalted realm of the gods is echoed, surprisingly, in Nietzsche, and led Otto to talk about 'breakthrough' in relation to the 'mad' god Dionysos (Lloyd, 1984 pp. 19–20; Kerenyi, 1976 p. 134).[18]

While this validation of disembodied frenzy has interesting implications for current debates, the suppression of men's distress has obvious resonance with feminist critiques of scientific psychology and psychiatry where, it has been argued, white, middle-class men established norms by projecting their 'inferior' qualities of vulnerability, emotionality, lack of control and so forth on to 'others' (Hollway, 1989 pp. 124–5). If we accept that an identification of hegemonic masculinity with reason has enabled men to act as 'the protectors and gatekeepers for this dominant vision of modernity', and that traditions of public masculinity have shaped the masks of sobriety, neutrality and 'normality' habitually worn by the exponents of progress, then postmodernity must move in a feminist direction, and men of reason may have something to learn from men with direct experience of being in crisis (Seidler, 1994 p. 19). If postmodernism is about confronting, unravelling or transforming the Cartesian dream of power, it must challenge the position of 'men' as self-appointed gatekeepers of both modernity and postmodernity. This might entail men becoming facilitators and caretakers rather than lawmakers, or becoming reflexive observers of much more closely entwined 'natural' and 'social' worlds.

Key elements of postmodernism, such as its challenge to rationalist assumptions about objective knowledge, its affirmation of the fluidity and constitutive power of language, and its celebration of diverse subjective realities, make it potentially congruent with the concerns of the psychiatric survivor movement (Beresford and Croft, 1998). Foucault's concept of discourse has been used to conceptualise self-advocacy as a pluralist critique capable of replacing bio-medical psychopathology (Wallcraft and Michaelson, 2001). Hermeneutic phenomenology – a mode of enquiry that sidesteps the quest for ultimate foundations, and treats interpretation as tentative and partial – is advocated as a way of attending to problems of meaning rather than to an ostensibly objective realm of 'facts' (Bracken, 2002 p. 206). Some practitioners have used post-modern perspectives in order to deconstruct their former positions of relative power within disciplines such as psychiatry and psychology, and open up ethical spaces in which people's own explorations of experience are validated (Church, 1995; Parker et al., 1995; Bracken and Thomas, 2001, forthcoming). In the following chapters I suggest that critical postmodern perspectives might help us approach men's emotional wellbeing in a manner that is both warm-heartedly optimistic and critically aware of differences in 'our' positioning in relation to, and orientation towards, hegemonic patriarchal power.

The making of a 'soft man'

One freezing evening in the winter of 1968/9, I went with a friend to see Ingmar Bergman's film *So Close to Life*, which turned out to be set in a maternity ward. Because I was quite needle-phobic, and already woozy from a heavy cold, I decided I'd made the wrong decision, and got up to leave. As I did so, a group of about five women turned and looked at me, and one of them commented, 'Typical man'. I remember feeling indignant, and quite confused by this unfamiliar experience of objectification. Such moments would become more common, and usually elicit a defensive silence or petitioning reply – 'I'm not/We're not all like that', or 'We suffer too'. By the late-1970s the word 'feminism' had entered my vocabulary. I remember a woman friend in Manchester saying, quite pointedly, 'Soft men are no good to us you know.' She wanted to know whether I was assertive enough to confront other men's sexism.

I was being challenged to find a distinctive voice, to become more of a 'doer behind my deeds', but wasn't sure I was up to it. After all, I'd been 'soft' for a long time. The first word I'd spoken, apparently, was 'pretty'. Once my three-year-old omnipotence had been disrupted by some difficult events – a fall necessitated a trip to casualty, and mum returned home after a three-month absence with a new brother (to mention two) – my coping strategy was to become 'good': sensitive, quiet, caring, imaginative and later studious. Most photographs show a fixed smile, a defensive reflex that persisted well into adulthood. In the spring of 1954 I was photographed as a six-year old sheriff, peeping out from behind a rockery in the badlands of suburban Kent, nervously pointing a toy gun at the camera. There were also some mixed messages. Mum may have enjoyed fitting me out as a cowboy, but she'd really wanted a girl who would share her love of ballet.

My precocious sense of social justice included a marked aversion to regimentation. When consulted about which grammar school I wanted to go to, I expressed a strong preference for the only one that didn't demand membership of either the boy scouts or a cadet force. Adolescence was an excruciating non-event. In retrospect, I seem to have been unconsciously refusing masculinity at a hormonal level. Driving across Europe as a student in the late 1960s, my fresh-faced andro-gynous looks caused predictable confusion. A group of Italian customs officers, who wouldn't have seen a young man with hair as long as mine, struck up an animated debate about my gender. They seemed genuinely puzzled.

My evident softness also troubled my father. One day, in my late teens, he asked me to come round to the garage with him, where he confided that he'd like me, as his eldest son, to have his Sam Browne army belt. Suppressing a gut-wrenching jolt of emotion, I said, 'I won't be needing that.' His reply, which seemed to combine incomprehension, exasperation and contempt, was that 'If Gerry came back today, he'd cut through your lot like a knife through hot butter.' I protested that Gerry wasn't coming back, and that what we were facing now was the atomic bomb.

Soon after moving to the north of England, my distress erupted. I'd already helped some friends in crisis, and knew I was in a more fortunate position than many, but at twenty-five, I thought I'd reached the end of the road. I cried quite a lot, screamed rather dramatically, and returned from an unforgettable visionary experience to find our dog licking my cheek. I would have gone on, but my excesses were putting a strain on tolerant friends – so much so that a woman living in the house forcefully reminded me that I was disturbing her young daughter, and warned that if I didn't pull myself together they'd have to have me 'taken away'. Because, at that point, I was far more terrified of psychiatry than distress, and was in a safe environment, I somehow managed to slam on the brakes.

Looking back, it does seem likely that my distress had released some of the impacted terror I'd absorbed, as if by osmosis, as part of my emotional inheritance. It may, however, also have functioned as a dramatic diver-sion from the need to talk about what was going on, or not going on, in my curiously frozen life. And for that to have happened, someone would need to have been listening and reassuring me that what I was feeling was not that unusual. With hindsight (this was 1973) I have a vivid sense of my younger self's hunger for libertarian rhetoric, and of how available discourse moved me towards the undoubtedly powerful and benign, but perhaps premature, 'breakthrough' experiences of that time, and paradoxically restricted my perspective on what might have been possible.

In the years that followed, I stumbled upon co-counselling, and began using it to work things out systematically. Only when I'd done this for a while did intimate relationship eventually become a possibility. Although self-help therapy was not a panacea – there was a tendency to romanticise regression and overvalue post-cathartic euphoria – it did give me a space in which I could gradually reclaim my body, and in the process become a bit more 'useful'. If I'd known about it earlier, or had been living in a culture in which young men could ask for help, and non-threatening, sensitive, well-informed support was readily available, I probably wouldn't have felt the need to erupt so disturbingly in the first place.

Part II

Four biographical sketches

Chapter 3

Genealogy and biography

How we become who we are

> The process of unmasking comes from questioning the seeming inevitability of traditional masculinity.
>
> (Jackson, 1990)

> The conventional model of biography production is one which can be likened to the effect of a 'microscope': the more information about the subject you collect, the closer to the 'truth' – the whole picture – you get . . . a more appropriate and less scientific metaphor to describe my way of working is to see biography as a 'kaleidoscope': each time you look you see something rather different, composed certainly of the same elements, but in a new configuration.
>
> (Stanley, 1992)

Each of the four men who are the chosen subjects of a series of critical biographical discussions in the next four chapters came to cultural prominence having produced significant work deconstructing the hegemony of reason. All four at some stage in their lives experienced distress or madness, and three of them published critiques of psychiatry. All are also, to varying degrees, contradictory figures, not least insofar as their widely differing emancipatory impulses were mediated by an unavoidable immersion in, and response to, the patriarchal institutions of their times. As previously noted, Foucault continues to exert a profound influence on contemporary challenges to psychopathology, and on surrounding debates about subjectivity and identity. Since his contemporaries regarded his *Madness and Civilisation* (1961/1967) as autobiographically motivated, I wondered to what extent this eminent philosopher could be said to have written from direct experience. Foucault's enthusiasm for Nietzsche, the huge influence of Nietzsche's Dionysian philosophy on postmodernism, his descent into madness, and recent reclamations of Dionysos as a model of masculinity, made me equally curious about the biographical experience of his nineteenth-century philosophical forebear. Given Nietzsche's notorious deliberations on the 'death of God', and Foucault's thoroughgoing critique of professional power and the medical gaze, I was fascinated to learn that both men had been expected to follow in the professional footsteps of their fathers and grandfathers, and go into the church and into medicine, respectively. Clearly both were responding to a very traditional patriarchal inheritance. Two further biographical chapters consider the stories of Antonin Artaud and Daniel Paul Schreber, whose declamations against psychiatry reflected nightmarish experiences of asylum life, and to some extent prefigure self-advocacy.[1] The published material surrounding their lives is reconsidered for the considerable light it casts upon the interface between the politics of gender and 'mental health'. Since both Artaud and Foucault located themselves within an intellectual lineage stemming from Nietzsche, it seems appropriate to assess their contributions to postmodern understandings of gender and distress using an approach that draws on Nietzsche's genealogical conception of identity; and to discuss them in chronological order, before moving on to Daniel Schreber.

The theoretical parameters of critical biography are established by Jackson, who builds on previous feminist, gay and anti-sexist men's life history work, and the social forms of autobiography developed by black African-American women, and by Stanley in her adaptation of postmodern ideas to feminist auto/biography. Rather than embarking upon a realist reconstruction of a biographical subject – a search for a true self that attempts to provide a complete, 'factual', truthful and neutral account of a fixed past – postmodern critical auto/biography produces a commentary on the intersection between social forces and the contingencies of individual lives. Where conventional biography masks both the fictive project of constructing lives and the social location of the biographer, critical approaches interpret plural and potentially conflicting voices from a particular and politically conscious perspective. The following discussions are necessarily based upon re-viewing extant biographies in order to foreground themes that have been overlooked or under-analysed (Jackson, 1990; Stanley, 1992).

As previously noted, writings about the 'private' biographical experiences of male theorists have traditionally been regarded as having, at best, only the most marginal relevance to understanding the production of their public work (Gane, 1993). Writing about men's experiences of distress and madness, on the other hand, demands attention to a whole set of issues surrounding the reclamation of suppressed and colonised histories. In relation to the three male theorists in question – all of whom were uncompromising individualists who resisted categorisation – there is clearly a need to account for the co-existence of powerlessness and power, to balance due sensitivity where they experienced oppression, with a need to critically interpret men's various investments in hegemonic values and practices.[2] Exploration of this Janus-faced both/and critical orientation is a key theme linking these biographical essays with the chapters discussing contemporary debates in the 'mental health' field.

Four lives

Before collapsing into 'madness', and then quiet incoherence, for the last eleven years of his life, Friedrich Nietzsche suffered from persistent ill-health and periods of intense despair. Whether or not we accept the consensus that attributes this collapse to tertiary syphilis, his personal fate certainly casts a bitterly ironic light upon his earlier introduction of the 'mad god' Dionysos into mainstream Western philosophical discourse.[3] Although Nietzsche made frequent use of the notion and imagery of madness as a trope, he had little interest in writing about it as a personal or social issue, but many who have done so, including both Artaud and Foucault, acknowledge their indebtedness to him; indeed Foucault, shortly before his death, went as far as to describe himself as 'simply a Nietzschean' (cited by Callinicos, 1989 p. 68). Given Nietzsche's apparently enthusiastic conformity with the masculinist conventions of his day there is also considerable irony in the recent adoption of Dionysos as an anti-sexist exemplar. Many feminists have, nonetheless, found elements in his work valuable (e.g. Daly, 1984; Irigaray, 1987/1993; Lionnet, 1989; Butler, 1990; Grosz, 1994; Brown, 1995). Although the appropriation of Nietzsche's work by Nazi ideologists has made him perhaps the most controversial of all major Western philosophers, a libertarian and negativist strand in his thought has also appealed to many on the left (Ascheim, 1992). In particular, he is widely recognised as perhaps the most important precursor of postmodernism. Best and Kellner simply comment that he 'took apart the fundamental categories of Western philosophy in a trenchant critique, which provided the theoretical premises of many poststructuralist and postmodern critiques' (Best and Kellner, 1991 p. 22). If one of the key themes of postmodernism, in terms of its relevance to understandings of men's 'mental health', is a willingness to engage with contradiction, to move beyond 'good' and 'evil', beyond a world of stereotypical 'heroes' and 'villains', then the life, work and legacy of Nietzsche arguably provides some valuable food for thought.

Antonin Artaud was an actor, writer, dramatist and acclaimed theorist of the theatre, and probably the first high-profile cultural figure of the twentieth century to take a radical stand against psychiatry. Like Nietzsche, he experienced his most intense period of 'madness' late in a relatively short life, but managed to survive long enough afterwards to declaim a lonely manifesto, culminating in a crescendo of choreographed screaming while performing a play written and recorded for, but banned as 'inflammatory, obscene, and blasphemous' by French radio (Barber, 1993 p. 157). Artaud was no politician, however, and denounced psychiatry as an artist rather than as an activist. Like Nietzsche, he struggled with intense physical affliction as well as distress, and wrote in a style characterised by flamboyance and excess; but, unlike Nietzsche, he was extravagantly expressive in his life as well. Artaud experienced quite extreme hardship, and at one point would not have been readmitted to an asylum had France not been occupied, and had he not been homeless and accosting passers-by with the formula 'Monsieur, the world has done me much harm. You are part of the world, so you have harmed me. Please give me five francs' (Hayman, 1977 p. 1).

Michel Foucault has been described as 'one of the most catalytic social theorists' of the twentieth century (Gergen, 1999). The discrimination and prejudice he faced as a young gay man in the Paris of the 1940s and 1950s contributed to distress which drove him to self-harm and suicidal obsession during this period (Eribon, 1993). His first major work, an acclaimed critique of psychiatry as 'a monologue of reason about madness', traces the historical exclusion of insanity in the Age of Reason during what he evocatively calls the 'Great Confinement' (Foucault, 1961/1971 pp. xii–xiii). Foucault wrote from a somewhat complex position, however, having also worked and trained for a few years as a psychologist. His later insights into the workings of power remain a source of inspiration for critics and activists.

Daniel Paul Schreber had been a high court judge before collapsing into 'nervous illness' and enduring a prolonged period of hospitalisation, during which he wrote and published an autobiographical memoir challenging the psychiatric dismissal of his supernatural experiences. After Freud wrote a commentary on the memoir, Schreber's story became perhaps the most celebrated of all psychiatric and psychoanalytic 'case histories'. A fourth biographical chapter discusses this appropriation of biographical experience, and looks at how the traditions and tenets of masculinity appear to have shaped Schreber's experience, the treatment he received, and the incorporation of subsequent interpretations within disciplinary discourse.

The genealogy of selves

The concept of genealogy, as developed by Nietzsche and adapted by Foucault, signals a particular way of approaching knowledge, history and subjectivity, but in this context the term also evokes a more or less direct line of intellectual descent in which Artaud can be seen as a linking figure in a loose male lineage of deconstructive thinkers. Since both Nietzsche and Foucault were scornful of the project of conventional biography, I was pleased to find some qualified encouragement for the distinctive contribution of critical biography where Nietzsche first introduces us to genealogy. It seems that he embarked upon writing The Genealogy of Morals in order to challenge the moral tradition of Western philosophy as derived from Socrates' adaptation of the Delphic oracular injunction 'know thyself'. Responding to the Apollonian assertion that 'the unexamined life' is not worth living, Nietzsche insisted, with characteristic candour, that the examined lives of philosophers were not worth living either, since Western philosophers had never actually examined themselves. The book opens with the statement: 'We knowers are unknown to ourselves, and for a good reason: how can we ever hope to find what we have never looked for?'

Unless knowers examine their own substance they must remain strangers to themselves (White, 1990 pp. 11–12; Nietzsche, 1887/1956 p. 149).

Nietzsche did regard the work of some thinkers as 'an instinctive biography of their souls', however, and a propensity to move between intimate personal confession and philosophical argument has led some critics to treat his books as though they were (in Goethe's phrase) 'fragments of a great confession' (Stern, 1979 p. 36). His last work was an autobiography which, insofar as it extravagantly parodies some conventions of the genre (most notably that of authorial modesty), and ironically inverts the Christian paradigm of essential selfhood, might be regarded as a precursor of critical autobiography. This is a complex, layered, self-protectively idiosyncratic text that has been cited as evidence of incipient madness, but also described as a 'text of rupture and fragmentation', which challenges the idiosyncratic prejudices of its readers (Nietzsche, 1888/1979; Lionnet, 1989 p. 20).[4] Some critics have been attacked for psychologising Nietzsche's every thought 'to the point where the entire work is reduced to a monstrous solipsism'. Nietzsche himself, at one point, commented on the 'vulgarity' of minds that demand personal experience, replete with sores and suffering, as evidence for the truth of an opinion (Stern, 1979 pp. 35–6, 41). It is important, however, to distinguish between objections to the reduction of philosophy to effects of psychology, pathology and personal circumstance, and the vehement policing of any reference to biography at all, that is quite common in the literature. The latter suggests an entrenched masculinist reluctance to engage with the personal, or to expose the male knower to any critical attention that might disturb the social hierarchy upon which his philosophical privilege rests.

Nietzsche's work has been identified as signalling an eclipse in our faith in the representational accuracy of language, and directing attention 'away from *what* was said . . . towards a genealogical critique of *who* said what was said, and on what the *reasons* were which had given rise to what was said' (Schrift, 1995 p. 29). Foucault has suggested that Nietzsche's sense of the word 'psychology' lay in this identification of the interpreter as the origin of interpretation. But for Nietzsche, the question '*who* speaks?' needs to be answered not by naming a subject, but by undertaking 'a genealogical enquiry into the type of will to power (life-affirming or life-negating) that manifests itself in speech or interpretation'. In place of the notion of an authentic self, Foucault adopts the Nietzschean project of creatively constructing oneself (Schrift, 1995 pp. 29–31; Nietzsche, 1887/1956). Theorists such as Derrida and Foucault, who elaborate on Nietzsche's innovation, have influenced contemporary poststructuralist and postmodern perspectives on auto/biography and identity (Denzin, 1989; Jackson, 1990; Church, 1995). These, then, are the kinds of terms within which genealogical method endorses critical consideration of biography.

Foucault developed genealogy as a method for 'diagnosing and grasping the significance of *social* practices' derived from the human sciences, and used it to demonstrate the pervasive and formative nature of the power of disciplines such as psychology and psychiatry (Dreyfus and Rabinow, 1982 p. 103, italics added). The genealogist, in this sense, becomes 'a diagnostician who concentrates on the relations of power, knowledge, and the body in modern society', without recourse to 'fixed essences, underlying laws, or metaphysical finalities' (Dreyfus and Rabinow, 1982 pp. 105–6). Genealogy looks at the effects of domination, at the contingency of errors and accidents, and at the minute changes that cumulatively lead things to be the way they are. For Foucault, following Nietzsche, it maps the detail of surface practices in order to side-step a widespread cultural belief in deep causation, taking an ever higher perspective from which 'depth' is rendered visible, 'an absolutely superficial secret'. Thus it exposes 'a body totally imprinted by history, and the process of history's destruction of the body' (Foucault, 1967/1984 cited by Dreyfus and Rabinow, 1982 p. 107; Foucault, 1971/1984 p 83).[5] Whereas official history projects the identity of protagonists as solid and unified, Foucault's genealogy, again following Nietzsche, makes no assumptions about an individual (or collective) subject shaping the flow of events. Its unmaskings and self-unmaskings depict the identities of significant figures as dissipated and discontinuous, and Foucault talks about '"subjectivation" as process, and "self" as relation', rather than using 'subject' to refer to a person, or form of identity (Deleuze, 1990 p. 127, cited in Schrift, 1995 p. 33). For this reason biography has been described as 'a very un-Foucauldian topic'.

At the beginning of The Archaeology of Knowledge, Foucault memorably demands 'Do not ask who I am and do not ask me to remain the same. Leave it to our bureaucrats and our police to see that our papers are in order' (Foucault, 1972 p. 17; see also Dreyfus and Rabinow, 1982 p. 104). Quite unlike Nietzsche or Artaud, both of whom had a strong tendency to represent themselves in their work, Foucault wanted to write 'so as to have no face', and is criticised for appearing 'to do his best to have no . . . human feelings' (Rorty, 1996 p. 13). If this self-concealing style, developed in an environment in which he found it necessary to mask both his sexuality and distress history, arouses curiosity about who this shifting, multi-faceted and contradictory 'knower' might have been, it also underlines the necessity of addressing the politics of writing about the 'described' lives of those of us already subject to normalisation (Halperin, 1995 p. 136). Making use of biographical accounts is also potentially somewhat more problematical in relation to Foucault because the first biography was being researched only five years after his death. My feeling, however, is that genealogical critical biography enables us to locate lives and works within a social and political context, without subjecting them to further microscopic examination in pursuit of essential truths. It has been suggested that genealogy 'opens up the possibility of . . . putting the genealogist in question', and might, ironically, reveal in Foucault a 'persistent and substantial' genealogical self, somehow exceeding its various masks and moments, its disguises and negotiations (MacIntyre 1994 p. 295).[6] If we are to claim Nietzsche and Foucault as key figures in establishing critical postmodern perspectives, it seems appropriate to direct genealogical enquiry towards these apparently neutral un-founding fathers, in order to look at how they themselves were formed, and at the relationship between their biographical experiences and the conceptual resources they bequeathed us.

In a late interview, Foucault argues that because the self is 'not given up to us' we have to 'create ourselves as a work of art', and that new forms of knowledge arise out of the ceaseless re-creation of oneself and one's life (Rabinow, 1984/ 1991 p. 351). This kind of processual understanding of selfhood is an important theme linking the first three lives under consideration, and recurs in discussions about the nature of 'madness'. It helpfully restores a degree of agency without reinstating a completely stable and consistent self, but has been criticised for its aestheticism and romanticism. Callinicos, for example, somewhat dourly objects that most people's freedom to make their lives into a work of art is severely restricted by the need to sell their labour-power (Callinicos, 1989 p. 90).[7] Flax notes that such formulations exclude any consideration of important social relationships. As already noted, she also points out that suspicion of the notion of coherent selfhood has only arisen now that women and people in other previously excluded groups have begun to re-member themselves as agents and subjects, a privilege previously only granted to a few white men (Flax, 1990).

Users and survivors of the psychiatric system are, of course, one of the long-excluded groups now asserting both individual and collective subjecthood. Given the nature of experiences of 'distress' or 'madness', the kinds of treatment too often endured, the appropriation of biography as case history, and the cultural devaluation of 'mad' identities, reclamation of agency and the reconstruction of identity are particularly sensitive issues in this context. Foucault's critique of confessional practices has obvious resonance here, and in the discussion of Daniel Schreber (Chapter 7 below) critical attention is primarily directed towards the successive manifestations of power-knowledge that have engulfed his life story. Drawing upon her work as an analyst (with people diagnosed as 'borderline'), Flax argues for the notion of a 'core', as distinct from a 'unitary', self. As we shall see, however, her suggestion that those who advocate a decentred self are naïvely unaware of the cohesion that protects them from 'a terrifying slide into psychosis' cannot fairly be applied to Foucault (Flax, 1990 p. 218). While it may be useful to envisage multiple, discontinuous or contradictory selves when deconstructing power relations, there are good reasons to be cautious about understandings of genealogy in which the dissolution of selfhood or agency becomes normative. In the context of distress and madness we need to acknowledge perspectives from which it can appear vital to celebrate selves that are not just coherent but stubbornly persistent. In relation to men and masculinities, on the other hand, we need to retain a sense of agency in order to ensure accountability (Jackson, 1990).

When arguing that men's appropriation of the realm of the mind has resulted in an unrecognised masculinity or maleness of knowledge, Grosz refers to

Nietzsche's insight that knowledge is an unrecognised product of bodies (Grosz, 1993). Seidler associates an identification between masculinity and reason with the ideals of modernity, and spells out the implications of this tradition by arguing that 'as men, we learn to live a lie. We learn to live *as if* we are "rational agents" . . . as if our emotional lives do not exist, at least as far as the "public" world is concerned.' Again Nietzsche is named as one of the first dissident voices to have questioned the terms of modernity, and Foucault's *Madness and Civilisation* is recommended for its historical account of masculinity's denial of 'unreason' (Seidler, 1994 pp. 19–20, xii). These explorations attempt a biographical reading of the origins of their theoretical innovations.

Although all four men whose life stories are discussed below came from relatively privileged backgrounds, each also experienced significant exclusion, and their otherwise elevated status arguably serves to underline the social costs associated with experiencing intense distress. Their experiences also remind us that the intense emotional charge of distress or madness doesn't necessarily move men in a pro-feminist direction. As histories of the present (biographical readings of the social), these studies are intended to raise questions about the interconnection between codes of masculinity, the forms taken by men's distress, and the traditionally male-dominated regimes of disciplinary power. Although these men faced a fairly monolithic form of hegemonic masculinity, my hope is that an account of their lived experience might illuminate our own much more variegated landscape of both gender relations and 'mental health' services, in some interesting ways. These chapters are followed by an extended exploration of the politics of biographical experience. By circumventing the search for ultimate truths about the essential nature of unitary selves, or about men and madness, and by focusing on processes of social construction and oppression rather than simply on the minutiae of lived experience, I shall be arguing that deconstructive critical biography (social readings of biographical experience) might facilitate careful discussion of the subjectivity of men whose lives have been harmed by normalising description. The practical potential of this kind of non-psychologising and non-medicalising approach to subjectivity is considered in Chapter 10 below.

Changing men?

When my turn came to suggest a theme for a meeting of our anti-sexist men's group, I chose a colour healing exercise. This entailed getting into pairs, centring ourselves, and taking turns to visualise a colour and 'pass' it through the palms of our hands to the hands of another man, who would then say which colour he'd received.* We were quite surprised, perhaps a bit spooked, by the accuracy with which we all seemed to be picking up these delicate invisible transmissions. Some will, of course, dismiss this episode as an outbreak of unreason, a collective delusion, but my understanding of what happened is that our success reflected the high level of trust we had painstakingly established by doing a lot of careful talking. In other words, it was not a trick, or a technical skill, that could be taken off the shelf and made to work in any circumstances.

But were such activities nothing more than cosy, or effete, self-indulgence? Some critics insisted that what we were doing was irrelevant to the lives of ordinary-decent-hardworking 'blokes'. In retrospect I certainly find the juxtaposition of that almost magically peaceful gathering of men, and my father's wartime exposure at about the same age to convincing approximations of hell, poignant. I now have a much clearer sense of how our bodies were both imprinted by, and enmeshed in the writing of, incommensurable yet intimately interwoven histories. At dad's funeral, a distant uncle was visibly shocked when I walked into the room, and said it was 'just like having Eddie coming in – you're just like him'. Although I found this timely observation both unexpectedly and profoundly pleasing, my life continued to be very different from my father's. During his married life, for instance, he had no close friendships with other men – in fact, no

* This came from a then recently published book, by a professor of nursing (Kreiger, 1979).

friends outside the family at all. I remember him becoming so embarrassed once, when two footballers hugged on the television, that he hurried out of the room. It was as though masculinity happened through him, its code of ingrained habits and assumptions remarked upon only in the breach. Relations between us mellowed considerably in his later years, but I was never able to talk to him in the way I would have liked about the strange new world that had my men's group in it.

Unfortunately, the atmosphere of relaxed openness in that group appeared to deter potential 'recruits'. One man, who came once and didn't return, said he'd assumed we were all gay. (This was a 'mixed' group.) Some initially rather awkward and obligatory hugging had paved the way for a much more relaxed and open way of relating, and because most of us were co-counselling, we were used to sharing quite intense emotional support with other men. But my recollection is that we also had enough experience to keep a fairly clear perspective on the political implications of meeting as members of a privileged group. We were hoping to change the world as well as our own lives, and most of us had been, were or soon would be engaged in the wider community. Coming together consciously as men, and learning to work together in new ways, informed the rest of our lives.

Chapter 4

Behold in me the tyrant of Turin!

Nietzsche, madness and postmodernism

> Ever since Copernicus man has been rolling down an incline, faster and faster, away from the centre – whither? Into the void? Into the 'piercing sense of his emptiness'?
>
> (Nietzsche, 1887/1956)

Nietzsche's work has been well described as containing 'a vast storehouse of suggestive themes, ideas, and categories'. Furthermore, his resolute resistance to systematisation, and a provocative and complex aphoristic style, coloured by hyperbole, invective, acerbic irony, paradox and dramatically shifting narrative viewpoints, have undoubtedly encouraged a 'protean fascination' with his legacy, and facilitated appropriation in the service of wildly incompatible causes, from feminism and bohemian anarchism to Nazism (Ascheim, 1992 p. 7). This intensely contradictory quality, both in Nietzsche's work and in the uses to which it has been put, is certainly troubling, and brings some of the key difficulties of an unbounded postmodernism into sharp focus.[1] Commentators tend to find themselves taking up positions in long-running controversies around accusations of misogyny and anti-Semitism, the implications of his consistently and robustly anti-democratic values, and a perceived irrationalism which some detractors have portrayed as evidence of 'madness'. Allison, who has been an influential advocate for a 'new Nietzsche', expresses concern that his reputation, though it 'rarely has any substantial bearing upon the content of his work', hardens contemporary prejudice against him. Nietzsche himself repeatedly asked for a 'generous' reading which recognised the perspectival nature of his texts, and the partial, provisional and circumstantial quality of any claims he was making (Allison, 2001 pp. 1, 80). But how generous can contemporary interpreters afford to be?

The clearest indication of the value of Nietzsche's work is that both postmodern theorists and their critics accord him a pivotal position as a dissident proto-postmodernist thinker who unmasked the primacy of Enlightenment rationality. Haar, for example, draws attention to the 'unique and inordinate privilege accorded him over a period of more than twenty years' by Derrida, who turned his normally 'ruthless and omnivocal cutting edge of deconstruction' away in the face of Nietzsche's authority alone (Haar, 1992 p. 53). Foucault is described as giving 'unstinting admiration' to Nietzsche, and came to define his intellectual project as a continuation of Nietzsche's. Deleuze evaluated Foucault's contribution in similar terms (Kumar, 1995 p. 130; MacIntyre, 1994 p. 297). Among the critics of postmodernism Callinicos concludes that poststructuralism owes an 'overwhelming' debt to Nietzsche, Giddens regards Nietzsche's 'nihilism' as a 'plausible starting point' for the challenge to foundationalism in epistemology, and Habermas responds to Lyotard by addressing 'Nietzscheanism', by which he means an excessively 'radical critique of reason' (Callinicos, 1989 p. 68; Hall *et al.*, 1992 pp. 369, 363, citing Giddens, 1990 pp. 46–53; and Habermas, 1987 pp. 336–40). Clearly, Nietzsche haunts debates both within and about postmodern social theory. I have already begun to argue for the far-reaching relevance of postmodern philosophical perspectives, of the figure of Dionysos, and of the genealogical method, to contemporary debates about gender and 'distress'. My hope is that a deconstructive reading of the relationship between Nietzsche's biography and the provocative storehouse of his life's work might cast new light on some questions about the conceptual material contained within it. I shall be focusing, in turn, on the effects of hegemonic masculinity, on a key biographical event, and on 'distress' and 'madness'.

Some difficulties with Nietzsche

But, first, I want to draw attention to some aspects of Nietzsche's thought that postmodern inheritors of his anti-foundationalist project must surely have found unpalatable. There has been considerable debate about the 'disturbing ease' with which Nazi ideologues were able to seize upon Nietzsche's 'immoral' vocabulary (Conway, 1994 p. 322). Deleuze mounted a spirited defence of Nietzsche on the grounds that the Nazis could only appeal to his work after 'mutilating quotations, falsifying editions and banning important texts', and that Nietzsche himself 'despised and hated' the Bismarckian regime, pan-Germanism and the anti-Semitism of his time (Deleuze, 1962/1983 pp. 126–7). Derrida, who was Jewish by descent, maintained that Nietzsche had been grossly caricatured but insisted upon a degree of complicity, while Allison admits that although 'few thinkers have been so maligned and abused as Nietzsche, fewer still have lent themselves to precisely this kind of interpretation' (Ascheim, 1992 p. 317; Allison, 1977/1985 p. xiii). Adorno and Horkheimer felt that Nietzsche's critique of Enlightenment contained the seeds of its own misappropriation, but still regarded it as a site of potential liberation in the darkest of times (Ascheim, 1992 p. 291). Some considerable difficulties persist, however.

Nietzsche's work became an important source of legitimation for Nazi eugenics, and hence for the policy of murdering people who were given the infamous psychiatric diagnosis 'life devoid of value' (Hill, 1983 p. 10). Ascheim finds 'no shortage of appropriate Nietzschean recommendations advocating what he called "holy cruelty"' (Ascheim, 1992 p. 243), and quotes a disturbing passage from *The Will to Power*:

> The biblical prohibition 'thou shalt not kill' is a piece of naivety compared with the seriousness of the prohibition of life to decadents: 'thou shalt not procreate!' – Life itself recognises no solidarity, no 'equal rights', between the healthy and the degenerate parts of an organism: one must excise the latter – or the whole will perish. – Sympathy for decadents, equal rights for the ill-constituted – that would be the profoundest immorality, that would be antinature itself as morality!
>
> (Nietzsche, 1968 p. 389)

Since this theme is echoed elsewhere in Nietzsche, it cannot be overlooked on the grounds that this was a distorted posthumous publication.[2] In *The Genealogy of Morals*, for example, we read 'The right to exist of the full-toned bell is a thousand times greater than that of the cracked, miscast one: it alone heralds in the future of all mankind' (Nietzsche, 1887/1956 p. 261). The irony here, of course, is not just that Nietzsche introduced us to, and identified with, the 'mad god' Dionysos, but that his own descent into insanity would have marked him out as a 'cracked bell' (Ascheim, 1992 pp. 243–4). This is the late Nietzsche, moreover, a writer profoundly aware of his own physical and mental vulnerability, whose warrior-ideal and disposition towards 'holy cruelty' were refracted through and, some would argue, forged out of intense personal pain (Pasley, 1978).[3]

Nevertheless, if we are looking for a theorist to help us reconceptualise responses to men experiencing 'distress' or 'madness' in the early twenty-first century, this is hardly an auspicious starting point. There is clearly a need to ask how far various aspects of Nietzsche's work were marked by the cultural prejudices of his time, and to consider what issues are at stake when theoretical concepts are transposed into radically different socio-political contexts. Even if we only intend to make indirect use of Nietzsche, through Foucault, these problems still need to be addressed. Clearly the relationships between biography, philosophy and political appropriation are complex, and there are some parallels with the debate surrounding Heidegger's direct transposition of the terms of his philosophy into a political affiliation with Nazism during the 1930s (Sedgwick, 2001 pp. 157–8; Polt, 1999 pp. 158–64). Postmodern 'generosity' acknowledges contradiction, before identifying and relating to those elements in a person that are constructive, and making selective use of the toolbox of their work. This said, there has undoubtedly been a tendency for deconstructionist readings of Nietzsche to evade uncomfortable aspects of his thinking (Warren, 1988 pp. 3–5; Ansell-Pearson, 1993). Although Deleuze and Guattari were sometimes referred to as the French Laing and Cooper, for example, Deleuze appears reluctant to discuss the difficulties that a proto-fascist strand in Nietzsche's work clearly poses for the politics of 'mental health' (Deleuze,

1962/1983, 1991).[4] Once again the need to ground postmodern social theory in relation to the experiences of oppressed groups is evident. Since much of the fascination of Nietzsche's writing lies precisely in its extreme heterogeneity, it is surely necessary to acknowledge that the potentially powerful emancipatory counter-currents within it emerged in tense juxtaposition with some deeply negative material.

For this reason I value Warren's argument that Nietzsche's neo-aristocratic political ideology should not be treated as merely metaphorical, and that it 'violates the integrity' of his critical postmodern insights, in particular his critique of metaphysics that clearly contradicts any resort to essentialist notions of genetic purity or to supposedly discrete and scientifically impartial categories such as 'degenerates'. Nietzsche sometimes uses the term 'will to power' in the context of a subtle critique of modernist metaphysical assumptions about free will, rationality, moral choice, the self and the 'doer', in order to explore post-metaphysical conceptions of subjectivity, agency and individuated power. At other times he writes as though 'will to power' denotes a universal underlying essence, a basic organic function that accounts for, and justifies, domination. Once we recognise this inconsistency between Nietzsche as philosopher and as polemicist (derived from the Greek *polemos*, meaning 'war'), it becomes possible to reject his evident enthusiasm for class- and gender-based domination, while still finding his philosophical insights into processes of domination invaluable. We can accept him as 'central to the transition from metaphysical to situated, modern to postmodern, ways of thinking about humans as agents', without masking the difficulties or invoking an uncritical generosity. Wondering how 'these two Nietzsches can coexist within the same body of thought', Warren points to a lack of interest in the categories of social analysis, and outlines a positive political vision, combining individuation, communal intersubjectivity, egalitarianism and pluralism, which remains consistent with Nietzsche's critical postmodern philosophy (Warren, 1988 pp. 1–3, 8–12, 208, 247). The question remains, however: Why was Nietzsche not more interested in the collective and relational aspects of individuation, or the prospect of an egalitarian postmodern politics? I want to consider the possibility that discourses of hegemonic masculinity may have been an unrecognised but decisive biographical influence, hardening his public political values against the kind of warmth and generosity he evidently shared, in the private domain, with some of his friends (Gilman, 1987).

Nietzsche and masculinity

Once we turn to accounts of Nietzsche's life and work in order to make gender issues more visible, motifs from an intensely traditional masculinity emerge as such an emphatic and pervasive presence that the failure of many accounts to conceptualise them as such is surprising.[5] In an early essay Nietzsche argued that struggle, contest and competition, known in Homeric Greece as *agon* (and the corresponding combative skills learned in war, in athletic competitions and in the arts), had allowed Greek culture to survive, flourish and develop the capacities of its people in unprecedented ways. He regarded Homer and Hesiod as key figures in establishing this agonistic culture and, in a narrative diametrically opposed to that of recent feminist accounts, contrasts it with the 'abyss of horrible savagery' of the pre-Homeric period (Allison, 2001 pp. 33–4, 61–2; Goodison, 1990; Baring and Cashford, 1991). Such a view was consistent with Nietzsche's personal experience. As a university student he acquired a duelling scar across the bridge of his nose, and this was prized as the insignia of noble manhood (Zeitlin, 1994 p. 2).[6] He was impressed and delighted that his grandmother, while carrying the child who would become his father, had been in the immediate vicinity of one of Napoleon's battles, and felt this gave him a personal connection with the Great Man (Gilman, 1987 p. 203). Nietzsche admired a 'Napoleonic masculinity' for its reassertion of aristocratic male mastery and suppression of 'modern' emancipatory ideals, and argued that higher cultures require violence (Ansell-Pearson, 1993 pp. 29–30; Warren, 1988 p. 188). He even identified violence as the hallmark of masculinity, specifying the 'fear-inspiring' as diagnostic of the '*man* in man'. When this was no longer developed, woman would 'degenerate', 'seize new rights, [and] look to become "master"' (Nietzsche, 1886/1970 pp. 167–9). His anti-feminism was often expressed in a militaristic idiom.[7]

The imagery of combat also permeated Nietzsche's philosophical thought. He famously referred to truth as 'a mobile *army* of metaphors', conceived of the body as an arena in which forces struggle for supremacy down to the cellular level, and defined *ressentiment* (resentment) as feminine, contrasting it with an immediate self-defensive reaction said to characterise noble masculinity (Allison, 1977/1985 p. xvi; Grosz, 1994 p. 122; Stringer, 2000). In *Ecce Homo* he proclaimed, 'I am by nature warlike. To attack is among my instincts . . . a philosopher who is warlike also challenges problems to a duel. The undertaking is to master . . . *equal* opponents' (Nietzsche, 1888/1979 pp. 16–17; and see Kaufmann, 1950/1974 pp. 386–7). Deleuze concluded, approvingly, albeit from a very different political perspective, that 'he made thought into a machine of war – a battering ram – into a nomadic force' (Deleuze, 1991 p. 149). Although Nietzsche's use of war as a metaphor for the interested nature of truth claims foreshadows Foucault's 'power/knowledge', and *agon* has been reclaimed as a prerequisite for pluralist democracy, these concepts obscure the association between war and masculinity, and the possibility of negotiating difference and disagreement in consciously collaborative ways.[8] Perhaps unsurprisingly, an agonistic spirit lives on in Nietzsche scholarship, which Dreyfus and Rabinow are not alone in characterising as 'a field of danger and strife, which we leave to others more fully armed' (Dreyfus and Rabinow, 1982 p. 106; also Patton, 1993 p. xii).

Nietzsche's persistent enthusiasm for militaristic masculinity undoubtedly encouraged the misappropriation of his work, and Ascheim (1992 p. 129) argues that his 'manly posture and his admonitions to live dangerously crucially affected turn-of-the-century attitudes towards a coming war'. Indeed, one of the earliest uses of the term 'postmodern' was precisely to encapsulate a Nietzschean sense of 'nihilism' reflected in the collapse of European values during the First World War, and the emergence of new 'postmodern men' who would incarnate militaristic, nationalistic and elite values (Rudolf Pannwitz, *Die Krisis der Euro-päischen Kultur*, 1917, cited in Best and Kellner, 1991 p. 6). These qualities were, of course, appreciated by Nietzsche's Nazi admirers, who celebrated him as a pioneer of the 'German rediscovery of the body', a critic of a 'decadent and feminised nineteenth century', and a champion of 'a new masculine warrior age'. The hard personality of the fascist *übermensch* would delight in dangerous living (Ascheim, 1992 p. 238; Stern, 1979 p. 99). Nietzsche's assertion that 'modern man' is ashamed of his instincts for cruelty, of his 'will to power', has also been deployed against fascism, however. Whitmont, for instance, empha-sised the excitement of violence and argued that a repetition of 'Hitler's mad-ness' would be more likely if murderous feelings were repressed (Whitmont, 1982/1997).[9]

The notion that masculinity is a performance of mastery and self-mastery, a conspiracy of agreement, conformity and collusion between men, which needs to be continually defended against all that is soft or 'feminine', has become commonplace. In repressing any sense of passivity, vulnerability and weakness, it is argued, men have traditionally displaced these qualities into 'contempt for women, and antipathy and loathing for excluded and subordinated groups of men'. Any process by which men come to recognise and accept their own 'multiple and conflicted identities', therefore, is potentially interesting in politi-cal terms (Segal, 1990/1997 p. xxix). Various authors, drawing upon psycho-analytic accounts, and often, but not always, working within the Foucauldian and postmodern traditions, have fleshed out this counter-discourse in response to what Connell calls the widespread gender ideology of an essential masculin-ity, rooted in the supposedly immutable and irresistible biological inheritance of men's bodies (Connell, 1995 pp. 9, 45; Frosh, 1994 p. 144; Kimmel, 1996; Segal, 1990/1997 p. xxx citing Butler, 1993; Bhabha, 1995). This flight from the feminine would appear to be epitomised in 'the male warrior ideal of the fascist imagination', where a 'controlled, emotionally bereft body – expresses revulsion and fear of the soft, fluid, and liquid female body', sensed as a quint-essential 'other', lurking inside, and threatening to disrupt its hardness. The male self seals off bodily pleasure and pain, locks away all feeling, and uses military discipline as a defence against 'the constant threat of disintegration' (Petersen, 1998 p. 54, citing Theweleit, 1989).

Nietzsche was no stormtrooper, however. A first spell in the Prussian army was curtailed by a riding accident, and a second, as a medical orderly, by diphtheria compounded by dysentery. He found his brief experience of the battlefront sobering, and became critical of Prussian nationalism, but continued to exalt the quality of 'hardness' in his writing. In *Ecce Homo*, for example, he says:

> any 'feminism' in a person, or in a man, likewise closes the gates on me: one will never be able to enter this labyrinth of daring knowledge. One must never have spared oneself, harshness must be among one's habits, if one is to be happy and cheerful among nothing but hard truths.[10]
>
> (Nietzsche, 1888/1979, p. 43)

At this late stage he even manages to reduce the otherwise extravagantly ecstatic Dionysos into an instrument of hardness: 'Among the decisive preconditions for a *dionysian* task is the hardness of the hammer, *joy even in destruction*. The imperative, "become hard", the deepest certainty *that all creators are hard*, is the actual mark of a dionysian nature' (Nietzsche, 1888/1979 p. 81). Although the hammer in question is the philosophical-geological one with which Nietzsche undertook his deconstructive *Götterdämmerung*, the distance between these professions of psychic rigidity and Hillman's bisexual figuration of Dionysos as archetype of undivided consciousness could be read as supporting speculation about the philosopher's sexuality (Conway, 1995, p. 32; Hillman, 1972). Nietzsche apparently once directed a friend towards a reference to the androgynous and strikingly feminine San Gennaro, saying that it revealed 'so much about me, which a hundred letters of friendship could not match' (Safranski, 2002 pp. 245–6). 'Hardness' also became the bulwark that Nietzsche's autobiographical 'psychologist', or unriddler of souls, felt he needed against introspection and pity during his struggle with emotional anguish, and when facing imminent mental collapse.[11]

Even Allison, who protests against an 'overly curious fascination' with Nietzsche's personal life, confirms that *Zarathustra* incorporates a personal engagement with Nietzsche's intimate concerns, about the validity and communicability of his philosophy, about his failing health, and not least about his emotional crisis following the breakdown of his relationship with Lou Salomé:

> This last *morsel of life* was the hardest I have yet had to chew, and it is still possible that I shall *choke* on it. I have suffered from the humiliating and tormenting memories of this summer as from a bout of madness . . . I am now being broken, as no other man could be, on the wheel of my passions. If only I could sleep!'[12]
>
> (cited by Allison, 2001 p. 115)

Nietzsche was speaking from experience when he wrote: 'the manifold torture of the psychologist who has discovered . . . the whole inner hopelessness of the higher man, this eternal "too late" . . . may perhaps lead him one day to turn against his own lot, embittered, and to make an attempt at self-destruction'

(Nietzsche, 1886/1970, in Allison, 2001 p. 171). At this point he developed the figure of the overman, his transformative image of a dancing 'new man', which Salomé read as a self-deification (Gane, 1993, citing Salomé, 1988). Nietzsche could hardly be accused of inexpressiveness, and although we may want to question his resort to the conventionally masculine notion of hardness, it should be remembered that protective withdrawal in the face of anguish is sometimes necessary and constructive. We should also distinguish between Nietzsche's personal injunction to become hard in the face of suffering, and his paradoxical use of the imagery of hardness in relation to what has become known as deconstruction.[13] In the 'mental health' field it seems particularly important to differentiate between deconstruction and 'joy in destruction', and to recognise the possibility that where deconstruction shades into an over-enthusiastic negativism this may be strongly configured by the entrenched emotional dynamics of hegemonic forms of masculinity.

We should not assume, however, that these emotional dynamics are so well understood that obvious summaries will suffice. In a critique of Theweleit's work, for example, Segal points out that fascism is not only about hardness, insofar as it also encourages the 'feminine' qualities of 'obeisance, even obsequiousness' in men (Segal, 1990/1997 pp. 116–21, citing Koonz, 1988). When fulminating against the conformity, passivity and habit-bounded morality of what he calls 'the herd', Nietzsche overlooks this facet of militaristic masculinity. Nevertheless, his distinctive innovations, in theorising plural and conflicted identities and mutable bodies, and in refusing to privilege minds over bodies, are widely acknowledged as significant first steps in the direction that Segal and other contemporary theorists of masculinity have taken (Grosz, 1994; Jackson, 1990). Nietzsche's view of the unitary self as a metaphysical fiction reflected his own conflicted sense of identity, and his work, much of which was written down while walking and is thus literally nomadic in origin, became a form of 'talking to oneself', a protracted argument between various voices. Hollingdale concludes not only that the mature Nietzsche loved his own company, 'for with no one else can he enjoy such good conversation', but that these were the very conditions his unusual creativity demanded (Hollingdale, 1965/1999 p. 116).

Some of Nietzsche's selves expressed decidedly unwarlike attributes. His long experience of health difficulties prompted a persistent and sometimes remorseless introspection, and an intense awareness of the significance of the body.[14] He was fond of dancing, and was described by one correspondent as 'very sensitive to the temperature fluctuations in human relations . . . easily irritable, easily offended, and vulnerable to positive or negative influences'. An emotional intensity became evident, for example, in 'monologues on Wagner, which began calmly . . . but soon accelerated into an avalanche of words that stirred up psychic depths and ended in tears' (Resa von Schirnhofer, in Gilman, 1987 p. 194). When a male friend sent him a picture of his newly born child, Nietzsche replied with a forthright declaration of vulnerability:

it was as if you were clasping my hand and gazing at me in a melancholy way . . . as if to say: 'how is it that we now have so little in common . . .', Oh friend, what a senseless withdrawn life I live! So alone, alone! So without 'children'!

(letter of 22 February 1884 cited in Hollingdale, 1965/1999 p. 116)

In this respect he seems closer to some early modern discourses of European masculinity that were no less hegemonic for permitting the public display of weeping and the expression of deep feelings of love between bourgeois men (Lupton and Barclay, 1997 p. 145).

As well as the tension, already noted, between the proto-postmodern philosopher and the polemicist, Nietzsche was exposed to conflicting discourses about gender, and an ambiguity about women and female imagery is evident in various contradictions between his lived experience and his writing, and between different texts. There is a striking contrast, for instance, between Nietzsche as radical exponent of the anti-Christian counter-doctrine of Dionysian sensuality, and the refined, considerate, exquisitely sensitive, withdrawn and reserved figure that emerges from contemporary testimony. This lonely libertarian, who was 'embarrassed by the bad manners of modern ladies' who make themselves 'conspicuous with loud talking and laughter', advised his mother not to read his books. Although his anti-feminist tirades, fuelled by a burning sense of loss and frustration, were already well known, he counted a contemporary feminist as a close friend for a few years from 1884 (Gilman, 1987 pp. 148, 159, 166–8, 197).[15] His penchant for describing truth as a woman, and describing his own creative process in terms of pregnancy, midwifery and childbirth, has attracted considerable commentary. Derrida writes 'one might imagine Nietzsche, who was easily moved to tears, who referred to his thought as a pregnant woman might speak of her unborn child . . . shedding tears over his own swollen belly' (Derrida, 1979 p. 65). For Ahmed, an image of the female body is appropriated in order to represent masculine philosophy's self-overcoming, a fantasy of 'becoming woman' in which any sense of female historical specificity is lost (Ahmed, 1998 p. 88).[16] But as well as looking at the literal envy here, Lionnet reminds us to pursue the metaphorical content, in which maternal space, depicted as a 'biocentric locus of energy and affirmation', encapsulates Nietzsche's insights about the embodied source of philosophical work, and about creating language that renders new experience visible (Lionnet, 1989 pp. 86–7).

The shadow of bereavement

Once we turn to Nietzsche's biographical evidence, a picture emerges from quite extensive evidence in which the death of his father when he was four years old stands out as a key event, casting its shadow across much of what was to follow.[17] Again I find myself surprised by the omission, from many accounts, of any serious consideration of the impact of this apparently seismic moment on the development of Nietzsche's thought, presumably because of the tradition of separating embodied biography from philosophical critique. My hope is that by reconceptualising biography away from the conventional linear image of a unitary self, towards a collection of stories about the social construction of complex and contradictory identities, it will be possible to explore the significance of such an event without lapsing into psychological reductionism, or 'trivialization' (as Kaufmann puts it, 1950/1974 p. 99).

In response to the question, 'how could Nietzsche as philosopher and Nietzsche as polemicist co-exist in the same body of work?' I have suggested that his polemical voice was responding to the demands of a very traditional and militaristic masculinity. In particular it conformed closely to the expectation of a rigidly gendered division between private and public realms, with the latter reserved as an arena for the 'manly' practices of *agon*, contest, competition and struggle. There would appear to be clear biographical antecedents for Nietzsche's lifelong adherence to just such a binary division of the world. His first four years were spent in the secure, peaceful and socially conservative surroundings of a rural rectory, complete with orchard and fishponds. His father, Pastor Nietzsche, became ill and died of 'softening of the brain' at the age of thirty-six, and during the following year, when the family had to move to the walled town of Naumburg, an infant brother also died. This meant that between the ages of five and fourteen, the young Nietzsche lived in an all-female household 'clasped to the bosom of a loving mother', with a sister, and initially two aunts, a grandmother and an elderly maid ever present.[18] Another upheaval occurred at the onset of adolescence, when he won a scholarship to the prestigious all-male public boarding school which he attended for the next six years. Hollingdale likens the regime there to that of 'a prison for persistent offenders', but nevertheless concludes that it was just what the young man 'required' (Hollingdale, 1965/1999 pp. 8, 18).[19]

Pointing out that Nietzsche was 'passionately attached' to his father, Hollingdale does argue that the death 'may have been the decisive event of Nietzsche's life.' Echoing aspects of the familiar 'families need fathers' discourse, he suggests that this early encounter with death, and the shocking disruption of a previously idyllic infancy, were probably what caused Nietzsche to abandon the utterly settled life of his forebears, and become 'chronically footloose' and 'homeless'. Nietzsche

> avoided as if by every instinct any commitment that might have fastened him to a particular place. He never married and never became a father himself, and eluded involvement with those institutions which provide most men . . . with a stable background to their lives.
>
> (Hollingdale 1965/1999 p. 8)

This sense of escaping patriarchal obligations is repeated, much later, when a friend responded to *Beyond Good and Evil* with the comment that 'what Nietzsche needs is to get a proper job' (Hollingdale, 1965/1999 p. 38). Since, as late as the 1850s, most men were still working in or near to the home, Nietzsche's experience as an 'orphan' might be expected to have set him apart from his contemporaries far more than would be the case more recently (Clare, 2001 p. 132).[20] Given his mother's lack of access to education and social influence, her academically talented son would have to move away from home, and break a family association with the Lutheran church dating back to the early seventeenth century, in order to satisfy his burgeoning intellectual curiosity. In that sense, Hollingdale's view that the death of his father left Nietzsche unable to 'settle down' seems reasonable. About the longterm emotional impact of his father's death we can only speculate, however, not only because of the historical distance, but because, for all post-Nietzscheans, there is no final psychological truth to be found. Any such discussion is necessarily perspectival, and infused by cultural discourse.

The absence of fathers has certainly become a prominent contemporary concern (Lupton and Barclay, 1997; Laquer, 1996). David Jackson opens the chapter of his critical autobiography on relations with his father with an enigmatic quotation from Nietzsche: 'What has the Man not been able to talk about? What is the Man hiding?' The answer he gives is that men have not generally been able to talk 'about the emotional histories of their relationships with their fathers (or lack of them).' In late or postmodern times, even when the father is alive and well, 'there is a frequent gap where the father ought to be'. He is somewhat detached and distant from the family group, and identified only in terms of his working relations (Jackson, 1990 p. 88).[21] One effect of this has been that 'over seventy mental health problems . . . have been blamed on mothers'. Contrasting markedly with the intensity of debate over 'maternal deprivation', a long-standing consensus has quietly assumed that fathers hardly matter at all in terms of their children's emotional development. Yet a son's yearning for an absent father is a widespread religious theme. In Christianity, the core image is of a son 'who never had a human father, never becomes a father, and dies on a cross lamenting his abandonment by the most powerful father of all' (Clare, 2001 pp. 161–2, 167).[22] It is hardly surprising, then, that Nietzsche, as a critically minded young philosopher, came to focus his deconstructive attention upon a Christian God, often portrayed as a perfect, but in the material sense, wholly absent, father.

Freud celebrated the supposed transformation to patriarchy, with the invention of paternity as a 'hypothesis, based on an inference and a premise', as a 'momentous step' that signalled a conquest of intellectuality over sensuality, and of the spiritual over the material, which would be enforced by the 'Moses' religion's' insistence on the invisibility of God. By pronouncing the name of God, the High Priest invoked ultimate authority, and established the dominance of speech over the material world (Freud, 1939 cited in Laquer, 1996 p. 178; and Frosh, 1994 p. 72).[23] For Lacan, the 'Name of the Father' both requires and enables entry into language, the world of the symbolic in which the male subject can constitute himself as One, against others. In this view, a lingering dread of disintegration, fragmentation and death remains, which can only be assuaged by turning to woman, or to God as 'ultimate guarantor of unified subjectivity'. Such a God underwrites male social dominance and 'the establishment of the Name/Law' of patriarchy (Jantzen, 1998 p. 49). Here, once again, we find a picture of masculinity as a project of self-control, demanding vigilance against ambiguity, denial of contradiction, management of vulnerability, and mastery of the 'feminine', which Nietzsche's critique of the fiction of a unitary self promises to undermine.

It has sometimes been argued that any original writer will elaborate so extensively upon biographical experience that there is little point in attempting to make connections between his or her 'work' and 'life'. In the case of Nietzsche, however, my sense is that traces of the overwhelming experience of the loss of his father are not difficult to find in key aspects of his proto-postmodern philosophy. Indirectly, the sharply gendered worlds of his formative years appear to have left him with a precarious sense of his own masculinity, and a markedly contradictory sense of selfhood. This biographical configuration is echoed in Nietzsche's concern with what he termed the 'subject-and-ego superstition', and in his exposition of the centrality of binary thinking in philosophical discourse which would become so influential when taken up by Derrida (Nietzsche, 1886/1970 p. 31; Jantzen, 1998 pp. 62–3; Schrift, 1995 p. 22).[24] It is striking that Nietzsche's personal restlessness was reflected both in an 'interim' philosophy of decentring, 'homelessness' and pervasive change and in a 'nomadic' style of thought that avoided any attempt at recodification (Deleuze, 1977/1985 p. 143). His preoccupation with transforming the effects of memory, and his insistence on working through his critique of morality and metaphysics at a personal level, would also prove influential. Since genealogy, in the conventional sense, traces the effects of power through patrilineal descent, his interest in the rewriting of histories also seems haunted by the emotional legacy of childhood loss.

From this perspective, the philosophical elaboration on the 'Death of God', which became pivotal to Nietzsche's proto-postmodernism, might be seen as the reworking of an image crystallised from personal grief, and the subsequent rejection of a very distinctive paternal inheritance. If we accept the continuing emotional significance, for Nietzsche, of the loss of his flesh-and-blood father, and the corresponding dramatic resonance of the 'death' of an invisible paternal deity, this reworking becomes, in effect, his most far-reaching piece of deconstructive genealogy. Given that such a conclusion would foreground a tense and uncomfortable inter-weaving between the gendered contingencies of intimate experience, 'external' social worlds and philosophy, and that an understandable suspicion of dominant psychologising discourse as a way of tracing such connections is compounded by a widespread absence of interest in the consequences of 'paternal deprivation', it is perhaps not surprising that it has been resisted.[25] Although some commentators argue that Nietzsche's loss of his childhood faith motivated his philosophical activity, or that his father's death instigated an inability to 'settle down', which, fortuitously, set him on the kind of unencumbered path his intellectual development demanded, I would contend that we are unlikely to understand why Nietzsche, and not some other philosopher, became 'the Lucifer match' that set this particular and powerfully panoramic image alight, without considering the impact of the loss of his father in early childhood (Sadler, 1995 p. 117; Hollingdale, 1965/1999 p. 116).[26] We might then also begin to understand the delightful irony that when the 'old artilleryman', who could 'fire a heavier cannon than any opponent of Christianity has ever dreamed of before', took aim at the religious tradition of his forefathers, he may also have 'hit' patriarchy by mistake (Levy, 1921/1985 p. 358).

Nietzsche insisted that the death of God, and specifically of the neo-platonic God of Being, the creator whose word, the logos, was said to have become flesh, removed any possibility of recourse to universal foundations, to absolute or transcendent grounds beyond human history. No longer could we look to an external metaphysical source for the authority of claims about truth and value, or pretend that religious, ethical and moral codes were anything other than social configurations regulating human activity (Allison, 2001). Nietzsche's argument that knowledge is perspectival and embodied, and his call for an abandonment of the quest for a 'privileged, epistemologically pure', God-like perspective, presage Haraway's critique of the patriarchal 'God trick', the pretence of writing from an omniscient and disembodied viewpoint (Conway, 1993 p. 114). After the death of God we would enter a transitional time, living under his shadow, and clinging to the habit of metaphysical thought, but attributing redemptive powers to surrogate beliefs in science, in moral causes or in totalising political ideologies. This would be an age of ambiguity, 'breakdown, destruction, ruin, and cataclysm', characterised by nostalgia and radical uncertainty, as we gradually responded to the reverberations of that most momentous event. Finally, as belief in divine creation, teleology, rational causation, the intelligibility of the world and the stability of identity came to be seen as lingering shadows on the wall of Plato's cave, a mature and transformed human subject could begin to emerge (Allison, 2001 pp. 97–100; Haar, 1977/ 1985 p. 14; Nietzsche, 1882/1974 p. 181).

Distress and madness

At this key point Nietzsche posed the radical question 'Must we not ourselves become gods?' What makes this question particularly resonant here is that Nietzsche chose to introduce his exposition of possible meanings of the 'Death of God' in the form of an allegory involving a 'madman', thereby opening up an analogy between 'madness', especially 'schizophrenia', and postmodern deconstruction that many others have since taken up. Nietzsche's madman runs into a market place, and provokes the dismissive laughter of a crowd of bystanders by incessantly crying out 'I seek God, I seek God'.

> The madman jumped into their midst and pierced them with his eyes. 'Whither is God?' he cried: I will tell you. *We have killed him* – you and I. All of us are his murderers. But how did we do this? How could we drink up the sea? Who gave us the sponge to wipe away the entire horizon? What were we doing when we unchained this earth from its sun? Whither is it moving now? Whither are we moving? Away from all suns? Are we not plunging continually? Backward, sideward, forward, in all directions? Is there still any up or down? Are we not straying as through infinite nothing? . . . How shall we comfort ourselves, the murderers of all murderers? . . . who will wipe this blood off us? What water is there for us to clean ourselves? What festivals of atonement, what sacred games shall we have to invent? Is not the greatness of this deed too great for us? Must we ourselves not become gods simply to appear worthy of it?
>
> (Nietzsche, 1882/1974 pp. 181–2)

The bystanders are shocked, not by the announcement that God is dead – they are modern non-believers who already take a godless world for granted – but by the intensity with which the madman proclaims the importance of the event. From their point of view the absence of God is no reason to be shaken to the core by terrible forebodings. According to Kaufmann, Nietzsche's prophetic gift consisted in experiencing his own 'wretched fate' so deeply that he could feel the 'agony, the suffering, and the misery of a godless world', thereby sensing the fate of a coming generation. In this passage Nietzsche prophetically envisages himself as a madman: 'to have lost God means madness, and when mankind will discover that it has lost God, universal madness will break out' (Kaufmann, 1950/1974 pp. 97–8; Nietzsche, 1887/1969).

A visceral quality in this account of violent disorientation, with its quite Oedipal-sounding insistence on the guilt of those left alive, transposes the death of God into a register of embodied experience that would be wholly consistent with an emotional investment by this most reflexive of philosophers in his theme. The apocalyptic urgency with which the 'madman' experiences and proclaims the significance of God's demise suggests a dramatic voice crafted for the express purpose of revisiting the sensitive legacy of childhood bereavement that was a key part of its writer's 'wretched fate'. Such an interpretation need neither reduce the writing to abreaction nor undermine the validity of Nietzsche's ambition to transmute introspection into the gold of philosophical understanding. How far such transmutation would help him on a personal level remains open to question, however. Indeed, since such passages locate transformative and redemptive personal anguish, to the point of madness, close to the heart of postmodern cultural transformation, their writing may well have exacerbated the long-standing sense of having a special mission that appears to have contributed significantly to their author's eventual breakdown (e.g. Hollingdale, 1965/1999 p. 115). Attention to the social formation of his various voices also suggests that this particular conception of madness is steeped in the traditions and tensions surrounding hegemonic masculinity.

With the earth unchained from its orbit around a sun of intelligibility, and darkened by a terrifying eclipse, a crisis of nihilism is ushered in. Nietzsche described nihilism as 'a passing pathological condition' of contemporary times. This 'most alarming of all guests' arrives insidiously, in states of gloom, which eventually develop into full-blooded terror at the exhaustion of all meaning, a perpetual twilight in which signification collapses. Haar likens this culturally mediated experiential condition to 'the onrush of a nightmare or . . . complete disorientation in space and time'. Because disorientation is complete, the *Stimmung*, or mood, of nihilism can change abruptly, manifesting in feelings of 'grand disgust', including self-disgust, or in contentment with emptiness, a con-viction that there is no longer any meaning worth searching for (Haar, 1977/1985 pp. 13–15).

According to Nietzsche, nihilism emerges when an impotent 'will to power' recoils from 'life', and proclaims that 'this world is worth nothing' in comparison with a 'true' Platonic world, with metaphysical attributes such as 'unity, stability, identity, happiness, truth, goodness'. Nihilism then proceeds through critiques of such constructions and values, which remain haunted by nostalgia for a 'true world', until the very dichotomy between 'being-in-itself' and appear-ance, truth and illusion, is finally rejected. At this stage appearance no longer refers to ultimate foundations. 'Everything is a mask. Any mask, once un-covered, uncovers another mask', and 'becoming' is recognised as an infinite play of interpretation. The purpose of nihilism becomes apparent when a 'consummated', 'ecstatic' or active nihilism affirms the creative destruction of all relations dependent upon metaphysical difference. A Dionysian perspective emerges, which celebrates the unity of oppositions, including that between creation and destruction, and proclaims a radical abolition of the 'true world' with its singular God and, by implication, all representatives of singular and arbitrary authority (Haar, 1977/1985 pp. 13–16). There is a strong sense, in all of this, that states of 'depression', chaos and craziness might be intrinsic to life's unfolding, and that personal pain and cultural change are profoundly con-nected. There is also a strong sense of the potentially visionary strand in 'mad-ness', that those deemed 'mad' might 'break through' and gain creative insight from the refusal of conventional 'truths' and totalising ideologies. But Nietzsche's life suggests that this can work the other way round as well, that a refusal of conventional 'truths', pushed too far, can precipitate destructive madness.

According to Heidegger, Nietzsche retold the story of metaphysics to the point where he was able to overturn and eventually 'twist free' of Platonism. This was a story of 'how the ground in which all would be anchored begins to drift away', a twisting free 'into a space lacking all the bounds, limits, measure, previously installed by two and a half millennia of western thought and language; into . . . an abyss.' (Sallis, 1991 p. 2). Moreover, Heidegger identified a biographical moment at which he felt Nietzsche had crossed both a philosophical and a personal Rubicon. In a letter written a year before his final collapse Nietzsche had spoken of reaching his 'high noon'. Heidegger noted that this peak was followed by a final creative year when 'everything about him radiates an excessive brilliance and in which therefore at the same time the boundless (*das Masslosse*) advances out of the distance', and that 'During the time when the overturning of Platonism became for Nietzsche a twisting free of it, madness befell him' (Heidegger, 1961 pp. 23, 233, cited in Sallis, 1991 p. 3). Ironically Nietzsche had once referred to metaphysics as a hegemonic delusion, and described the whole of Western history since Plato as a 'madhouse' (Warren, 1988 p. 101).

Heidegger's perception of a close, and seemingly causal, linkage, between the final overcoming of metaphysics and descent into madness has important implications, and the boundary tension of such moments reverberates throughout subsequent discussions, both about 'distress/madness' and about the need to somehow ground an otherwise unbounded postmodern social theory. Interestingly, Nietzsche offers a characteristic theoretical insight into these questions when he argues that we think the way we do not because we are unified rational subjects, but because we are, in his intentionally provocative social Darwinian terms, 'herd animals', with shared habits and collective linguistic norms. Rather than directly representing an objective world, language expresses our need to conceptualise our environment in terms of representations, in order to survive. Far from facilitating access to a fixed external reality, 'Reason' actually falsifies the evidence of our senses (Sedgwick, 2001 pp. 70–3). Nietzsche insists, however, that this metaphysical 'error', the supposition that language about reality corresponds to things-in-themselves, is initially necessary and helpful, a view closely echoed, for example, in Butler's postmodern description of the temporary totalisation of categories within identity politics as a 'necessary error' (Butler, 1993 p. 230). The most significant, persistent and, no doubt, necessary of these pervasive 'errors' is that of belief in an I-substance, a subject, the 'enabling fiction' or 'helpful fantasy' of Nietzsche's 'doer behind the deed' (Warren, 1988 p. 129; Grosz, 1994 p. 126).[27] The question arises, then, as to why, in the throes of his decisive breakdown of 1889, Nietzsche was no longer able to heed his own insight into the necessity of consciously making certain philosophical 'mistakes', of accepting the sustaining illusion of a core voice.

Missing from these various accounts of Nietzsche's response to the Western metaphysical tradition is any sense that the tradition has been rooted in an emphatically gendered mind–body dualism (Heidegger, 1961; Haar, 1977/1985; Sallis, 1991; cf. Lloyd, 1984; Plumwood, 1993; Spellman, 1999). Once this is accepted we can trace various ways in which masculinity characteristically exaggerates the 'errors' of metaphysics. Jackson, for instance, talks about the construction and representation of men as rational subjects in biographical accounts that trace the trajectory of a 'lonely male hero', using energy, determination and will-power to pursue a 'rising arc of progress' towards public glory. He memorably describes a 'sky-rocket narrative' in which this arc ascends 'from a usually spluttering start . . . in a curving loop to burst, in the performance climax, into a flowering cluster of exclamatory stars'. Crucially, this is a narrative in which public achievement takes absolute precedence, and concern about personal relationships or emotional wellbeing are consigned to a devalued private realm. Nietzsche's claim that he had been 'the opposite of a heroic nature', that he had never struggled towards a goal, is flagrantly contradicted by his burning sense of mission, and by the corresponding comprehensiveness, and hyperbolic crescendo, of his philosophical ambition. However much he might appear to satirise these qualities in *Ecce Homo*, they are markedly present, and consistent with the masculinist expectation of a 'rising arc' towards a 'performance climax' of public achievement (Jackson, 1990 p. 19; Nietzsche, 1888/1979 p. 35).

Of course, the intensity of Nietzsche's final philosophical flowering may well have been sharpened by foreknowledge of the imminence of terminal illness. Hollingdale asserts that Nietzsche's sense of mission kept him alive in the face of increasing health difficulties, and that his exaggeration of the significance of his mission was a response to increasingly desperate illness (Hollingdale, 1965/1999 p. 217). Others, however, argue that it was his 'masochistic self-discipline', expressed in a prodigious work rate, destructive self-criticism and an inadequate diet, that rendered his personal mission unsustainable, and fuelled the final breakdown (Stern, 1979; Hayman, 1997 p. 46). During an earlier period of emotional crisis, Nietzsche had devised the quintessentially autobiographical concept of 'self-overcoming', which appears counter-cultural in the context of Western philosophy for valuing reflexivity. In privileging a process of systematic liberation from any 'fetters' of convention that constrain individuality, and in moving beyond self-scrutiny to a 'dangerous' testing of all limits and proscriptions, however, it also seems coloured, albeit paradoxically, by unrecognised discourses of masculinist radicalism (Allison, 2001 pp. 176–7). This ostensibly creative impulse, to leave the 'home' of familiar values and seek ever greater self-determination through transformative and 'overturning' systems of valuation, is strikingly self-referential, but for good reason. The Nietzsche who decided to 'experiment' in this way was the author of *Zarathustra*, who had 'almost choked' on an unbearable morsel of life, was painfully isolated, and urgently needed to overcome the 'fetters' of intense love and hatred following an emotional crisis.

Nietzsche's retreat into hermetic reflection was understandable, given that he had been ostracised and was in poor health. The traditional injunction against any public sharing of vulnerability by and between men, though perhaps less uniformly observed in Nietzsche's day, would almost certainly have constrained both his response to being emotionally overwhelmed and his friends' ability to offer him the kind of support he needed. In this sense he was arguably limited by values and conventions of masculinity that remained beyond 'the utmost limits of [his] imagination', and still await substantial overturning more than a century later (Allison, 2001 p. 177). Such defiant and paradoxical advocacy of liberation through individual experience amounts, ultimately, to a refusal to 'revalue' the realm of human relationship, and suggests that Nietzsche's newly found 'generosity of spirit' constituted only a partial cure. Perhaps the enabling fictions, that he had been the doer of his own deeds and that others he had been close to were in some sense, at least, subjects, with coherent and persisting identities, simply became too painful to sustain. His exposition of 'self-overcoming' nevertheless constitutes an early acknowledgement of the social construction of memory and emotional subjectivity, and remains an influential and potentially creative response to isolation and distress.

One of the distinctive ways in which Nietzsche coped with his illness and loneliness during this period was to converse with what he called his 'free spirits', 'shadows' or 'good Europeans'. These were imaginary interlocutors with whom he could conduct self-conscious philosophical dialogues, invisible companions and familiars he could laugh and chatter with or 'send to the Devil when they become tedious' – compensation for the friends he lacked (Allison, 2001 pp. 175–6).[28] Voices have long been a favourite diagnostic sign of incipient madness, and some commentators have seized upon an earlier passage, written when Nietzsche was twenty-five years old, for this reason. 'What I am afraid of is not the frightful shape behind my chair but its voice; also not the words, but the identifying unarticulated and inhuman tone of that shape. Yes, if only I could speak to it' (cited in Hayman, 1997 p. 45). Describing this as 'an outcrop of delusionary language', Hayman evokes a contorted substratum of essential craziness awaiting further exposure. He stresses the 'emphasis on voice', and goes on to attribute Nietzsche's final madness to an eventual loss of 'editorial control' over voices in his head, conceiving these in Jungian terms as repressed elements erupting into hallucinatory independence (Hayman, 1997 pp. 45, 54). Nietzsche had long insisted that the question 'who?' demanded genealogical enquiry into the nature of the 'will to power' being expressed, rather than the naming of a subject, but when friends began to receive letters signed 'Dionysos' or 'The Crucified One', this was interpreted as a key sign of incipient madness (Schrift, 1995 p. 30). There is further irony here, both because for Heidegger the name 'Nietzsche' became paradigmatic of the 'problematic of the name' and the question of unity in Western metaphysics, and because Nietzsche's sense of the multiplicity of selfhood arguably supports contemporary pluralistic approaches that demedicalise problematic voice hearing (Derrida, 1995 p. 59; Romme and Escher, 1993).

Nietzsche's symbolic abandonment of his own signature appears to have coincided with a retreat into grandiloquence, though the 'inspired clowning' that accompanied this undoubtedly compounds the difficulty of interpreting his missives. One morning he tearfully flung himself around the neck of a cart horse that was being beaten, then collapsed and was taken back to his lodgings.

The increasing strangeness of subsequent letters moved friends to seek psychiatric advice.[29] Not surprisingly, they were advised that he was indeed mad, and should be taken to a clinic. Nietzsche was duly deceived into making the journey from Turin to Basel under the pretence that receptions had been laid on for him, together with pageants and music festivals.[30] Yet another irony arises at this point, in that amidst the playful and rather desperate bombast, there was more than a grain of truth about the enormous posthumous influence of Nietzsche's work. Subsequent philosophers, notably Heidegger who situates him 'on the crest' of occidental metaphysics, echo the extravagance of his own claims (Derrida, 1995).[31] Undoubtedly driven by a masculinist imperative to excel in the domain of the father, to emerge victorious from the field of *agon*, Nietzsche had yearned for public affirmation, and paradoxically, perhaps experimentally, assumed the mantle of an almost forgotten god. With a tangle of contingent circumstances conspiring against his expectation of a triumphant 'performance climax', he chose to embrace not paternal Apollo, the formgiver, but Dionysos, the 'mad' god of dismemberment and renewal. 'Twisting free' of metaphysics, he spiralled into lonely chaos, then confinement, regression and oblivion. During this process, unfortunately, no one appears to have reminded him that an extravagant crescendo of personal success would have amounted to an absurd exaggeration of the metaphysical 'error' of 'subject-and-ego superstition' that his proto-postmodern voice had once so carefully elucidated.

Predictably, there are discrepancies between various contemporary as well as subsequent commentaries in the extent and timing of Nietzsche's 'madness'. While some dismissed his entire output on the grounds of irrationality, others, notably some of the women who knew him in his later years, categorically deny that there were any signs of impending breakdown.[32] Accounts inevitably draw upon available discourses about both gender and madness. There is a strong tradition, for example, that 'nervousness is the penalty of genius'. One commentator, writing in 1921, observes that 'Nietzsche's nervous system was not as perfectly balanced as that of a boxer or cricketer' (Levy, 1921/1985 pp. vi–vii). More recently, by contrast, Yovel finds hermeneutic value even in Nietzsche's final declamations, arguing that some major preoccupations (including opposition to anti-Semitism) became 'illuminated by the high beam of madness', albeit in distorted form (Yovel, 1994 p. 223). Whereas most authors emphasise the need for extreme caution when reading the play of forces, masks and voices at work in Nietzsche's hieroglyphic aphorisms, there is a tendency to discard critical subtlety once descent into 'madness' has been diagnosed. In an otherwise fascinating account of this period, Hayman, for instance, interprets Nietzsche's habit of calling himself the Kaiser, and his comment that he was 'Friedrich Wilhelm IV last time', as evidence of confusion about his identity, despite having previously informed us that he had not only been born on the birthday of King Friedrich Wilhelm IV, but named after him. Neither does he elaborate on the possibility that the philosopher's continued singing and screaming might have been, in part at least, a response to the way in which he was being treated (Hayman, 1980 pp. 339, 14, 337).[33]

Nietzsche was detained in the clinic at Basel for a week and then transferred to the asylum at Jena, where his mother could visit him regularly. Because of her financial circumstances he was admitted as a second-class patient, and would be confined there for just over a year. Not surprisingly, he soon became enraged at his new situation, frequently screaming and hardly sleeping, despite tranquillisers. The hospital routines, the summer heat, and other people irritated him (Hayman, 1980). A former medical student recollects a lecture at which the famous psychiatrist, Professor Otto Binswanger, presented 'Professor Nietzsche' to an audience of students who were clearly unaccustomed to being addressed by an inmate of such high social standing. Wanting to demonstrate disturbances in his patient's gait, Binswanger asked Nietzsche to walk about the room. When he responded 'slowly and lazily', the psychiatrist admonished him: 'Now, professor, an old soldier like you will surely be able to march correctly!' Thereupon Nietzsche's 'eyes lit up, his form straightened up, and he began to pace . . . with a firm stride' (Gilman, 1987 pp. 222–5). Binswanger took no interest in what the 'professor' had been writing, however. In February 1890 Nietzsche's mother moved to a flat in Jena, where he initially visited her, and then moved in. Jettisoned from a male-defined public realm in which he could no longer survive independently, he was returned once again to the maternal 'bosom' and a world of 'feminine' domesticity. In May they moved back to the same house in Naumburg that he had left at the age of fourteen, and his mother would spend almost all of her time caring for him, until she died, seven years later (Hollingdale, 1965/1999 p. 245).[34]

Nietzsche's story demonstrates that the line marking 'madness' is drawn differently by different people, not least according to their social position, and degree of investment in the gendered codes of public rationality, and that eventually a consensus emerges with sufficient collective power to proclaim a social Rubicon. Although Nietzsche himself had 'loved to emphasise [that] there are no normal persons at all', he was increasingly perceived through a conceptual lens of reductive diagnostic language, that effectively constrained the kinds of 'help' available to him (Gilman, 1987 p. 205). During this all too familiar process, the complexity and subtlety of multifaceted lives and events become condensed into a culturally and institutionally sanctioned story. Interpretations harden and polarise into a binary hierarchy of metaphysical absolutes – sanity and madness, reason and unreason, normality and abnormality – that progressively conceal the human drama actually unfolding, and mask the constructed nature of the discourses of dominant rationality. Even when visiting him in the asylum, two of Nietzsche's closest friends independently suspected, with some consternation, that he was only feigning madness, and was, once again, playing with 'self-concealments' and 'spiritual masks'. Their confusion was not surprising perhaps, given that he had once written about the Greeks simulating madness and praying for delirium (Hayman, 1980 p. 341). Some aspects of

Nietzsche's descent into madness, particularly the intense and sometimes inspired improvisation on the piano, and the child-like 'clowning', dancing and gesticulation, were, after all, closely consistent with his Dionysian philosophy, and self-declared status as an initiate of the 'mad' god.[35] But what he says about Dionysos is of more than biographical interest.

Tragic wisdom

In *The Birth of Tragedy*, his first major work, Nietzsche had constructed Apollo and Dionysos as contrasting figurations of two experiential principles, conceived as 'formative forces arising directly from nature', and divine patrons of complementary arts.[36] Demanding self-control, self-knowledge and moderation, Apollo was concerned with light, beauty, order and form, and 'must incorporate that thin line which the dream image may not cross under penalty of becoming pathological'. He embodied unshakeable confidence in the principle of individuation, but also the 'full delight, wisdom, and beauty of "illusion"'. Dionysos brought 'an ecstatic reality, which takes no account of the individual and may even destroy him, or else redeem him through a mystical experience of the collective'. This god of masks continually threatened rupture and renewal. His rapture came with 'narcotic potions' or the surging onrush of spring, and was celebrated by the Bacchic chorus, by St Vitus's dancers, and by the song and dance of medieval carnival. Nietzsche scorned the 'benighted souls' who label such phenomena as 'endemic diseases', but have no idea 'how cadaverous and ghostly their "sanity" appears as the throng of revellers sweeps by' (Nietzsche, 1871/1956 pp. 21–4). Tragedy reconciles these forces. In tragic culture, wisdom supplants science. 'This wisdom, unmoved by the pleasant distraction of the sciences, fixes its gaze on the total constellation of the universe and tries to comprehend sympathetically the suffering of that universe as its own' (Nietzsche, 1871/1956 pp. 111–12).[37] Where the wordless Dionysian chorus evokes an abyss from which individuality must continually be reconstituted, Apollonian imagery, by simultaneously revealing yet concealing, allows us the necessary detachment to make present that which cannot be represented, and to make bearable that which cannot be borne. Here, once again, we find the metaphor of an underworld journey. Tragedy gives us 'the means whereby a good crossing can be made, back from the Dionysian to the everyday, a crossing like that made by Er, back from Hades'. After making us 'tremble at the edge', it discloses the abyss as sublime, and leads us back from pessimism towards affirmation (Sallis, 1991 pp. 92–8).[38]

In tragedy, moreover, we assent to the destruction of the hero, as paragon of the will, 'since he too is merely a phenomenon' (Nietzsche, 1871/1956 p. 102). Nietzsche's Dionysos, a god who is dismembered yet eternally reborn, within the world rather than beyond it, epitomising and celebrating the dissolution and fragmentation of will, seems momentarily at least to converge with contemporary accounts of the 'mad god' as anti-sexist exemplar. But this very recognition that the solidity of the hero is illusory, a tiny cosmic irony, signals the possibility of an excessive celebration of dispersal, an engulfing ecstasy of asocial liberation that radically erodes any remaining awareness of the survival value of metaphysical 'error', and especially of coherent selfhood. When the late Nietzsche returned to the *Birth of Tragedy* he found some of it 'saccharine to the point of effeminacy'.[39] Having come to identify with Dionysos as 'will to power', the entire creative force, he now regarded Apollo, not as a complementary disposition, a 'fraternal' agency 'to be developed in strict proportion', but as the sublimation of that primordial Dionysian substratum (Hollingdale, 1965/1999 p. 85; Nietzsche, 1871/1956 pp. 141, 6). Whether this turning away from the paternally framing, restraining and image-building Apollo, in favour of a Dionysian 'primary man' of revelry, enchantment, sensuality and disintegration, but also potentially of 'monstrosity' and intoxication, followed or precipitated Nietzsche's madness, this was evidently a dangerous identification. The implications of an unmediated allegiance to such a principle, in terms of the persistent link between masculinity and violence, are self-evident, particularly if coupled to cultural values of the kind espoused by Nietzsche.[40]

Nietzsche's Dionysian recognition of mystery as a fundamental aspect of reality, as more than just a gap in our understanding, remains important, however, not least in relation to his challenge to dominant Enlightenment assumptions about rationality, and 'the square little reason' of scientists that was already underpinning a nascent scientific psychology (Sadler, 1995 pp. 137, 26). His rediscovery of Dionysos, a god of chaotic fragmentation, laceration and madness, but also of ecstasy, shape-shifting ambiguity and survival, is also interesting because of its influence on mythopoetic attempts to re-envision masculinity. But in the context of writings that advocate attention to men's emotional lives in response to long-standing feminist claims that the privileging of mind over body, and reason over emotion, is a hallmark of masculinity, Nietzsche's masculinist and anti-modernist reading of Dionysos may seem, at the very least, surprising (Seidler, 1994). It reminds us that our understandings of modernity and postmodernism, and of 'inner' voyages and therapeutic projects, are necessarily situated within particular values and assumptions. Despite his innovatory insights into the body and emotional life, Nietzsche's contribution now looks progressive only where his critical intellect established a deconstructive framework, thereby 'overcoming' an intense personal investment in the habitual values, the embodied language of feeling and thinking, of contemporary 'herd', or perhaps 'pack', masculinity. Given his sustained enthusiasm for hegemonic values it indeed seems astonishing that he generated such a potentially rich conceptual resource for subsequent deconstructive critiques.

It seems, from the foregoing exercise in critical biography, that the unacknowledged strictures of masculinity played a significant part in influencing the contingencies of Nietzsche's personal life, and hence the 'work' wrought from it. In particular, hegemonic values informed Nietzsche's personal crises, his experiences of loss, his solitary struggle with persistent health difficulties, and the 'hardening' not only of his polemics, but also, eventually, his philosophical attitude. Warren's reconstruction of a positive political vision commensurate with Nietzsche's preoccupation with life-affirmative individuation, and grounded in community, relatedness, egalitarianism and pluralism, implies a need to retain both his insight into the value of metaphysical 'error' and his conception of a 'tragic spirit' in which the two dispositions represented by Apollo and Dionysos are interwoven, generating a supplementary wisdom (Warren, 1988 p. 241; Allison, 2001 pp. 30–1; Sallis, 1991). Safranski, in similar vein, laments Nietzsche's failure to develop his own recurrent idea of a bicameral system of culture (Safranski, 2002 p. 200).

Nietzsche's late identification with Dionysos rather than Apollo foreclosed the possibility of envisioning an integrated masculinity, and symbolised an opening of the floodgates of experience, a personal journey beyond the orbit of self-restraint, and past the point where madness can be transmuted into tragic wisdom. It seems that people who recover successfully from periods of 'madness' are, unlike Nietzsche, able to cope with, or even benefit from, the seductive mystery of non-rational perception by affirming qualities such as patience, consistency and a degree of sobriety that often comes from valuing domestic responsibilities. Such people tend to have personal projects, and develop a sense of purpose, a 'horizon' that is practical as well as interesting and worthwhile (Chadwick, 2002). Nietzsche's lack of any sustained and sustaining commitment to other people, and the wild inflation of his personal horizons, meant that he had precious little grounding or capacity for moderation when it really mattered. Unlike his own formula for 'self-overcoming', Greek tragedy was conceived as a collective remedy against isolated suffering, a communal realisation of the capacity of experiential art to transform unspeakable pain and remake human worlds.

One way of pulling these strands together might be to counter the long silence of psychological discourse on the emotional contribution of fathers by reimagining a post-patriarchal Apollonian principle alongside the reconstructed Dionysos of Hillman and Rowan. Despite its corruption within patriarchal cultures, the function of framing, giving form, perspective, definition, stability, beauty, warmth, light and a necessary illusion of internal coherence, remains one that men need to embody.[41] In relation to fatherhood this necessarily entails negotiating horizons that are always already encrusted with ideology. In Nietzsche's case the earth had been unchained from its orbit around an Apollonian sun, or the sun had been eclipsed, and horizons radically destabilised by the symbolically resonant death of a paternal God. This primal rupture arguably instigated a cumulative loss of faith in 'Apollonian' processes that proved pivotal both to his post-metaphysical philosophy and to his experiences of distress. If we accept the implications of Nietzsche's insights into the complexity and constructed nature of subjectivity, however, we should be correspondingly cautious about making simple cognitivist and voluntaristic assumptions about the cultural effects of mythopoetic remythologising.

Rather than attempting to unravel contemporary diagnostic discourse, and the contingencies that formed the embodied complexity of Nietzsche's lived experience, I want to emphasise some broadly recognisable themes from his story. Firstly, I hope to have shown that critical readings of biography can focus, for instance, on men's relationship with their fathers, as an intimate encounter with patriarchal power, rather than as an expression of individual psychology. Secondly, in terms of biographical readings of the social, Nietzsche's story casts interesting light upon ways in which public masculinity has historically shaped men's experiences of distress and 'madness', informed institutional responses, and constrained processes of recovery. Since our capacity for integrity, commitment, accountability, even our 'sanity', may depend upon an ability to construct stories powerful enough to orchestrate the boundary tension between dissonant desires, voices and selves, an ability to engage with the helpful fantasy of personal coherence may be of much more than theoretical value. Yet this vital practice of self-containment becomes problematical for men, especially when recovering from personal crisis, if the only accessible narratives of coherent male selfhood are variations on the theme of hegemonic masculinity, and the only criteria for legitimacy, value and meaning are those of public prowess and domination. Nietzsche's story epitomises contradiction, ambivalence and complexity, and the 'generosity' he asks from his readers, and that may be needed in order to read past his deeply unattractive anti-democratic polemics, in some ways mirrors the critical generosity needed to relate constructively to the manner in which some men respond to experiences of distress or madness.[42] There are also issues around gender in relation to 'caring', and the complexity and difficulty of relationships with family, friends and the wider world, that still have a familiar ring about them. Thirdly, in terms of biographical reading of theory, I have argued that Nietzsche's investment in hegemonic masculinity may account for the marked discrepancy between his politics and his influential deconstructive philosophy. I also identify an association between a certain impulse towards visionary transcendence, paradoxically consistent with a gendered over-valuation of disembodiment in the Western metaphysical tradition that Nietzsche challenged in his writings, and the genealogy of unbounded malestream postmodern theory. In various ways, then, Nietzsche's story can be read as a history of the present.

In *Ecce Homo*, Nietzsche wanted simultaneously to distinguish his life from his books *and* to show the impossibility of being anything other than the body of work he produced (Lionnet, 1989). His insistence that creativity is situated, and that selfhood and writing are layered and plural, enables us to side-step this Dionysian conundrum. As a political polemicist, he relied on a universalising metaphysics of domination, yet remained very much a man of his time (Warren, 1988). As a proto-postmodern philosopher, however, Nietzsche's mad-sounding claim that he was a 'posthumous' figure seems amply justified by the treasure that critically generous readers continue to find among the conceptual legacy he bequeathed to subsequent generations.

Chapter 5

The scream of life itself?

Language and power in the life of Antonin Artaud

An exemplary madman?

> Let us leave textual criticism to graduate students, formal criticism to
> aesthetes, and recognise that what has been said is not still to be said; that
> an expression does not have the same value twice, does not live two lives;
> that all words, once spoken, are dead and function only at the moment
> when they are uttered.
>
> (Artaud, 1938/1970)

> All these pages are leftover icicles of the mind. Excuse my absolute freedom.
> I refuse to make distinctions between any of the minutes of myself. And I
> don't recognise any maps of the mind.
>
> (Artaud, *Here Where Others* . . . in Hirschman, 1965)

The work of Antonin Artaud, writer, visual artist, performer, dancer, film actor,
theatre director and actor, traveller and 'destroyer of languages', continues to
'ricochet strongly through contemporary culture' long after his death in 1948
(Barber, 1993 p. 2). He has been called a 'modern master', a pioneer, even a
prophet (Esslin, 1976 pp. 10–11). Such hyperbolic assessments may well have
been influenced by Foucault's celebration, in the closing pages of *Madness and
Civilisation* (1961/1967), of Artaud, alongside Nietzsche and Van Gogh, as an
exemplar of madness as a fundamental experience, an absolute Otherness. In
this early work, Foucault suggests that the 'sovereign enterprise of unreason'
might open up a 'total contestation' of Western culture; and, echoing Nietzsche's
turn away from Apollonian processes, he looks for this opening where madness
effects an absolute break with the work of art. In what Dreyfus and Rabinow
describe as an early 'flirtation with hermeneutic depth', he asserts that madness
itself draws an absolute ontological boundary, 'the exterior edge, the line of dissolution, the contour against the void'.[1] Much as Heidegger had located the
cusp of Nietzsche's madness at the crest of Western metaphysics, Foucault
accords Artaud an exalted position for having journeyed closest to that point

where some unspecified yet utterly profound truth about the human condition might be revealed. Artaud's *oeuvre*

> experiences its own absence in madness, but that experience, the fresh courage of that ordeal, all those words hurled against a fundamental absence of language, all that space of physical suffering and terror which surrounds or rather coincides with the void – that is the work of art itself: the sheer cliff over the abyss of the work's absence.
>
> (Foucault, 1961/1971 p. 287)

In this blurring of conventional boundaries between life and art, madness enjoys a paradoxical victory through a radically enlarged conception of art, so that a world expecting to measure madness through psychology now has to measure itself against the 'mad' excess of Artaud's work (Foucault, 1961/1971 pp. 278, 286–9; Dreyfus and Rabinow, 1982 pp. 11–12).

Derrida, in his essay 'La Parole Soufflée', takes issue with the appropriation of Artaud's madness as a 'case' in both clinical and critical (literary or philosophical) discourse, where the specificity of his life experience has been 'silenced by the totalising operation of the exemplary'.[2] He has in turn been accused of treating Artaud in much the same way, however, using his urgent ambivalence towards language to illustrate the 'parasitical' strategy of deconstruction, which must necessarily use tools fashioned from within the logocentric tradition it seeks to disrupt. Although Derrida insists he isn't looking to 'extort hidden truth from a life experience that refuses to signify', he 'does not avoid the danger of exemplarity' and even finds '*the very essence of madness*' in Artaud's project (Derrida, 1967/1978; see also Pireddu, 1996 pp. 44–6). The same issue also arises when Deleuze and Guattari use Artaud as a model for their conception of a 'schizoanalytic' mode of thought and being (Dale, 1997 p. 591; Atteberry, 2000 p. 716). I want to explore this marked tendency to regard a particular kind of male madness as exemplary in an anti-heroic sense, and to consider the life and work of Antonin Artaud in the context of his positioning within this kind of discourse.

Artaud and Nietzsche

Since there are some striking parallels between the lives of Nietzsche and Artaud, and since Artaud explicitly regarded Nietzsche as an influential predecessor in a tradition of dissenting and misunderstood artists, we might expect some of the same issues to arise in relation to their respective biographical experience. I will begin, therefore, by reviewing some of these similarities. The lives of these two men overlap chronologically, but only just. By the year 1896, when Antonin Artaud was born, Nietzsche was alternating between 'dreadful excitability' and mute prostration, having finally retreated beyond the reach of those closest to him. Like Nietzsche, Artaud would experience chronic ill-health, document his suffering in impressive detail, and reconceptualise the human body accordingly, before dying in equally tragic circumstances. Like Nietzsche, he lived a relatively short but intense life, in which a prodigiously productive late burst of creativity was impelled by the knowledge that there was little time left.[3]

Both men experienced incarceration, and of course both became the focus of considerable subsequent popular, cultural and academic interest (Hayman, 1980 pp. 352–3; Ward, 1999 p. 130). Both men also became absorbed in solitary experimentation upon themselves. For Artaud this took the form of constant explorations of his own body and senses, his breathing and his voice. Where Nietzsche had written about the value of intoxication for creativity, Artaud experimented with drugs such as opium and peyote in order to investigate altered mental states. Like Nietzsche, Artaud wanted to transcend social restrictions that limited mental and bodily experience, and to reinvent what it might mean to be human (Ward, 1999 p. 129). Like Nietzsche, Artaud regarded his work as intensely autobiographical. As early as 1925, before the age of thirty, he proclaimed that 'where others aspire to create works of art I do not want anything apart from showing my spirit . . . I cannot conceive of a work of art as distinct from life' (Esslin, 1976 p. 12). Both men described their writing in visceral terms. Where Nietzsche 'wrote in blood', Artaud described his work as 'waste matter from myself, scrapings off the soul' (Allison, 1977/1985 p. xiii; Hayman, 1977 pp. 139–40). Curiously, however, he was also similar to Nietzsche in managing to combine ferocious public rhetoric with an 'exceptionally mild' and 'sweet natured' manner in his private life (Esslin, 1976 p. 109).[4] Both men, at various times, also expressed the prevailing cultural assumption that a sensible woman could be found to look after them while they got on with their life-long creative endeavours.[5]

Both men had an intensely religious upbringing, and for both, the death of God opened up possibilities for a transformed spirituality. As with Nietzsche, some commentators find qualities in Artaud that might have made him a shaman or prophet.[6] Where Nietzsche continually opposed the Western metaphysical tradition in philosophy, Artaud, with comparable vigour and single-mindedness, directed his critical energy against the scourge of representation, a theme that would be taken up by Derrida (Derrida, 1967/1978). For Artaud, the term 'metaphysics' had positive connotations, signifying an examination of inner worlds, and contemplation of the mysterious source of human existence. Such metaphysics was habitually concealed by intellectual language, and by preoccupation with mundane matters, but could be approached with 'the spirit of profound anarchy which is the basis of all poetry', or by working directly on the body (Artaud, 1970 p. 71; Esslin, 1976 p. 81; Hayman, 1977 p. 79). Derrida regarded his move away from psychological theatre towards a rediscovery of religious and mystical meaning as a challenge to the secularising trajectory of the West (Derrida, 1967/1978 p. 243).[7] Artaud came close to Freud, however, in seeking to distil articulate speech into 'hieroglyphic' imagery of dream-like quality, though his priority was to forge language into a physical medium that could shatter and then 'manifest', even if recovering its shock potential meant relinquishing the capacity to signify what was being summoned (Esslin, 1976 p. 81; Derrida, 1967/1978; Artaud, 1938/1970). His performative metaphysics of fragmentary incantation would be inherently unsuited to the grounding of truth claims, and hence very different to the hegemonic metaphysics of Western idealism. As with Nietzsche, such a perspective would make for a tense encounter with psychiatry.

The Theatre of Cruelty, masculinity and language

Comparing him with Nietzsche, Esslin describes Artaud as 'a romantic vitalist, a believer in the healing power of the life force', the power of instinct, body and emotions, against rationalism and rarefied abstraction. But where an early Nietzsche located the origins of theatre in the capacity of Apollonian clarity, measure, and reason to moderate the turbulent, passionate but inarticulate Dionysian force, Artaud, who describes theatre in very Nietzschean terms, 'rejected the Apollonian element altogether', and identified entirely with 'the dark forces of Dionysian vitality with all their violence and mystery' (Esslin, 1976 p. 80).[8] It is hardly surprising, therefore, that his work, like that of Nietzsche, is replete with violent imagery. Artaud is best known for his conception of a Theatre of Cruelty, distinguished by an emphasis on the ability of theatre to act physically upon a crowd of spectators using actions comparable with, though 'sublimated' into subtler forms than, direct physical assault. The proximity to actual violence here becomes clear in an injunction that that an actor should 'use his emotions in the same way that a boxer uses his muscles', and that 'once launched into his fury the actor needs infinitely more virtue to stop himself from committing a crime than an assassin needs courage to commit his' (Artaud, 1938/1970 p. 89; Esslin, 1976 p. 82).[9] It is important to note, however, not least with his subsequent 'madness' in mind, that Artaud acknowledged the risks inherent in such a strategy, and was clear, at least in terms of intention, about the distinction between 'cruelty' and violence.

Whereas Nietzsche envisaged an endless succession of masks, Artaud adopted a discourse of therapeutic depth in which masks would be torn away, 'impelling us to see ourselves as we really are'. Yet he was clearly not expecting to expose static essences. The purpose of incantation was 'to benumb, to bewitch, to arrest our sensibility', to open up a deeper, subtler, more magical state of perception, 'to generate stupendous flights of forms'. He felt that theatre should act upon us 'after the manner of unforgettable soul therapy', and memorably deployed the lurid anatomical metaphor of the plague. Theatre is 'collectively made to drain abscesses'. It works like a healing poison, 'a revenging scourge, a redeeming epidemic', fomenting a crisis that can only be resolved by death or 'drastic purification'. 'Final balance' can only be attained through destruction. In particular, theatre 'urges the mind on to delirium'. Madness, specifically a madness that confronts murderous rage and the extremities of experience, is a necessary stage in this unforgettable therapy (Artaud, 1938/1970 pp. 70–1, 64, 21–2). So confident was Artaud in the purgative power and 'purity' of illumination in a theatre 'where violent physical images pulverise [and] mesmerise the audience's sensibilities', that he defied his (generically male) spectator, once outside the theatre, 'to indulge in thoughts of war, riot, or motiveless murder'. The success of this alchemy would depend significantly on the 'affective athleticism' of his actors, amounting to an almost tantric 'mastery' over the passions.[10] Whereas a murderer's fury is released in the act, and 'exhausts itself', the actor's fury 'remains enclosed within a circle', progressively denying itself as it is expressed, so that it 'merges with universality' (Artaud, 1938/1970, pp. 62, 88–90, 16).

The use of generic male pronouns throughout would have seemed unremarkable when Artaud was writing, but many subsequent commentators still overlook the implications of his gender-blind exhortations to direct considerable dramatic fury at an undifferentiated audience. Any experiential exploration of the charged and necessarily unstable boundaries of violence must now be seen in the context of feminist understandings that show men to be 'the experts . . . specialists' and 'major *doers* of violence' (Hearn, 1996 p. 99). In *The Theatre and its Double* Artaud seemed to be expounding a soul therapy for himself, but set out a method that reduced human communication to an all-or-nothing binary choice between the invasive sensory overload of total encounter or complete withdrawal (Artaud, 1938/1970). All the nuances of interpersonal relationship would be lost in a cathartic carnival. Much of his material has an excremental quality, and he wanted to approach the work of detoxification at a collective and cultural, rather than individual, level but his manifesto remained apolitical, and paradoxically insensitive to the needs of vulnerable people.[11] We would now be looking, for example, for some recognition that a man processing rage should not expect to be regarded unquestioningly as simply a victim, however badly he may have been hurt. Recent understandings that men's social power can include individual powerlessness, and that men's pain needs to be located in the context of men's aggregate power, appear relevant here (Kimmel, 1998). If men's rage often conceals socially proscribed tenderness, Artaud's insistence on an angry cataclysm might be regarded as concealing a marked reluctance to admit any vulnerability, or express the softer and supposedly 'feminine' emotions (Seidler, 1994). But, as with many men who experience intense distress, he may well have had compelling personal reasons for such avoidance.

Given that Artaud's life story became something of a paradigm of medicalisation, his resort to therapeutic language in the theatrical manifestos is unsurprising. It also seems likely that the quite disturbing and quintessentially tragic preoccupations he brought to bear in the few plays he either wrote or recommended for their 'cruel' quality were the smoke from some intractable, if obscure, biographical fires. Prominent among these preoccupations was incest in all its forms, not least between brothers and sisters. The sense that emotional injury drove his later mental distress is compounded by recurrent nocturnal imagery of being sexually assaulted by 'malicious demonic figures' that persisted throughout his later years. So vivid and threatening did this imagery become that he would try to protect himself from it by struggling, screaming and dancing (Barber, 1993 p. 93).[12] Like Nietzsche, Artaud was also exposed to the reality of death at a very early age. Only two of his eight siblings survived infancy, and a few months after the death of a three-day-old brother, the four-year-old Antonin suffered a bout of illness so severe that he was not expected to survive.[13] Like Nietzsche, curiously, he was then left with a sister, with whom he developed a close and mutually protective relationship, and because his father was often away, was 'surrounded for most of the time by females' (Hayman, 1977). As with Nietzsche, difficulty with an absent father figure also seems to have been a major theme.[14]

Unlike Nietzsche, however, Artaud developed his distinctive ideas about language through a protracted struggle with the medium. Such was this struggle that he took the paradoxical step of coining a term, 'unpower' ('impouvoir'), to refer to 'the inability to ever make . . . language one's own' (Atteberry, 2000 p. 718). This new concept emerged during Artaud's formative correspondence with Jacques Rivière, conservative editor of the prestigious Nouvelle Revue Française. Artaud, then an aspiring young poet, argued for the greater vitality and value of the fragment, or 'failed' text, as opposed to the whole or 'successful' poem. His own intensely autobiographical offerings were 'exceptional in their willed upheaval and contraction of the language of poetry and the imagery of the self' (Barber, 1993 p. 20). Artaud accused language of imprisoning thought by reducing the particular to the level of signification, and hence generalisation, and experienced thought and language as a dispossession, a violation of his uniqueness. Far from reflecting the 'impotence' of 'having nothing to say', however, 'unpower' signified and celebrated a force of inspiration suffused with an awareness of the impossibility of ever fully understanding its own origins, or the nature of the voice that would speak it. Artaud was particularly fascinated by what Derrida terms 'glossopoeia', a form of language that neither imitates nor names, but keeps returning to the moment before articulation (Derrida, 1967/1978 pp. 176, 240).[15]

In the correspondence he surrendered himself to the editor's 'judgement' and repeatedly asked for forgiveness, yet clearly hoped to demolish the entire metaphysical and religious tradition of judgement upon which Rivière's position rested. Rivière responded by rejecting the poems, but offered to publish the correspondence instead, anonymously. Artaud was furious: 'Why attempt to put on a literary level a thing which is the scream of life itself?' His wild 'shreds', detailing the painful cerebral processes of creativity, must be exposed, so that their fragmented sounds could be given breath and life (Barber, 1993 p. 20; Atteberry, 2000). The correspondence was finally published on 1 September 1924, and on 7 September, Artaud's father died. During a lecture given twelve years later, in Mexico, Artaud recalled:

I lived to the age of twenty seven with an obscure hatred of the Father, of my own father in particular, until the day when I saw him die. Then, that inhuman rigour, which I had often accused him of oppressing me with, fell away. Another being left that body. And for the first time in our lives, my father held out his arms to me. And I, always restless in my body, I understood that all through life he had been made restless by his body, and that there is a lie to being alive, against which we are born to protest.

(Artaud, 1976 vol. 8, p. 146)

His exchange with Rivière soon attracted the attention of Breton, and shortly after the funeral the leading Surrealist invited him to join the movement.[16]

This sequence of contextual events is interesting when considered in relation to discussions about the development of Artaud's orientation against language. Derrida's observation, that although 'cruelty' was not necessarily about sadism and bloodshed, there was 'always a murder' at its origin, in particular, a parricide, is potentially significant in this respect, though the murder in question is clearly a patricide. 'The origin of the theatre . . . is the hand lifted against the abusive wielder of the logos, against the father, against the God of a stage subjugated to the power of speech and text' (Derrida, 1967/1978 p. 239). In the process of evicting God from the theatre, it seems, a cruel father, 'another being', had to be confronted among Artaud's memories and imaginings. This kind of process is suggested by a transition in the way in which he presents his beliefs about language. In his letters to the paternalistic Rivière, Artaud had somewhat apologetically advocated a perpetual negation of structure. This refusal to 'fix' language remained a central preoccupation, but once he joined the Surrealists, Artaud became much more resolute and angry about the issue, urging them to use language that was 'scathing and glowing, but glowing in the way that a weapon glows'. Here, of course, he is very close to Nietzsche's conception of language as an arsenal of weapons, useful for precipitating violent upheaval.[17]

But whereas Nietzsche often used 'cruelty', even 'festive' cruelty, in a physical and emotional sense, Artaud developed the term in a manner reminiscent of Nietzsche's notion of 'hardness' (Ascheim, 1992 p. 243). For him it signified 'an unforgiving and rigorous struggle for the *measure without measure*, a refusal to allow the self to relax, to settle into any determinate mode of thought or expression'. Failure to be 'cruel', in this sense, would allow language to solidify into the paralysing codes of *parjuger*, the prejudgement he associated with the written word, and with the 'judgement of God', a repressive structure separating us from the force of life and from the world (Atteberry, 2000 pp. 733–7). For Artaud, then, a 'festival of cruelty' would be a space opened up by transgression, in which the distance of representation, with all its 'footlights and protective barriers', is collapsed in favour of 'absolute danger . . . without foundation'. There would be no message, no interpretation, no repetition, nothing to see. Spectators would become actors, in an experience of presence, force and life

(Derrida, 1967/1978 pp. 244–5). But before experiencing the presence of life, they must be confronted with a truly Nietzschean outpouring of creative destruction. Violent imagery would be deployed in the service of deconstruction, yet rendered paradoxically synonymous with a profound, though intolerant and intensely dualistic, affirmation. At times Artaud wants to kill in order to cure. 'He who does not smell of a smouldering bomb and of compressed vertigo is not worthy to be alive' (Hirschman, 1965 p. 158).

The presence of this disturbing element in the discourse of two formative male theorists of deconstruction, and their enthusiastic conception of language as weaponry, suggests common influences within a social landscape significantly shaped by gender systems that consistently validate the expression of men's anger (Connell, 1987 p. 140; Flax, 1990 p. 138). The prominence within their respective counter-discourses of the symbolic death, or eviction, of a distantly omnipotent God, and the possibility that much of the impetus to destroy and reconstruct may have emanated from a desire to 'murder' an absent, and painfully remote father, appears consistent with this. Moreover, the intensification of their eschatological pronouncements, as the conventional trappings of maturity, for various reasons, evaded them, seems to confirm the intractable and visceral nature of their hunger for radical renewal.[18] Artaud's oeuvre culminated in an extraordinary radio play whose title, To Have Done With the Judgement of God, clearly foregrounds this lifelong theme. Still vehemently committed to fracturing the processes of signification and representation, he orchestrated an impressive cacophony of invented language, multi-layered voices, percussion, screaming and laughter, in a recorded performance of various texts dealing with his main preoccupations.[19] One of these was devoted to a mocking denunciation of the diagnoses and definitions of insanity upon which various God-like psychiatrists had based their judgements about him (Barber, 1993 pp. 151–5).

Clinical and critical discourse: unpacking some 'case' history

While emphasising the probability of linkages between personal experience and the virulent nihilism that pervades Artaud's work, I want to reassert the importance of attempting to talk about emotional injury without colluding in psychologising and medicalising discourses. Because Artaud's entanglement with these discourses was so intimate, spectacular and destructive, because they have become insidiously constitutive of our sense of our selves, and because they have been appropriated even within ostensibly 'critical' discourse, this will necessitate some careful unpacking.[20] Their widespread adoption also exacerbates the problematic ambivalence of mainstream postmodern social theory about appeals to experience.

In 'La Parole Soufflée', one of two essays on Artaud in Writing and Difference, Derrida argues that critical commentary that sets out to protect the value of a work from psychomedical reduction, ends up being just as reductive, since it also treats the work as a case. An 'adventure of thought' becomes a mere example of 'a structure whose essential permanence becomes the prime preoccupation of the commentary' (Derrida, 1967/1978 pp. 170).[21] But before we allow Derrida's observation about an omnipresent urge towards parricide to close our discussion about Artaud's use of language, it should be remembered that his essays on Artaud are both haunted by the unacknowledged presence of Lacan and Freud.[22] The psychoanalytic theory of Lacan is of particular relevance here, having been proposed, in response to 'La Parole Soufflée', as a means of attempting 'to partake in Artaud's psychotic discourse by following the surface movement of its signifiers, a trajectory with many distortions and no secrets' (Pireddu, 1996 pp. 47–50). Lacan's view of schizophrenia as a 'linguistic disorder', in which the signifying chain of meaning crumbles, also has a broader significance, having been adopted as a metaphor for the postmodern condition (Sarup, 1996 pp. 96–7). I want to critically evaluate the impact of clinical discourse, therefore, by looking at how Lacan's work has been used to approach to the 'case' of Artaud.

Pireddu advocates Lacanian psychoanalysis on the basis that it attempts to interpret 'psychosis' by means of establishing 'a network of relationships that do not involve any depth', and by attending to shifting positions in language, rather than by imposing arbitrary fictions and then claiming to understand. Like Freud, Lacan understood psychosis in terms of a lack of censorship. By means of 'foreclosure', 'the psychotic rejects an unbearable representation as if it had never reached his ego', and the 'ego', at the mercy of the 'id', constructs a deluded view of the world. Lacan's distinctive contribution was to identify 'the foreclosure of the Name of the Father' as the origin of psychosis, a move that resonates unmistakably beneath Derrida's references to parricide.[23] According to Pireddu, Artaud faced an acute impasse in constantly wanting to use the laws of language to convey pre-linguistic and inherently incommunicable experiences of 'jouissance', to 'partake simultaneously in the real and the symbolic'. He was unable to circumvent the necessity of repetition, yet unwilling to abandon the quest for non-repetition, and his frustrated desire to belong to the symbolic, if only in order to challenge it, expressed resistance to Oedipalization and 'repudiation of the paternal yoke'. Artaud wanted to use the 'naked language of theatre' in order to embark upon an 'infinite regress', to reinstate 'true beauty' and unmask the void of nature. The stage would become a 'pre-symbolic' space, where he could 'condense the life of flesh into an inscription', and 'transgress the ordinary limits of art and the word', in order to create a 'real' language. Signifiers would be incarnated into characters, and thus treated, in Kristeva's terms, as the 'true real', a move regarded as typical of 'psychotic discourse'. In the end, after a 'titanic struggle' against language and its difference, however, Artaud resorted to painstaking record keeping, encoding his work in 'musical scores' and texts, so that writing ultimately retained its power as the 'master code' (Pireddu, 1996 pp. 52, 56–62).

However evocative and plausible this kind of interpretative framework may initially appear – Lacan's description of the reproduction of patriarchal power and, in particular, his conception of the symbolic as 'a set of meanings that define culture and are embedded in language' has been important for some feminist and pro-feminist psychoanalysts – a number of difficulties arise with the use of Lacanian theory, in terms of the politics of both gender and 'mental health' (Mitchell, 1974/2000; Frosh, 1994).[24] The repercussions of his ideas for understandings of 'madness' have often been overlooked, however. From the viewpoint of perspectives critical of psychopathology the difficulties may prove insurmountable, but here too there could be a positive element. Lacan's view that each individual must take up a position in the social order by 'inscribing' themselves within a chain of cultural signifiers, or risk psychosis, has the latent merit of locating madness in relation to processes of linguistic and cultural exclusion, specifically from the norms of patriarchal culture (Frosh, 1999 pp. 216–17).[25] By linking 'psychosis' in men with the ongoing trauma of metaphorical castration, and with a failure to repudiate the 'feminine', Lacan appears to be reaffirming the familiar association and overlap between the historical exclusions of women and those deemed mad as non-rational outcasts from the 'Cartesian dream of power' (Scheman, 1996). When coupled with his insistence that even 'normal' selves are decentred and founded upon a 'delusional' image of integrity that holds disintegrating forces at bay, this seems, at first sight, a constructive and non-medicalising perspective that could generate empowering interpretations of the kind of 'madness' that Artaud experienced (Frosh, 1999 pp. 142–5).

Some of the difficulties with Lacan that undercut this promise also arise from his reliance on Freud, however. Far from inspiring cultural transformation, Freud's use of the vividly tragic story of Oedipus has arguably served to reinforce oppression. Although it may be fruitful to explore the familial construction of rigid sexual differentiation, normative heterosexuality and hegemonic rationality, the 'Oedipal struggle' and the 'Name of the Father' are both problematic reference points. Use of these powerful rhetorical devices, even as descriptions of how patriarchal authority is sustained, carries some important implications. For example, although Freud invoked the Oedipus myth to dramatise his contention that every son must live with an unconscious desire to kill his father and marry his mother, this is a story of extreme paternal violence and abuse (Claire, 2001 p. 168).[26] Any interpretation of it that depicts a young boy's rage towards his father as an innate and defining characteristic not only exacerbates the likelihood that abusive fathers will be let off the hook but risks perpetuating the very emotional damage that psychoanalysis purports to elucidate.

Lacan's formulation of psychosis replicates this fundamental problem, effectively leaving 'the psychotic' in a position similar to that of Freud's pre-Oedipal child. Responding to the apparent frequency of the theme of paternity in delusions, Lacan noted that events which evoke the idea of symbolic paternity often served as a catalyst for psychosis. The individualising momentum of psycho-analysis turned his gaze towards the discourse of those whose emotional injury had forced them to 'foreclose' the entire notion of paternity, at the expense however, of investigating the operation of patriarchal norms and conventions, or the actions of actual fathers (Jantzen, 1998 p. 53).[27] Having recognised this danger, we can begin to consider whether our need to understand the formation of male subjectivities means that there may still be a case for adapting some elements from psychoanalytic explanations, rather than rejecting them out-right.[28] Before we borrow such conceptual clothing, we need to be confident that we are not thereby tacitly assenting to oppressive clinical practice, or abetting medicalisation. Any resort to psychoanalysis when talking about the lives of 'mad' people is likely to be contested, with good reason. Whether we regard 'madness' as a dimension of difference, or see it purely as a social category instituted or legitimated by clinical discourse, this is politically sensitive terrain. Ostensibly scientific psychoanalytic terms such as 'paranoid', 'narcissistic', 'hysterical' or 'neurotic' are suffused with pejorative connotations, and belong with the burgeoning psychiatric discourse that emerged from the same origins within the nineteenth-century asylum, and that has been repeatedly critiqued and rejected from within the survivor movement (Plumb, 1993; O'Hagan, 1996; Pembroke, 1994/1996; Wallcroft and Michaelson, 2001; Foucault, 1961/1971).

It should be possible to talk about the self-absorption of a man such as Artaud without encapsulating this within the universalising and totalising structuralist parameters of 'narcissism', not least since he himself came to reject psycho-analytic commentary, and the associated notion of secret interiority (Derrida, 1967/1978 p. 242). When Artaud turned to psychoanalysis at the age of thirty-one, he wrote to Dr Allendy: 'I have a fundamental need for someone like you. There is something rotten inside me, a sort of fundamental defect in my psyche, which prevents me from enjoying what destiny offers me.' After a short series of sessions he reported feeling 'a sort of prostitution, of shameless-ness', in letting his consciousness be 'penetrated . . . by an alien intelligence' (Hayman, 1977 p. 72). Because of the horrific ill-treatment he was later sub-jected to, it becomes difficult to question whether this rejection was, even in part, the product of a conventional masculine defence against introspection. Artaud may, of course, simply have been acutely sensitive to the nuances of power involved in such a relationship. After his experience of incarceration, he would radically reverse his ideas about doctors and patients.

> So it is that I consider
> that it's up to the everlastingly sick in me
> to cure all doctors
> – born doctors by lack of sickness –
> and not up to doctors ignorant of my dreadful
> states of sickness

to impose their insulintherapy on me,
their health for a worn out world.

(Hirschman, 1965 p. 193)

The most serious difficulty with Lacan as a source of inspiration for discussions about Artaud, however, undoubtedly stems from his psychiatric background. Artaud's period of incarceration began when a trip to Ireland, undertaken as part of his mounting preoccupation with imminent catastrophe and global upheaval, which he would personally direct, was curtailed by his arrest on vagrancy charges. He was duly deported, and after a disturbance during the voyage was put in a straitjacket. At the General Hospital in Le Havre he was left in the straitjacket for seventeen days, and then admitted to an asylum in Rouen. After his mother's intervention he was transferred to the Henri Rouselle clinic at the Sainte-Anne Asylum in Paris, and was held there between April 1938 and February 1939. As director of this clinic, Lacan was responsible for diagnosing patients and arranging for their transfer to other institutions, and there seems to have been considerable contact, as well as mutual hostility, between the two men. During this period, Artaud was diagnosed as chronically and incurably insane, and was contemptuous of the conditions under which he was held (Barber, 1993 pp. 9, 99).[29]

Neither Derrida, who admittedly only alludes to Lacan while advocating absolute resistance to clinical exegeses, nor Pireddu, who explicitly recommends Lacanian psychoanalysis as the key to interpreting Artaud's 'psychotic discourse', mentions this historical detail, which may only seem crucial to those informed by the politics of 'mental health' (Pireddu, 1996; Derrida, 1967/1978). Perhaps Derrida was unaware of it, and only knew the seemingly reconstructed Lacan who was later associated with the anti-psychiatry movement. Even if the encounter had not taken place, however, Lacan's initial training still casts a shadow across his later work on subjectivity and language.[30] From perspectives critical of psychopathology, the term 'psychotic',[31] however reformulated, remains an arbitrary fiction, one of the key terms used to legitimate the right and duty of psychiatry alone to treat certain individuals (Parker et al., 1995 pp. 101–2). It effectively condemns victims for their injury – remember Artaud's nocturnal imagery of being sexually assaulted by demonic figures – by marking them as alien. In critical discourse its unexamined use has clearly worked against the force and coherence of Artaud's published self-advocacy, retrospectively reducing his work to an effect of symptomatology, and erasing his considerable contribution as an agent, thinker and writer. Far from avoiding the theft of Artaud's words, Pireddu surely secures their classification within a Lacanian clinical taxonomy, as a 'case' of psychotic discourse, unambiguously confirmed by the omnipresence of an unacknowledged father metaphor (Pireddu, 1996).[32]

Insofar as they depend upon borrowings from clinical discourse, such accounts negate the value of ambivalence, contradiction and liminality, and undermine

Artaud's capacity to open up 'cruel' existential terrain by negotiating tense and protracted explorations at the boundaries of thought, language and consciousness. His own subtle concept 'unpower' grasps this well, whereas terms such as 'psychotic discourse' or 'thought disordered' can only caricature and close down such processes. 'A world expecting to measure and justify madness through psychology must justify itself before madness', not simply, as Foucault demanded at the close of *Madness and Civilisation*, through the excess of Artaud's work, but by recognising the contribution of his intellect as well (Foucault, 1961/1971 p. 289). Ironically, the early Foucault's celebration of Artaud's madness as radically Other (and Derrida's surprising claim to have identified the very essence of madness in his project) may well have compounded the constraining impact of medicalisation on this madman's reputation. As with Lacan's closely comparable description of a mysterious essential femininity, characterised by inexpressible 'jouissance', anyone characterised in this way is 'charged with introducing difference', yet deemed unable to speak (Flax, 1990 p. 106). For all his eloquence about the cultural production of madness and the broken dialogue between reason and madness, Foucault chose not to close his historical treatise with an examination of the specific ways in which exemplary 'madness' had been socially constructed in the lives of Nietzsche, Van Gogh or Artaud. Despite his obvious sympathy, his analytical method meant that he neither mentioned Artaud's ferocious initial objection to being designated 'mad' nor cited his influential reclamation of 'authentic madness' (Foucault, 1961/1971 pp. xi–xiii).

Making an example of 'poor M. Antonin Artaud'

Derrida regards Foucault's insistence that 'madness is the absence of a work' as the fundamental motif of *Madness and Civilisation*, and continually associates madness with silence, in terms redolent of Artaud's struggle with thinking and writing. This leads him to conclude that

> The misfortune of the mad, the interminable misfortune of their silence, is that their best spokesmen [sic] are those who betray them best; which is to say that when one attempts to convey their silence *itself*, one has already passed over to the side of the enemy, the side of order, even if one fights order from within it, putting its origin into question.
>
> (Derrida, 1967/1978 pp. 34–5, 54, 36)

Leaving aside the question of Foucault's claim that there was a singular historical 'Decision', when madness was excluded from the world of reason, the dangers inherent in accepting a binary framework that continually reinforces this schism, and of conflating essentialised madness with an essentialised mad person, are epitomised here.[33]

Derrida seems so excited by Artaud's 'stratagem', his howling articulation of 'the meaning of an art prior to madness *and* the work, an art which no longer yields works, an artist's existence that no longer . . . gives access to something other than itself', that he too ignores the texts against psychiatry. However much an 'existence that refuses to signify . . . an art without works, [or] a language without a trace' may confound both critic and doctor, Artaud did speak, did produce 'works', and did signify. When Artaud says, for example, that he was 'writing for illiterates', Derrida recognises this as a careful reference to his fascination with non-Western civilisations that show how 'the most profound and living culture' can flourish without writing (Derrida, 1967/1978 pp. 174, 188).[34] Yet Artaud's late writing, forged from and articulating his asylum experience, is surely as valid as the earlier theorising about the difficulty of language. Any unquestioning acceptance of Artaud's declaration that 'what you took to be my works were only my waste matter' effectively amplifies a powerful voice within him that subverts his own increasingly hard-won moments of lucidity – and silences another that insists upon 'cruelty' as an exercise in consciousness (Derrida, 1967/1978, p. 182; Barber, 1993 pp. 7, 23). Derrida effectively endorses an essentialist and totalising assumption that 'mad' people are always, and only ever, 'mad', and are therefore unable to speak as subjects. Once we look at how Artaud's madness was actually constructed, at what he experienced as a result of that construction, and at what he had to say about it, the implications of such a position become glaringly apparent.

Firstly, of course, Artaud experienced the almost 'interminable misfortune' of being forcibly silenced in some far from subtle ways. The timing of his hospitalisation, during a period approaching the high water mark of incarceration of those deemed mentally ill, and coinciding with the Second World War, was hardly auspicious. After the fall of Paris in May 1940 inmates were on starvation rations, and those like Artaud who were deemed incurable risked deportation to Nazi concentration camps. An estimated forty thousand psychiatric patients died of cold and malnutrition in France between 1940 and 1944 (Macey, 2000 p. 149). Since the story of how he came to be incarcerated and detained for eight years and eight months is detailed in various biographies, I want to focus here on the issue of his extremely noisy 'silence'.[35]

Artaud reportedly became lucid again within two months of his initial 'collapse', but withdrew into almost monastic isolation in response to what had happened to him. In August 1939, some six months after his admission to a fourth institution, the very large Ville Evrard Asylum on the outskirts of Paris, he turned his attention towards reformulating his identity.[36] Feeling humiliated by his earlier failure to establish a reputation in the male-dominated public world of Parisian literary society, he announced the death 'from sorrow and pain' of Antonin Artaud, the writer, and adopted his mother's maiden name. Significantly, the new and 'virginal' Antonin Nalpas hardly wrote at all. Then, in February 1943, a friend from the Surrealist movement managed to arrange his transfer to Rodez, a hospital outside the officially occupied zone, where he came under the 'care' of the head psychiatrist, Gaston Ferdière (Barber, 1993 pp. 102, 105). Artaud expected Ferdière to be his liberator, and for a while his hopes seemed to be justified.[37] According to Barber, however, Ferdière soon came to 'detest' Artaud's habitual humming, gesturing and spitting, all of which was intended to protect him from unseen demonic figures. When challenged about this, Artaud quoted his published ideas about 'affective athleticism', and argued that he must have always been sick because his theatre direction 'consisted of nothing other than that'. Ferdière was unimpressed, and declared him 'violently anti-social, [and] dangerous for public order and people's security', though in the absence of any record of his patient seriously harming anyone, or any possibility of appeal, and in the context of the mayhem of war, this seems somewhat harsh (Barber, 1993 p. 106).[38]

In June 1943 Ferdière decided to employ an innovatory treatment from the armoury, and I use the term advisedly, of modernist psychiatry. At that time electroshock (or ECT), applied without anaesthetic or muscle relaxant, was still regarded as something of a panacea. Artaud had fifty-one treatments over an eighteen-month period, the third of which broke a vertebra in his back, 'forcing him to walk in a bent over position'. Each shock was followed by a coma of between fifteen and thirty minutes, and then, upon waking, a period of disorientation that caused him intense anguish. Ferdière dismissed this as merely a 'sub-anxiety' and thought it 'even desirable', since it obliged the patient, who had been 'reduced to nothingness, who has been totally obliterated, to build himself up again' (Hayman, 1977 p. 128).[39] In September 1943, towards the end of his electroshock ordeal, and under great pressure from Ferdière, Artaud finally abandoned the name 'Antonin Nalpas' four years after adopting it, and returned, grudgingly, to the 'name of his father', and to his former identity as a writer. It was a time of dramatic upheaval, in which he alternately embraced and then virulently rejected the religious belief that had been so important to him as a young man. Determined to avoid further electroshock 'torture', Artaud began to affect a deep attachment to his family, and claimed always to have been a royalist and patriot. He resumed his intellectual work, including adaptations of one of Ferdière's favourite texts, the Humpty Dumpty chapter from Lewis Carroll's *Through the Looking Glass*. He also produced a series of powerful drawings, particularly of suffering and dismembered bodies, and from early 1945, with great persistence, taught himself to write forcefully and fluently once again, in a language that erupted from 'a tetanus of the soul'. By the end of his incarceration his output was 'torrential', and he was re-establishing his notoriety, an achievement which ironically made him something of a trophy patient. The psychiatrists at Rodez duly claimed that his improvement exemplified the therapeutic potency of electroshock, but Barber points out that Artaud's creative capacity only returned strongly once the shock treatment had been stopped. Bizarrely, the elderly Ferdière would weep at literary gatherings whenever the subject of Artaud's subsequent rage towards him was raised (Barber, 1993 pp. 106–18).

All of this is interesting, of course, in relation to Lacan's theory that a man must inscribe himself into the patriarchal language of the symbolic, or go mad. Artaud had been enticed out of his defensive withdrawal and then coerced into rekindling a previously 'obsessive' desire to create 'a great, all-consuming work', to achieve public recognition by means of a spectacular, if defiant, performance climax (Jackson, 1990). He had always been intensely ambivalent about this kind of desire, of course, and at various points in a highly unorthodox career had dramatically undermined his own cause by giving public lectures in which he became ostentatiously provocative, directing vitriolic invective towards an initially sympathetic audience. His preoccupation with bringing difficult and often disturbingly explicit material into the public domain meant that conventional success was likely to elude him (Barber, 1993 p. 86). It is also interesting, incidentally, that Sylvia Plath, who had comparable experiences with ECT in 1953, likened it to possession by an electric god who acted specifically as a male muse. For her it was like being born again of man, fathered rather than mothered, purged of female vulnerability, and hence freed from constraint as a creative agent (Showalter, 1987 pp. 216–19; Plath, 1963).[40] A second difficulty, then, with the notion that the 'mad' are cursed with an intrinsic silence, and that any who attempt to communicate that silence are condemned to betray themselves, is amply demonstrated by the poetic lucidity and integrity of the testimony of survivors such as Plath and Artaud.[41] Because the notion of incommunicable madness can so easily slip into dangerous caricature, it is also important to stress Artaud's self-advocacy, and his belief that madness encoded a message for, and about, society.

After his release from hospital he only lived for another two years, but this was a prolific period. In Van Gogh, the Man Suicided by Society (in Hirschman, 1965) he wrote about the 'authentic madman' as someone 'who prefers to go mad in the social sense of the word, rather than forfeit a certain higher idea of human honour'. He (sic) is 'a man that society does not wish to hear, but wants to prevent from uttering certain unbearable truths'. Artaud's argument that 'a sick society invented psychiatry to defend itself against the investigations of certain visionaries whose faculties of divination disturbed it', is said to have decisively inspired Laing (Artaud in Hirschman, 1965 pp. 137, 141; Barber, 1993 p. 141; Hayman, 1977 p. 144).[42] Contrary to Derrida's notion of madness as incommunicable 'silence', Artaud now energetically celebrated the agency, courage and choice involved in going mad, understood as an act of commitment to pure vision and 'unbearable' truth. There is also a strong sense here that the moment of disturbance of madness is a social phenomenon, and an implicit suggestion that the silences of madness often conceal the silences of abuse. Although Artaud has no interest in disaggregating the notion of society, he writes evocatively, for instance, that Van Gogh 'did not die of a condition of delirium proper/but of having bodily become the field of a problem' (Hirschman,

1965 p. 139). He is not just concerned with a pantheon of exceptional predecessors, however, and goes on to assert that 'in every demented soul there is
a misunderstood genius that frightens people'. Psychiatry functions as social
censorship, 'a kind of Swiss Guard', put there to 'sap the rebellious drive that
is the origin of all geniuses' (Artaud, in Hirschman, 1965 p. 144). Artaud thus
democratises the discourse of exemplary madness, and turns it into a rhetorical
device in the context of his coruscating reply to psychiatric diagnosis, and the
appalling conditions he experienced and witnessed.

Gendered expectations

Because Artaud was subjected to such devastating 'prejudgement', and because
his voice came to epitomise survival, many commentators, wary of 'being
inscribed amongst the guilty', have been reluctant to look beyond this energetic
identification with the tragic theatricality of martyred genius (Atteberry, 2000
p. 715). But since psychiatrists had undoubtedly encouraged Artaud, at various
points in his life, to regard himself in this way, even his chosen form of
resistance was informed and invaded by a version of therapeutic discourse.[43]
Once we turn away from the necessary error of a pure politics of 'mental
health', it also becomes apparent that Artaud's identity as 'mad genius' was
socially constructed, well before his incarceration, in the context of a gendered
biographical trajectory that was spinning painfully out of control. Since considerable tensions and opportunities arise at the boundary between the registers
of 'mental health' and gender, the process of 'turning' our attention between
these viewpoints may be of considerable theoretical and practical importance.
In the former register, the focus falls upon the oppression and vulnerability of
men like Artaud, and the prevailing tone is one of generosity, informed by the
political imperative to believe what people who have been deemed mad are
saying. In the latter register, the focus shifts towards a concern with men as a
dominant group that has evaded deconstructive attention. The prevailing tone
is one of critique, informed by the knowledge that a substantial, and invisible,
minority of men behave violently or abusively, and tend to be devious
(Hearn, 1996). Although there are significant overlaps and areas of commonality between the politics of 'mental health' and feminism, it is interesting to
reflect upon various readings of Artaud, and the biographies, in the context of
the lively creative tension between these two sensibilities.

Despite his apparently intense ambivalence about the practical realities
entailed in any quest for public recognition, the dramatically self-absorbed
ambition of Antonin Artaud, as anti-hero and great artist in waiting, was
undoubtedly an important element in his tragic personal trajectory. Two biographers identify the 'catastrophic' closure of his play, The Cenci, after a seventeen-
day run (in May 1935) as a crucial biographical turning point. This turned out
to be his last opportunity to realise the vision of a Theatre of Cruelty, and to
establish himself as a working director on the Paris stage. Critical rejection

and financial disaster ended his dream of accomplishing an 'all-consuming work', the project that Ferdière would later coerce him into reviving, almost as a condition of release from Rodez. Now characterised as mad and ostracised from literary circles, Artaud aptly described himself as 'on the verge of the abyss'. In 1937 and 1938 he embarked upon his fateful journeys to Mexico and Ireland, which became an increasingly destructive flight from human reciprocity, in the direction of lonely messianic enthusiasm and apocalyptic vitriol (Hayman, 1977 p. 99; Esslin, 1976 p. 42; Barber, 1993 p. 73). Given that unforgivingly competitive codes appear to have defined even the ostensibly countercultural circles he moved in, it is hard to see how Artaud might have resolved his anguish about this costly yearning, particularly perhaps if it resonated with the painful presence and prolonged absences of his father in childhood. Far from supporting a move in this direction, most of the formal 'help' he received was clearly intended to enforce conformity with hegemonic values. Furthermore, since hegemonic masculinity, according to Connell, often involves the creation of fantasy figures expressing qualities that most men cannot hope to attain, this would be tantamount to reinforcing the very state of longing that had arguably precipitated Artaud's crisis (Connell, 1987).

Noticing that almost all of the men attending mythopoetic retreats, or reading *Iron John*, identified with the prince in the fairy tale, Kimmel concludes, in somewhat absolute terms, that men speak from 'a place of gnawing, yawning anxiety, a place of entitlement unfulfilled'. He sees this strong sense of identification with an heir to the throne, a figure who is entitled to absolute power over others, as central to the project of male subjectivity (Kimmel, 1998 p. 65; Bly, 1991). This is interesting in relation to Artaud's sense of himself as an undiscovered prodigy, and indeed, only two years before *The Cenci*, he had identified strongly with the figure of Heliogabalus, who had become emperor of Rome at the age of fourteen.[44] The notion of entitlement clearly needs to be handled with sensitivity, however, when referring to men who, as occupants of 'Othered' positions in relation to hegemonic forms of masculinity, have some urgently appropriate claims to make (Hearn, 1998). As we have seen, Artaud's oppression as a psychiatric patient centred upon a grotesque drama in which a markedly paternalistic psychiatrist coerced him into readopting his relinquished sense of masculinist entitlement, and re-embarking upon a melodramatic 'performance climax' which would combine genuine achievement with poignant parody. The significant element here, once again, is an over-investment in the pursuit of public achievement at the expense of other people, personal relationships and emotional wellbeing, not the undoubted value of an artistic identity or career as a space in which unorthodox vision and critical insight can flourish. When Artaud spoke as an 'authentic madman' he was claiming important and legitimate entitlements, but this voice was always interwoven with one or more voices constructed around the presumption of male privilege.

Postmodern and poststructuralist accounts would emphasise that such tensions are inevitably present in the subjectivities of marginalised men. The voices of men who are users/survivors of psychiatry or who experience distress will always contain contradictory strands, some of which resist dominant masculinist formations, and some of which collude with or accentuate them. Artaud's unwavering commitment to exploring the non-rational (Kristeva's (1977/1980) poetic language of the 'semiotic'), and the unsettling experience of 'unpower', his revaluation of madness, and his respect for non-Western and supposedly primitive indigenous cultures clearly ran counter to the prevailing norms of his day. Ironically, however, his belief in public displays of cathartic anger, his over-valuing of negation, and his unremitting assault on representation could readily be accommodated within the strategies of hegemonic masculinity. An enlivening but perpetually marginalised substratum of furious art, wrought from the overheated symbiosis between protesting sons and apparently civilised fathers, even the sacrificial exile of some of those sons from the domain of reason, may, after all, be essential to the regeneration of patriarchal authority. Far from constituting a mode of resistance capable of overturning the old order, male 'madness' of this kind may sharpen hegemonic reflexes that seek to siphon off disturbance by sanitising vision, silencing inconvenient testimony and censoring dissent. Artaud's story would seem to indicate that the path towards mad excess locks protest within an individualistic cycle of desperate gesture, ironically compatible with the dynamics of masculinity. If this is the case, Foucault's pre-poststructuralist depiction of the distress flares of Artaud's 'madness' as a 'lightning flash' that might open up a 'total contestation' of Western culture begins to look questionable on more than theoretical grounds (Dreyfus and Rabinow, 1982 p. 11).

Derrida's response to Artaud reflects the reluctance of mainstream postmodern critics of Enlightenment to challenge hegemonic forms of masculinity that have long sustained conceptions such as universal reason (Seidler, 1994 p. 207). With the benefit of hindsight it seems astonishing that he could have followed Nietzsche and Artaud in recognising the metaphorical richness of the image of a distantly omnipotent male God, but still not specified its salience in relation to masculinity. Yet this message appears to have been latent, as if only barely repressed, and waiting to break through the notoriously opaque and elaborate surface of his rhetoric. We are now perhaps better placed to reconsider Artaud's project in the context of an understanding that what Derrida identifies as the 'irreducible secondarity' of the speaking subject derives from a cultural field that is gendered. We might, for example, respond to Artaud's characteristically graphic question 'Do you know anything more outrageously faecal than the history of God?' – by identifying the God-like habit of appropriating life for 'works' whose primary purpose is that of display and domination as a hallmark of masculinist discourse (cited by Derrida, 1967/ 1978 pp. 178, 182). We might then envision a cultural field where co-operation and non-violence replace the social relations of 'theological machinery', so that it becomes possible to conceive of works that are both benevolent in conception and generous in performance, and readings that are not entirely motivated by malice or theft. In doing so we might ponder the kind of experiences that drove Artaud into a posture of such absolute suspicion, and thank him for drawing our attention, by default, to the potential fragility and constructed nature of the relatively easy sense of integrity and coherence that many of us take for granted. Furthermore, now that feminist understandings make clear the unconscious complicity of Nietzsche, Artaud and Derrida with a hegemonic order that, despite their formidable deconstructive acumen, they were unable to conceptualise, we might also argue for a greater sense of the limits of our own, and other people's, reflexive awareness.

The impulse to use aspects of Artaud's life as an 'example' may say more about the social location and intent of various commentators than it does about the difficult and complex figure in question. Despite the difficulty of reading biographical experiences that have already been so thoroughly enmeshed in the interpretative nets of disciplinary power, I don't share Artaud's view that his 'life' and 'work' were inseparable, or that any move towards generalisation amounts to theft or appropriation, and I have aimed for a critically generous reading taking account of the politics of both gender and 'mental health'. My contention is that the stories surrounding Artaud's life can usefully be read in relation to a tendency to romanticise a certain kind of male madness, and as epitomising the necessity of looking at men's pain, as well as, and in the context of, men's power. His experiences of modernist psychiatry remind us of the need to focus on the extent to which hegemonic masculinity still shapes that discipline, and on the question of how 'mental health' services return men, not necessarily to war, but back into patriarchal cultures of domination, rather than becoming overly preoccupied with the internal worlds of wayward sons. But the political imperative to respect the privacy and autonomy of men subjected to intrusive diagnostic and administrative scrutiny needs to be balanced against the need to counter a powerful tradition of reticence about men's 'private' inner worlds, and open up discussion about the nature, social construction and human costs of men's distress or madness. Unless we attempt to understand the contradictory and complex ways in which hegemonic masculinities can call tortured male subjectivities into being, it will remain difficult to discuss the potentially threatening aspects of some men's distress without recourse to a language of pathology, psychological reductionism or privatising blame.

Chapter 6

Deconstructing sovereignty
The post-revolutionary toolbox of Michel Foucault

The purpose of history, guided by genealogy, is not to discover the roots of our identity, but to commit itself to its dissipation. It does not seek to define our unique threshold of emergence, the homeland to which metaphysicians promise a return; it seeks to make visible all those discontinuities that cross us.
(Foucault, 1984)

It does not require any very strenuous effort to discredit the views of an ideological adversary when that adversary has already been branded, in the eyes of some portion of one's readership, at any rate, as a madman or a pervert.
(Halperin, 1995)

In his early essays Foucault privileges a grouping of 'mad philosophers' whose transgressive explorations of language appeared to constitute a counter-tradition against the optimism of the Enlightenment and its human sciences (Bouchard, 1977 pp. 18–19). In *Madness and Civilisation* (Foucault, 1961/1971), Nietzsche and Artaud are exalted to the point where they seem to function as 'tutelary deities' in his pantheon (Macey, 1993 p. 103). We might reasonably expect such fascination to be grounded in some compelling commonality of biographical experience, but at first sight Foucault's 'lives' look somewhat different from those of his favoured predecessors. Although Foucault came from a relatively privileged class background, and gained entry to the exclusive Ecole Normale Supérieure (ENS), he also encountered the realities of oppression as a gay man. Largely because of this, it seems, he endured a period of suicidal distress, during which, we now know, he repeatedly self-harmed.[1] Unlike Nietzsche and Artaud who both descended into madness later in life and for whom public recognition was largely 'posthumous', Foucault recovered and went on to pursue a distinguished career, first in cultural centres run by the diplomatic service, and then in academia. For much of his life, therefore, he had to negotiate simultaneous social inclusion and insidious marginalisation, and it was this contradictory positioning that fuelled and informed his hugely influential philosophical investigations into the operations of power.

Significantly, Foucault trained in psychology as well as philosophy, even studying with the same eminent psychiatrist he had consulted as a patient, and then working for a three-year period in the same hospital. Sainte-Anne also happened to be the hospital where, only ten years previously, Artaud had been incarcerated in a clinic run by Lacan. Not surprisingly, Foucault described his writings on madness and sexuality as 'twin projects' (Macey, 1993 p. 354). The books on madness came first, followed, after some twenty years of rumination, by *The History of Sexuality* (1976/1978), a sequence that reflects biographical contingencies, and is in turn reflected in differences in style and theoretical development. There are important common themes, however, which highlight the linkage and overlap between the histories of exclusion of 'madness' and 'homosexuality'. In particular, Foucault treated both as effects of discourses that constitute reason and heterosexuality, respectively, as normative, and discussed them in terms of relations rather than as natural realities. His critique of reason has been regarded as a precursor to the grounding axioms of queer theory,[2] and his *History of Sexuality* is of considerable interest in relation to the politics of 'mental health' (Halperin, 1995 pp. 39–40).

Foucault's biographers have had to negotiate his deconstruction of the concept of the author as a function of discourse, as well as the politics of writing about lives already subject to normalising description. Halperin, moved to passionate identification with Foucault because of the *ad hominem* demonisation of his work, regards any biographical writing about him as, at best, an occasion for embarrassment. At worst, to compose a biography of Foucault is 'to convict oneself, in effect, of having understood nothing about either Foucault's life or his work'. He nevertheless concludes that Foucault's acute and constantly revised sense of his own social location, and consequent ability to respond politically to changing discursive and institutional conditions, make his life as much and perhaps even more of a model for subsequent scholars and activists than his work (Halperin, 1995 pp. 129, 7). During the years when Foucault was establishing his career, his public reticence about the periods of depression and about his sexuality tells us more about the society in which he was living than about his 'most profound self', or any innate personality, of course.[3] He was certainly resistant to the conventional project of biography, which imposes a linear trajectory upon a unified authorial subject, and had good reason to be suspicious of intrusive personal enquiry. Against this, however, Eribon points out that Foucault did provide much information in interviews, and once proposed jointly editing and contributing to a collection of interviews with intellectuals about how their work arose (Eribon, 1991).[4]

Although Foucault objected to repetitive enquiries into what an author may have revealed about their innermost self, he also criticised those who were willing to denounce power in their adversaries but never analysed 'the mechanics of power' in themselves (Foucault, 1980 p. 116). Macey finds encouragement in his comments that 'each of my works is a part of my own biography', and that 'the work includes the whole life as well as the text' (Macey, 1993 pp. xii–xiii).[5] If we are attempting to understand forms of normalising power that are sustained through processes which impact pervasively upon our sense of selfhood, attention to subjectivity arguably becomes a crucial enterprise, ripe for recasting in anti-essentialist and genealogical terms. Sometimes the link between life and work is both obvious and poignant, as, for example, when following Nietzsche, Foucault situated genealogy in relation to the body, understood as the locus of a dissociated self: 'a volume in perpetual disintegration', and an inscribed surface of events bearing 'the stigmata of past experience' (Foucault, 1971/1984 p. 83). Although he ended his discussion of the 'author-function' with the provocatively rhetorical challenge 'What matter who's speaking?', his own new questions about speaking positions within discourse constitute a powerful response to this, and support the contention that genealogists themselves can and should be put in question, and that in some senses Foucault needs 'turning against himself' (Bouchard, 1977 p. 138; MacIntyre, 1994 p. 295; Grimshaw, 1993 pp. 66–7).[6]

Unlike Nietzsche and Artaud, Foucault developed a detailed theorisation of the social operation of power. He was politically active and wanted to fashion discourses, including a genealogy of psychiatry, that would be politically effective.[7] Readers were invited to open his books as if they were 'little toolboxes', and 'make use of such and such a sentence or idea, of one analysis or another, as they would a screwdriver or a monkey-wrench, in order to short-circuit or disqualify systems of power' (Eribon, 1989/1991, p. 237). As part of this borrowing Foucault explicitly anticipated critiques of the systems of power from which his own writings emerged, and therefore came close to recognising that the matrix of biographical experience beyond his 'work', that his work was part of, might be of interest to the critical reader. In a final interview, he even suggested that each of his books could be approached as a 'field of experience', by reinserting an occluded autobiographical dimension (Miller, 1993 p. 31). I would see any difficulties with the extant biographies as indicating a need to reconceptualise biography, and be clear about the politics of writing it, rather than abandoning interest in men's subjective experience.[8] Since this is a sensitive issue in the 'mental health' field, and since postmodern approaches to the political uses of experience differ from those rooted solely in identity politics, it is one I shall return to (Foucault, 1975/1977 p. 228). My immediate concern is that any such account needs to be orientated towards a respect for the person, informed by what they, though not necessarily they alone, have to say, and towards understanding, short-circuiting and transforming systems of power that conspire to diminish or injure.[9]

This chapter looks at how an understanding of the interweaving of biographical strands and discontinuities that informed Foucault's work might suggest new perspectives on the uses we make of it. I am particularly interested in tracing a subtext linking masculinity, madness and power, and using it to reassert the value of critical and non-psychological approaches to subjectivity as a site where domination meets resistance. At various points the discussion becomes doubly genealogical because of the marked resonances between both the works and contingencies linking the lives of Nietzsche and Foucault. These connections between the prophets of the 'Death of God' and the 'Death of Man' appear to confirm refusal by rebellious sons as a theme within main- and malestream postmodern theory, and illuminate the gendered intellectual inheritance that informed Foucault's theorisation of power. I conclude the chapter by discussing the contradictory influences that shaped his writings on madness.

The Name of the Father

I was surprised and fascinated to find that in 'The Father's No', an early essay written shortly after Folie et Déraison (Madness and Civilisation), Foucault takes up the question of biography in terms that resonate closely with some of the key themes that have previously arisen in relation to Nietzsche and Artaud. In it he reviews a psychobiography of the poet Hölderlin, written by the psychoanalyst Jean Laplanche. Foucault's interest in Hölderlin centres upon the relationship between experience and text, and madness and art. Dismissing the assumption in psychological discourse that the meaning of a work can be traced directly, through an unbroken chain of signification, to a series of events, he wants us to look instead at 'the way in which a work gradually discloses the open and extended space of schizophrenic existence' (Bouchard, 1977 p. 71; Muldoon, 1995). Having entered this caveat, he follows Laplanche's use of Lacan's masculinist theory of 'psychosis', and foregrounds a formative series of biographical events in Hölderlin's early life. Interestingly, the poet's father died when he was two years old, and two years later his mother married another man who also died when the poet was only nine, leaving him with 'delightful memories'.[10] As we have already seen, Lacan argued that psychosis is linked with the absence of a father who should function as 'third party' in an Oedipal triangle, and who (after Melanie Klein) 'is not only the hated and feared rival, but the agent whose presence limits the unlimited relationship between the mother and the child'. His world-defining paternal Law and initially constraining speech – 'The Father's No' of the essay's title that is said to give rise to language and to the 'exclusion and symbolic transformation of repressed material' – also protects the child from its fantasy of being devoured by the mother (Bouchard, 1977 pp. 81–2).[11]

Although the younger Foucault adapts Lacan's account of the gap left by the father's absence, he appears to endorse its deterministic and essentialist message:

> To be able to say that he is missing, that he is hated, excluded, or introjected, that his image has undergone symbolic transformations, presumes that he is not 'foreclosed' (as Lacan would say) from the start, and that his place is not marked by a gaping and absolute emptiness. The Father's absence, manifested in the headlong rush towards psychosis, is not registered by perceptions or images, but relates to the order of the signifier.

The 'no' through which this gap is created does not imply the absence of a real individual who bears the father's name; rather it implies that the father has never assumed the role of nomination. . . . It is toward this 'no' that the unwavering line of psychosis is infallibly directed. As it is precipitated inside the abyss of its meaning, it evokes the devastating absence of the father through the forms of delirium and phantasms and through the catastrophe of the signifier.

(Foucault, in Bouchard, 1977 p. 82)

This passage, recalling the imagery of a 'sheer cliff over the abyss of the work's absence' from the discussion of Artaud in the closing pages of Madness and Civilisation, clearly locates the breach between madness and the work in the context of a psychoanalytic discourse that attributes (men's) madness to an interruption of the male prerogative of naming, of using 'rational' language to define the world and distance masculinity from all things feminine (Foucault, 1961/1971 p. 287). Foucault then considers a period when Hölderlin, prefiguring Nietzsche, devotes himself to confronting paternal absence, and reworks his material until 'the burning proximity of the divine is transformed into the distant radiance of the unfaithful gods', whose dying is marked and witnessed by the arrival of Christ-Dionysos. Since the death of God, language has assumed 'a sovereign position', emanating from a place no one can speak of. Within this strongly Nietzschean overarching context, every work becomes 'an attempt to exhaust language' (Bouchard, 1977 pp. 82–6).[12] This theme is repeated across Foucault's often literary and densely mythopoetic writings from the early 1960s.[13]

One way of approaching these texts is to situate them in relation to the death of Foucault's father in 1959, when the philosopher was in his early thirties, and just before the publication of his first major book.[14] Loyal Foucauldians have energetically resisted this kind of reading, partly and understandably because political opponents have dismissed Foucault's work as an expression of the 'never fully articulated personal agenda' of a bizarre individual (Jones and Porter, 1994 p. 28). However, given that the literary Foucault of this period specifically argued that in a post-theocratic world language can only be fashioned into a work when directed against the absence of a paternal god, it seems particularly appropriate to consider work produced in the aftermath of that death, in those terms. Any such readings of the 'open and extended' space of biographical experience and its formative context, that avoid the temptation of securing an 'easy passage' between event and meaning, would seem to be consistent with his own perspective.

Bereavement is perhaps the most radical of all the many and various discontinuities that cross us, and though we should be wary of universalising constructions, it is often a profoundly unsettling process. Understandings may fluctuate wildly as seemingly arbitrary and perhaps bewilderingly cruel events unfold. Latent emotion can become dramatically exposed, as the limits of ordinary experience rupture. Under such disorientating circumstances, a gradual and painstaking search for meaning can become a central preoccupation. Foucault, already silenced about his distress history and sexuality, and having to pass as 'normal' on both counts in a markedly patriarchal environment, is likely to have wanted to protect this site of tender introspection from inappropriate public scrutiny. This would have been doubly advisable given that medical discourses enforce hegemonic codes in relation to bereavement by interpreting distress, and any expression of the softer emotions beyond certain bureaucratically permissible limits, as evidence of 'mental illness'. Though we do not know, and do not need to know, much about Foucault's immediate personal response to his father's death, the process of facilitating a sufficient opening of sensitive terrain such as this, while avoiding intrusion, remains central to the complex interface between the politics of masculinities and 'mental health'.

At times of bereavement, which can come close to, or overlap with, madness, we often turn for insight and solace to the protectively elliptical and supposedly 'feminine' languages of art and poetry. It is interesting then, that Foucault, at this time, turns to literature, and frequently adopts an intensely lyrical style. His essays, dealing with the vivid imaginal worlds of 'mad' poets, writers and philosophers, brim with labyrinthine argument, decorated by occasional clusters of language that sparkle, even in translation.[15] They resemble jewel caskets more than toolboxes. But in reworking this material there is a sense that Foucault is, quite understandably, struggling for mastery over elusive and potentially treacherous terrain. Evocative imagery about death and the negotiation of loss is much in evidence. The conclusion of his 1961 thesis ('Introduction to and Translation of Immanuel Kant's *Anthropologie in pragmatischer Hinsicht*') for example, includes the following resoundingly valedictory passage:

> for man, in his finitude, is not separable from the infinity of which he is both the negation and the herald. Is it not possible to conceive of a critique of finitude which would be liberating with respect to both man and the infinite, and which would show that finitude is not an end, but that curve and knot of time in which the end is the beginning?
>
> (cited in Macey, 1993 p. 89)

Near the close of *The Birth of the Clinic*, we find him in similar vein, writing 'it is death that fixes the stone that we can touch, the return of time, the fine, innocent earth beneath the grass of words' (Foucault, 1963/1973 p. 197).

The Birth of the Clinic was the only major new book Foucault published during this period, and despite the obscurity of its subject matter, a historical study of the evolution of modern clinical medicine, it introduces some important analytical motifs into his work (Foucault, 1963/1973 p. ix). Foremost among these, the concept of the gaze prefigures later discussions of surveillance, and is often regarded as focal in relation to his analysis of modern forms of power.[16] An opening declaration, that 'this book is about space, about language, and about death; it is about the act of seeing, the gaze', therefore suggests that the ontological questions pursued in 'The Father's No', will (or perhaps, could) be grounded in an understanding of social power, yet to be developed. Eribon notes Foucault's comment that, like his other books, this one 'had its birthplace in personal experience', and wonders in passing whether it was about settling accounts, or paying the respects he had been unable to convey when his father was still alive (Eribon, 1991 p. 152). Since three previous generations of men in the Foucault family had all been doctors, it would inevitably bear traces of personal history, even had it not been written shortly after the death of Dr Paul Foucault. It is not surprising, therefore, that the debate about the personalisation of Foucault's work has surfaced around it.[17] Although we cannot know whether Foucault consciously crafted a personal subtext, a shadowy crosscurrent, charged with possible subjective meanings, occasionally seems to ripple the dense analytical surface of his intellectual archaeology. For example, when he traces both medicine and poetic language to 'the same profound law', this looks very much like a gesture of reconciliation on the part of a son who has broken with the patriarchal lineage of his family (Foucault, 1963/1973 p. 198).[18]

Like Artaud before him, Foucault not only said that he hated his father, but also refused to use his father's name, becoming Michel instead of Paul-Michel to all but his immediate family. Given that all three previous generations of doctors had also been called Paul, this effectively signalled a rejection of powerful paternal expectations that must have contributed to early difficulties with a reputedly remote and authoritarian father.[19] Since *Birth of the Clinic* focuses on the significance of wresting knowledge about life from the dissection of dead bodies, and the recently deceased Dr Foucault had been a surgeon, it seems inconceivable that anyone close to Foucault could have been unaware of an intimate subtext in the book. Foucault's influential suggestion, in the concluding section, that medicine is significantly involved in the fabrication of individual experience and identity at 'a very deeply embedded level' is strongly consistent with this possibility (Foucault, 1963/1973 p. 196; Armstrong, 1997 p. 22).[20] For Foucault, a distinctive characteristic of modern power, based on discourse, surveillance and the gaze, is that it is constitutive.

If the father, a skilled exponent of the medical gaze, his 'absolute eye' attuned to what Foucault describes as the perceptual and epistemological structure of 'invisible visibility', was unable to welcome his son's sexuality, then there is considerable irony in the many passages elaborating upon the notion of the gaze. For example, 'The aim of the anatomists is "attained when the opaque envelopes that cover our parts are no more for their practised eyes than a transparent veil revealing the whole and the relation between the parts"' (Foucault, 1963/1973 pp. 165–6 citing Marie-Françoise Xavier Bichat).[21] The traditionally 'feminine' coding of this metaphor of concealment contrasts with the stereotypically male imagery of the toolbox that, for whatever reason, Foucault favoured when describing his work. Once the veil is circumvented and the 'visible invisible' finally exposed to scientific perception, it turns out to be no less than 'the forbidden, imminent secret: the knowledge of the individual'. Empowered by its access to this knowledge, medicine comes to occupy a pivotal place in the constitution of 'the sciences of man', those sciences of modernity that render 'man' an object of positive knowledge. In his later work, Foucault identifies sexuality as focal to this process (Foucault, 1963/1973 pp. 170, 197, 1976/1978). Central to the ironic potential of such passages, of course, is Foucault's own analysis of the formative part played by psychiatry in constituting the notion of homosexuality, and thereby facilitating social control, but also the articulation of a 'reverse' discourse of resistance, and even arguably, of dissent beyond it (Foucault, 1976/1918; Halperin, 1995 pp. 56–60). Had the 'speaking eye' of medicine seen and – albeit normatively – named what the medical patriarch from Poitiers was unable to acknowledge in his own son? Had the father's failure to 'nominate' contributed towards his son's distress?[22] Whatever passed between father and son, testimony from Foucault's homosexual contemporaries confirms that the harmful effects of medicalising discourses may in any case have been sufficient to propel the young Foucault towards a critical engagement with psychology and psychiatry (Eribon, 1991 pp. 27–8).

At this point I should perhaps re-emphasise that my purpose in raising these questions is not to establish a totalising and reductive psychological commentary about the essential truth of Foucault as unitary subject that might unlock an ultimate meaning for this text. What interests me here is the relationship between sons and fathers as an intimate and intense instance of negotiation with what Foucault has enabled us to understand as constitutive power. I am proposing that an account, however unavoidably partial, subjective and incomplete, of the immediate social context in which a work was formed, of the intersection between discourses and voices in play at its inception, might helpfully inform any borrowing of the various 'tools' within it. The relevance of Foucault's discussions of the gaze, and of the evolution of disciplines whose project is to reveal and thereby construct individuality, in the context of a newly omnipresent form of normalising power, is widely recognised, and positively invites genealogical enquiry of this kind. I now want to look at this body of theory, and at its paradoxical inattention to violence, in relation to critiques of masculinity, before considering some further biographical contingencies surrounding its production.

Power reconfigured: a political anatomy of masculinity?

According to Foucault, the development of modern disciplines made possible the gradual emergence of a new configuration of power, so that 'after the Enlightenment . . . power no longer emanated from the patriarchal or sovereign negative imperative: "no! thou shalt not"' (MacCannell and MacCannell, 1993 p. 210; Foucault, 1980 pp. 139–40). In place of the king a 'machinery of furtive power' began to function 'like a faceless gaze that transformed the whole social body into a field of perception: thousands of eyes posted everywhere'. Under such a regime, symbolised in the iconography of the Panopticon, with its invisible 'eye of power', individuals would effectively police themselves, and 'become the principle of [their] own subjection'.[23] In a 'reversal of the political axis of individualisation', the examination and description of individuals, now conceived as 'cases', becomes a method of domination, augmenting or supplanting previous, originally violent means of inducing and perpetuating a radical internalisation of instinct in the interest of social conformity.[24] Nowhere is this more evident than in relation to the supposed animality of madness (Foucault, 1975/1977 pp. 192, 203, 214; 1961/1971 pp. 74–8). Foucault's relentlessly claustrophobic historical account of the evolution of 'carceral society' in *Discipline and Punish*, which fittingly opens with a description of the gruesome public execution of an unsuccessful regicide, thus revisits terrain covered in Nietzsche's *Genealogy of Morals*; and his new political anatomy (a term bearing resonances from *Birth of the Clinic*) can be seen as a political anatomy of nihilism, a critique directed against the negation of life (Haar, 1977 p. 15; Allison, 2001 pp. 193–4, 230–2).

Nietzsche's account of an earlier historical transformation appears to have been motivated by his desire to recuperate Dionysian wildness from Christian (or Buddhist) inhibition, and by a certain nostalgia for feral social violence. His distinctly ungenealogical 'hypothesis' for the origin of bad conscience posits a polity founded by act of violence, in which ruthless oppression by a 'warlike pack' forces members of a populace to sublimate their instinctual power (Nietzsche, 1887/1956 pp. 219–21).[25]

> Hostility, cruelty, the delight in persecution, raids, excitement, destruction, all turned against their begetter. Lacking external enemies and resistancies, and confined within an oppressive narrowness and regularity, man began rending, persecuting, terrifying himself, like a wild beast hurling himself against the bars of his cage. This languisher, devoured by nostalgia for the wild, who had to turn *himself* into an adventure, a torture chamber . . . became the inventor of 'bad conscience'.
>
> (Nietzsche, 1887/1956 p. 218)

Butler sees Foucault's account of disciplinary power as an attempt to rewrite Nietzsche's doctrine of internalisation in terms of a model of inscription, in which an expanded interior world of 'the soul' is produced as a 'surface signification' on the body, albeit one that 'perpetually renounces itself as such', so that, for instance, prisoners' bodies are compelled to signify prohibitive law as if it were their very 'essence, style, and necessity' (Butler, 1990 p. 134). Foucault is explicit, however, that it is 'the beautiful totality of the individual' which is neither repressed nor altered by the social order, but carefully fabricated in it (Foucault, 1975/1977 p. 217).

Foucault sometimes seems to share Nietzsche's enthusiasm for the historical cruelties that he catalogues, and in a strongly Nietzschean conclusion to

Discipline and Punish privileges the 'the necessity of combat and the rules of strategy' as a ubiquitous organising force behind the diversity of carceral mechanisms (Foucault, 1975/1977 p. 308). While there is undoubtedly a need to recognise the realities of conflict, and the interested nature of truth claims, this unquestioning reaffirmation of Nietzsche's public *agon* comes close to normalising violence.[26] Interestingly, the transition from sovereign to disciplinary power is personified for Foucault by Napoleon, a figure whose single gaze loomed over an entire empire and whose attributes epitomised an ideal of masculinity for the polemical Nietzsche. For various reasons, then, the pervasive presence of Nietzsche behind this text suggests the potential value of reading it in relation to assumptions about an apparently asocial and instinctual masculinity, in some ways akin to 'madness', and with a corresponding dynamic of containment and transgression.

Discipline and Punish is replete with unacknowledged imagery of gender, not least in the figure of the soldier that functions as a galvanising image, modelling the definition and production of 'docile bodies' in a newly enlightened world of 'Man-the-Machine'. His upright and regimented male form appears to replace 'the body of the king' in an imaginary anatomy of masculinity, announcing 'the birth of meticulous military and political tactics for the control of bodies and individual forces within states', as disciplinary modes of power infiltrate all others (Foucault, 1975/1977 pp. 216, 136, 168). Surveillance and inspection become pivotal, as recruitment in the service of such states requires the overt or covert screening of each individual as a potential madperson, pervert or criminal. If masculinity is a – presumably hierarchical – process of 'homosocial enactment', demanding constant vigilance and mutual evaluation, 'an intense scrutiny of its own boundaries' in order to repudiate difference and ambiguity, then the Panopticon seems an obvious symbol for this aspect of its historical project (Kimmel, 1994 p. 128; Frosh, 1994 pp. 103–4; Weeks 1985).[27] But the construction of paradoxically docile masculine individuals probably relies as much upon the management as upon the repudiation of 'instinct'. Public discourse, perhaps increasingly, fabricates an idealised image of masculine agency, whether through physical strength, wildness, reason or consumer choice, as if *these* were men's interior essence, an image that (as in the case of the obsequious fascist) often masks collusive weakness, and reverses Nietzsche's picture of pallid 'bad conscience' in which an ethic of altruistic sympathy has to be superimposed over seething instinct (Butler, 1990 p. 136).

As carceral networks proliferate, a diffuse and furtive paternalism begins to constitute normality and madness through the theoretical reach and disciplinary practices of masculinist psychology and psychiatry. Foucault's notion of political anatomy also resonates with Lacan's versatile concept of 'imaginary anatomy', and his assertion that the unified body image of 'normal' individuals is a precarious achievement that needs protection against the threat of disintegration.[28] In 'psychosis' Lacan claimed to have found 'the fundamental alienation constitutive of our experience', which he analysed in the context of his theory of a mirror stage (Rajchman, 1985 p. 21). Conversely, the concept of imaginary anatomy has been described as 'crucial in explaining the sympto-matology of psychosis' (Grosz, 1994 p. 44). Despite its internalising dynamic and medicalising focus, the idea of an imaginary anatomy becomes potentially interesting if we reconsider Foucault's metaphor of a prodigiously productive panoptic machine in relation to his earlier theme, the social production, rather than treatment, of 'mental illness'. If, in a world of disciplinary surveil-lance, madness, inflamed by a vivid sense of actual and possible persecution, or driven to transgress symbolic paternal limits, seems to reveal the 'paranoid' nature of the ego, this will surely be because both have been forged within the same configuration of power. (See Grosz, 1990 pp. 38, 47 on Lacan's account of the ego.) We don't need to accept Lacan's theorisation, however, to picture embodied masculinity, constructed around the concealment of intractable fears and instabilities that madness might expose.

Writing about the moral treatment of those deemed insane at the end of the eighteenth century, Foucault famously asserted that the English Quaker reformer William Tuke and French Doctor Philippe Pinel 'liberated' asylum inmates from their chains only to inaugurate 'a gigantic moral imprison-ment' based on self-restraint inculcated by exposure to observation, that only Nietzsche, Artaud and a few other gifted madpersons would successfully defy in the lightning flash of their work.[29] Moreover, this new reign of reason was modelled on the patriarchal family, a 'parental complex' in which the authority of the physician depended upon his becoming Father and Judge, Family and Law', and the madman was treated as a minor under 'family tutelage'. Hence the 'profanations or blasphemies' of madness came to be constructed as 'an incessant attack upon the father', just as, according to Nietzsche, expressions of instinct had been construed as rebellion against God the Father under a pre-modern regimen of religious 'bad conscience' (Foucault, 1961/1971 pp. 278, 272, 252–4; Nietzsche, 1887/1956 p. 226). Foucault argues that this historical rearrangement of institutional power not only revived the prestige of the patri-archal family but prefigured psychoanalysis, shaping its claim to explain 'the meaning and destiny that supposedly marked all of Western culture and perhaps all civilisation' through the Oedipus myth. Since psychoanalysis retained the 'structure' established in the nineteenth-century asylum, it accumulated quasi-divine powers to construct and preside over the turbulence of instinctual life, but remained 'unable to hear the voices of unreason' (Foucault, 1961/1971 pp. 253, 278).[30] Interestingly, it has been suggested that Freud's formulation of his Oedipal theory enabled him to 'mediate the crisis of mourning his father's death'. Freud wrote that the death of a father is 'the most important event, the most poignant loss, of a man's life', but his letters reveal a conviction that Jacob Freud had been a serial abuser, in which case he would effectively have been exonerated by his son's abandonment of the seduction theory (Spreng-nether, 1995 pp. 150–3).

Forrester draws attention to Foucault's later argument in *Will to Knowledge* that the repressive hypothesis of psychoanalysis, and its concomitant identification of power with the patriarch as lawgiver, was generated precisely at a time when 'patriarchal law was being . . . supplanted by the positive mechanisms of power-knowledge. "We must not forget that the discovery of the Oedipus complex was contemporaneous with the juridical organisation of the downfall of the father"' (Forrester, 1990 p. 309, citing Foucault, 1976/1978 p. 130).[31] Subsequently, the notion that neurosis is intimately associated with 'a failure in relation to the father' has been a persistent theme within psychoanalytic theory. He then asks:

> Are we to assent to the implication in Foucault's argument, that this Nietzschean crisis of authority of the law and its makers is the mythical skein under which is played out the 'true' relations of the individual to power? . . . Can we, finally and definitively, declare, not only that God is dead, but also that we have begun to sketch out the historical conditions which made possible his exact, clinical and scientific murder?
>
> (Forrester, 1990 p. 310)

As a means of evoking overarching power structures, however, the delicate idealism of this 'image of a mythical skein' risks veiling both the brutal textures of systematic domination that Foucault is already accused of overlooking, and the historical function of discourses about masculinity in crisis (Hartstock, 1990 p. 169; Kimmel, 1987). In his analysis of the asylum Foucault had situated this downfall of the private patriarch relative to public and professional patriarchal power in the context of a symbiotic relationship between the patriarchal family and evolving disciplinary discourses and institutions.

Feminist critics have accused Foucault of neglecting the specific disciplinary practices that engender a greater docility in female bodies (Bartky, 1988; Ramazanoglu, 1993). While welcoming some aspects of his account of a constitutive mode of power, they identify an explanatory gap between its detailed treatment of the 'capillary' level of micropolitics and a cursory acknowledgement of overarching patterns of domination which leaves 'the immensity of the consolidation of men's power' unacknowledged (Ramazanoglu and Holland, 1993 p. 260).[32] Foucault's desire to avoid prescription meant that he didn't set out to provide either an internally consistent or global definition of power, but his oracular rhetoric, at once authoritative and cryptic, undoubtedly causes difficulties.[33] While his docile soldier signals a masculine passivity and conformity that Nietzsche had both tragi-comically embodied and conspicuously overlooked, the prevalence of men's social violence slips from view (Foucault, 1976/1978; MacCannell and MacCannell, 1993 pp. 210–13).

Foucault's account of disciplinary power also emphasises the coercion of bodies at the expense of any sense of the importance in more recent times of ideology, however defined, in reproducing the cultural ideals, and corresponding internalised imagery, of masculinity.[34] His emphasis on the importance of tactics and strategy is nonetheless consistent with Connell's understanding of hegemonic masculinity as 'a configuration of gender practice which embodies the currently accepted answer to the problem of the legitimacy of patriarchy'. The notion that this is marked by successful claims to authority rather than by direct violence converges readily with Foucault's description of a new form of power that prefers to avoid overt displays of violence. If Connell is right in saying that violence is a measure of imperfection in a system of domination, then the establishment of 'disciplinary' regimes which largely efface it as public practice would seem an obvious aspiration for and solution to the problematic legitimacy of modernist masculinity (Connell, 1995 p. 84). Foucault comes close to developing a gendered account of disciplinary power as an adaptive manoeuvre, in which patriarchal authority annexes 'feminine' concerns such as attention to subjective interiority and the art of listening, and fashions them into mechanisms of control. His critique of psychoanalysis appears to demonstrate that the interests of masculinity can be served by claiming an 'anti-repressive' trajectory in which promises of progress rest, in part, on the knowledge and power of 'caring' professions and institutions. Freud's abandonment of the seduction theory and formulation of the 'truths' of the Oedipus complex, effectively shoring up patriarchal authority and diverting attention from perpetrators of sexual abuse, is a complex case in point (Masson, 1984/1992).

According to Spivak, Foucault was neglectful of the realities of imperialism that underpinned the historical development of new mechanisms of power in the West, whilst perpetuating older modes, sometimes combined with new ones, 'elsewhere'. His accounts of the clinic, asylum and prison even 'seem like screen allegories that foreclose a reading of the broader narratives of imperialism' (Landry and Maclean, 1996 pp. 219–20). Part of the problem here is perhaps that the core counter-narrative of *Madness and Civilisation* – with its critique of the Enlightenment 'liberation' of asylum inmates, and its curious leap from Pinel and Tuke to Freud – can seem to suggest that physical repression was rendered all but obsolete by the 'gigantic *moral* imprisonment' (italics added) facilitated by modernist psychiatry.[35] We need only look at Artaud's account of his experiences, as opposed to Foucault's romantic appropriation of them, to see that this would be a seriously misleading impression, and that in the asylum too, violence continued to be deployed alongside newly constitutive disciplinary modes of power. Indeed, the twentieth century witnessed burgeoning incarceration as well as the atrocities facilitated by Nazi psychiatry. Similarly, the core counter-narrative of *Discipline and Punish*, tracing a progressive abandonment of physical methods of punishment in the West, might give the impression that Foucault was unaware that clandestine torture had been routinely practised in Paris during the 1957–61 Algerian War (Macey, 2000 p. 348; Lennon 2001). How then might recourse to social biography help illuminate these important but problematic later formulations on the omnipresence of power?

Writing and life

Several biographical strands appear to contribute to the emergence of his new position. Firstly, the mid-1970s saw a shift in the political landscape of the French left, and Foucault, who was not alone in distancing himself from Marxism, was now critiquing class warfare, and the attendant fascination with political violence and a 'racist' urge to eliminate adversaries. Interestingly, he endorsed the conclusion of former Maoist André Gluckmann that this totalitarian impulse implicated everyone and was not something external, by commenting that he was not invoking 'a new Dionysos beneath Apollo' (Miller, 1993 pp. 290–1, 296–7).[36] Although Miller portrays this as a departure from Nietzsche, it could be seen as a move towards the pre-postmodern Nietzsche who offered 'a philosophy of power that does not enclose it within a political theory'. Foucault was now elaborating what Rajchman calls a post-revolutionary politics. Critical of the tendency in revolutionary discourse to treat some version of 'the people' as signifying our real social nature, and as constitutive of who, or what, should be sovereign, he wrote 'in political thought and analysis, we still have not cut off the king's head' (Foucault, 1976 pp. 88–9; Rajchman, 1985 p. 64).

A second biographical strand arguably associated with Foucault's new view of the omnipresence of power was that he had just emerged from various subjectively important experiences that seem to have functioned as personal rites of passage. Foucault's biographers agree that he found California, with its large and organised gay community, almost utopian. Here he 'finally achieved a reconciliation with himself . . . was happy in his work . . . [and] happy in the pleasures of the flesh.' (Eribon, 1991 p. 316; Macey, 1993 p. 458). In 1975 one of his hosts recommended a trip to Death Valley, where he might feel 'suspended among the forms hoping for nothing but the wind'. The words were from Artaud's account of his experiences with peyote in Mexico in 1936, and Miller quotes from a memoir written by one of Foucault's two companions during a nocturnal LSD trip in the desert.[37] The only experience he could compare this with was the 'experience of truth' attained in his various sexual encounters with strangers in San Francisco. In the long silence that followed he apparently said that he was very happy, had achieved 'a fresh perspective on himself', and now understood his sexuality (Miller, 1993 pp. 246–51).

Although Miller has been robustly criticised for the luridness of his speculation about Foucault's participation in gay S/M subculture, his account of this period does establish that the resulting personal insights preceded a radical revision of the work on sexuality. Hundreds of pages of drafts were shelved in favour of a small essay on method proposing a new 'analytics' of power, and declaring: 'we must at the same time conceive of sex without the law, and power without the king' (Foucault, 1976 p. 91, quoted in Miller, 1993 pp. 251–2, critiqued by Halperin, 1995 p. 148). It seems appropriate, therefore, to link the philosopher's exploration of sadomasochism, conceived as a move away from phallocentric masculinity, with his subsequent writings, and timely that he now challenged what he called the 'repressive hypothesis',[38] and the corresponding 'juridico-discursive' representation of power as monarchical, centralised, and working only through negation (Halperin, 1995 pp. 89–90; Macey, 1993 p. 369; Dreyfus and Rabinow, 1982 p. 129). At this juncture it became clear to Foucault that there was no transhistorical and cross-cultural sexuality, and that while sex, like revolution, and perhaps 'madness', appears to function as a repository of truth beyond power, it is always already imbued with power, albeit of a more insidious kind. Moreover, since power seems to work through prohibition more obviously in relation to sex than anywhere else, the effect of the juridico-discursive model of power here can be regarded as exemplary, and illustrative of its hold on our political thinking (Foucault, 1976 p. 90; Sheridan, 1980 p. 180).[39] Noting that the appeal of this new model of power to radical gay activists might surprise many left-liberal male critics who felt that Foucault was undermining political agency, Halperin argues that 'nothing communicates the sense that power is everywhere more eloquently than the experience of the closet' (Halperin, 1995 pp. 16, 29).[40]

During this period there is a palpable sense that a once omnipotent organising image, that of the body of the King, is disintegrating. The philosopher's vision does seem to have been transfigured in the sense that it would no longer be refracted through the limiting discourse of the Law of the Father. For Eribon, the distinctive force of *The Will to Knowledge* lies in the implicit break Foucault makes with Lacanian psychoanalysis. The notion of the 'Law' positively and internally constituting both desire, and the lack that institutes it, now appears as firmly rooted in a monarchical conception of power as are theories of repression and censorship that externalise power (Eribon, 1993 p. 272; Foucault, 1976 pp. 85–6). The imperious 'father's "no"', towards which an 'unwavering line of psychosis' had once seemed 'infallibly directed', is finally discarded, unmasking an altogether more complex, unstable and unsettling image of power relations as slippery, paradoxical, sometimes reversible, always inescapable and apparently subject-less (Foucault, 1977 p. 82; also for example 1980 pp. 141–2). Yet paternal prohibition, envisaged as a pervasive cultural discourse endlessly reworked in diverse settings rather than as a transcendental structure enshrined in the foundational myth of Oedipus, hardly seems an 'emaciated' form of power, and still, surely, constructs power in starkly negative terms, by making it conditional upon a lack of 'femininity' – reciprocity, care, nurture or love.

If Foucault's new model of power was grounded in biographical experience, its complex origins must lie, in part at least, among intimate truths whose fine detail has rightly remained protected from public scrutiny. I have argued that interest in the subjectivities of men remains valid and necessary, that we should converse and speculate around the edges of private terrain, but when bringing language into such 'penumbral' places, we need to recognise the inherent limitations of representation that so fascinated Foucault for a while

(Foucault, 1963/1973 p. 169; Bouchard, 1977 pp. 51, 86). Any such genealogical speculation here will inevitably become freighted with the charge of subsequent history, since it was at this point, ironically, that Foucault introduced
the power/knowledge dyad, a conceptual 'tool' that gets close to the heart of
the politics of 'mental health'. Power/knowledge refers to a proliferating configuration of practices, techniques of knowledge, and relations of power, applied
to the examination of individuals, conceived as originating in the confessional
and evolving into an array of rituals of 'scientific' truth. It appears that Foucault
developed his critique of a therapeutic incitement to seek and disclose ever
more intimate truths in the hope of liberation, after experiencing a series of
apparently decisive insights into the formation of his own subjectivity, and
describing these in terms of 'truth', and even 'a sort of psychoanalysis' (Macey,
1993 pp. 340, 371). But he seems to have found 'technologies of the self' that
were relatively free from the interpretative frameworks of power/knowledge we
inescapably internalise. Whatever the content of these experiences, it appears
that Foucault was now at last engaged in unravelling the formative effects,
on both subjectivity and thought, of having attended Lacan's seminars, and
assimilated the conception of a 'phallic gestalt' centred upon an assumption of
masculine privilege (Schneider, 2001 p. 8). A key element in the insights of
this period may well have been a realisation of the depth and extent to which
processes of power/knowledge and regimes of truth had become ingrained
within his own sense of selfhood.

Despite the apparent difficulty of doing so, I want to persist with the
unpostmodern-sounding suggestion that Foucault's writings are more or less
haunted, albeit less transparently so than those of Nietzsche, by the seemingly
endemic patriarchal 'wound' of unacknowledged grieving for a distant father.
It should be possible to trace connections between the ubiquitous imagery of
the king and the figure of the father without either compressing their complexity to the point of caricature, or claiming undue ease of passage between 'life'
and 'work'. Foucault understood the potential intimacy of exchange between
writing and selfhood, developing a Nietzschean sense of the importance of
'elaborating one's own life as a personal work of art', as well as seeking to transform himself though knowledge wrested from writing (Kritzman, 1988 p. 49;
Rabinow, 1994/2000 pp. 131, 208ff., 232). One reading of Foucault's late
account of an ostensibly benign form of disciplinary power might therefore be
that it reflected, but also helped fashion, a gradual process of autobiographical
'self-overcoming' in relation to memories of the absent presence, and then
present absence, of his bullying father. If victims of intimidation commonly
focus upon an inspecting gaze, rather than directly contemplating the troubling
prospect of violence, it is possible that Foucault's surprising reticence about the
function of violence might have been related to some personal history (Mac-
Cannell and MacCannell, 1993 p. 215). In a late interview he recalled an
adolescence in which 'the menace of war was our background, our frame of
reference . . . our private life was really threatened', and even describes this as

'the nucleus of my theoretical desires' (Kritzman, 1988 p. 7).[41] Perhaps growing up in the shadow of a remote and violent man was what turned this generational inheritance into a personal quest for him, shaping his portrayal of a masculinist political anatomy characterised by invisible surveillance and ubiquitous coercion, in which rebellious passion must be curbed by moral imprisonment?

In a contemporary essay on globalisation, the figure of the king re-emerges as 'King Rumpel', depicted as 'powerful, pitiless, and armed to the teeth'. His realm is 'raw capital, his conquests emerging markets, his prayers profits, his borders limitless, his weapons nuclear'. Interestingly, Arundhati Roy then observes that 'to even try to imagine him, to hold the whole of him in your field of vision, is to situate yourself at the very edge of sanity, to offer yourself up for ridicule' (Roy, 2002 pp. 129–30). This terrible image, wrought from insight into the machinations of macro-systemic abuse, and the immanence of orchestrated violence, which is of course all too often pivotal in precipitating madness and distress, contrasts with Lacan's internalised 'imaginary anatomy' – the coherent and paternally derived self-image we are said to need as protection from the brink of 'schizophrenia'. One of the dangers inherent in attending to the early formation of subjectivity is that we become diverted into a will to truth about the nature of an individual's 'real self', rather than unravelling a story of encounters and negotiations with power. Critical biography nevertheless contends that our responses to the reality of overarching structures of domination are partially but influentially shaped by our cumulative experiences of them, and that our knowledge of power will remain unnecessarily circumscribed until we look at how our various voices were socially formed (Jackson, 1990). This kind of perspective appears to have informed Foucault's analogy between the operations of power in the fields of sex and politics, and enabled him to move between personal reflection and a wider theorisation of power, without limiting the former to an exercise in psychological self-discovery, and the latter to a formulaic exposition of disembodied structures and ideologies.

A coloniser who refused?

In the concluding section of this chapter I want to look briefly at some of the wider influences that shaped the voices with which Foucault wrote so influentially, both directly and indirectly, about the politics of madness. Invoking the Jewish Tunisian theorist Albert Memmi, Hartstock characterises Foucault as a 'coloniser who refuses'. Although he exists in painful ambiguity, Foucault ultimately writes from the position of the dominator and 'understands the world from the perspective of the ruling group'. He makes some important contributions, but because he renders systematic power relations and social structures invisible, and makes domination hard to locate, his work is inadequate, 'even irrelevant to the needs of the colonised or dominated' (Hartstock, 1990 pp. 165–9; Memmi, 1967).[42] Ironically, Hartstock arrives at this somewhat harsh conclusion using Edward Said, whose influential *Orientalism* draws on

Foucault. While I have some sympathy with negative responses to Foucault, I would argue that some of his contributions, such as his insistence that there is no political space beyond power, are of vital relevance to any political challenge to structures of domination. Since the metaphor of colonisation is often used within the politics of 'mental health' it seems doubly appropriate to ask how far Foucault's contribution to the field can be understood as that of a 'coloniser who refuses'.

In *Madness and Civilisation*, Foucault famously asserted that the language of psychiatry was 'a monologue of reason about madness', and that the performative power of its practices owed less to knowledge generated in its factories of 'illness' than to the paternalistic moral authority around which those institutions had been constructed (Foucault, 1961/1971 pp. xii–xiii; Kritzman, 1988 p. xxi). Because the book had a considerable influence on the British anti-psychiatry movement this can be seen as a key political contribution, but Foucault made no attempt to apply his critique directly to contemporary instances of psychiatric oppression until the later interviews. Here, for example, he argued that Soviet psychiatry was a continuation, not a distortion, of the fundamental project of a discipline that had intervened in 'public hygiene', questions of public order, as early as 1830 (Kritzman, 1988 pp. 181–2). The masculinist tradition that shaped the young Foucault's academic writing would certainly have discouraged direct engagement with contentious issues.[43] In a prevailing climate of discrimination, he could only make oblique references to personal experience, including his activism, but his recourse to writing 'histories of the present' shouldn't be taken as indicating any lack of interest in the issues of his day. He was able to alternate between formal academic language and a much more immediate style when discussing practical agendas in interviews and pamphlets.

For Hartstock, the central issue is that the creation of 'Others' depends upon the simultaneous construction of a 'transcendent and omnipotent theoriser', but as well as being manifestly, and often actively, supportive of the decolonisation of marginalised groups, Foucault clearly rejected such a role (Hartstock, 1990 p. 163). His concept of the specific intellectual, who would focus upon a particular sector in order to expose the daily detail of oppression, facilitate political debate, and work upon 'regimes of truth', was contrasted with the traditional role of the universal intellectual who sets out to enlighten by proclaiming general truths (Sheridan, 1980 p. 222). The GIP (Groupe d'Informations sur les Prisons), a loose 'cultural weapon' improvised by Foucault and Daniel Defert in 1971, was intended as a testing ground for this form of subversive intellectual work based upon personal involvement, and Dr Edith Rose, a prison psychiatrist at Toul, who reported on appalling conditions and the 'extreme frequency' of suicide attempts and self-harm there, is cited as exemplifying the approach (Miller, 1993 pp. 187–93). Because Foucault strongly opposed any attempt to speak for others, the GIP was also intended as a forum through which the voices of prisoners could be heard describing their mistreatment. He noted, however, that whereas exploited groups had always recognised and resisted their oppression, the willingness of professionals to speak out about practices and power structures they were implicated in was a new phenomenon (Macey, 1993 p. 269).

Foucault talks about 'an insurrection of subjugated knowledges' that have been disqualified as naïve, low ranking and inadequate in comparison with dominant knowledges, and contrasts the knowledge of psychiatric patients with that of medical practitioners. Far from demeaning these particular local and 'popular knowledges', as Hartstock suggests, he celebrates their irreducible diversity, and advocates a union of erudite knowledge and local memory as a way of emancipating them, not least from subjection within formal, unitary and scientific theoretical discourses.[44] While proclaiming the 'strange efficacy of localised anti-psychiatric discourses', he alerts activists against the temptation of recolonising their own liberated, and necessarily fragmented, knowledges within such overarching schema (Foucault, 1980 pp. 80–7). Hartstock argues that Foucault is only able to conceive of the intellectual as someone who works alongside those struggling for power, rather than being fully and directly involved (Hartstock, 1990 p. 165). It is certainly striking that in the lectures he gave in January 1976, close to the publication of The Will to Knowledge, there is still very little sense of a speaker whose personal experiences and engagements might be relevant either to his critical contributions or to his relationship with disqualified knowledges. This disappearance of the personal conforms to the demands of dominant masculinist 'colonial' discourses, and reflects Foucault's contradictory and silenced subjectivity. The admission of marginalised voices into institutions of 'erudite knowledge', particularly as survivor researchers, is an important but recent development for which Foucault's formulations arguably prepared the ground.

Reflecting on his work in one of the later interviews, Foucault expresses regret that it had been taken by some simply as 'a sign of belonging', of being 'on the "good side", the side of madness, children, delinquency, sex'. The real work begins once we try 'to turn off these mechanisms that cause the appearance of two separate sides, by dissolving the false unity, the illusory "nature" of this other side' that we identify ourselves with (Kritzman, 1988 pp. 120–1). Rather than negating emancipation, the intention here was surely to draw attention to the tendency of broad political categories, such as 'woman', 'black', 'gay' or 'mad', to function as what Nietzsche had termed 'necessary errors', insofar as they conceal the complexities of power. While Foucault's later writings on sexuality show that this kind of postmodern perspective need not depend upon the relative luxury of speaking as a dissenting colonial, it is noteworthy that his altogether more hybrid speaking position in relation to psychiatry had produced the dramatic dualism of Madness and Civilisation. In that early work, moreover, the very clarity of demarcation between reason and madness arguably served to obscure other axes of power, in particular the patriarchal nature of the nexus of domination he was beginning to elucidate in the figure of the asylum physician.

Though the biographies contain quite detailed information suggesting that Foucault's early experiences of distress and involvements with psychology were profoundly formative, he managed to avoid becoming either a psychiatric inpatient or a fully fledged 'mental health' professional. Rather than emerging from a symmetrical splitting between devalued 'Other' and transcendent theoriser, his writings on madness draw upon direct but atypical experience of both positions, as well as being strongly coloured by his sexuality and class background. Though the young Foucault's distress was clearly serious, his encounter with services was about as different from that of Artaud as could be imagined. His consultant surgeon father arranged for him to see Jean Delay, an eminent psychiatrist with literary interests, with whom he subsequently chose to study and work, and developed a lasting friendship (Eribon, 1991; Macey, 1993).[45] Foucault's direct personal experience would, in terms of currently prevailing identity politics, qualify him as a survivor of self-harm, but only marginally as a service user. He is perhaps such an interesting and provocative figure, however, largely because he evades easy categorisation, and sets out a constructive challenge to the assumptions of revolutionary liberation politics based on a track record of activism, and a wealth and diversity of personal experience that was riven with contradiction. One effect of this was undoubtedly that he produced a body of work whose impact has often depended upon mediation through other voices. For this reason Foucault's influence on professionals and academics has been stronger than on the survivor movement.[46]

The young Foucault seems to have entertained the possibility of crossing the consulting room floor and joining the colonisers. His active interest in psychology began on arrival at the ENS, where students were exposed to liberal psychiatry and were taken to hospitals, including the Sainte-Anne, where they would see patients and listen to medical presentations. Foucault obtained various qualifications including a diploma in pathological psychology, and his first book was influenced by the Pavlovian approach then promoted within Marxist circles. In his mid-twenties he worked in a voluntary capacity, as a trainee, both at the Sainte-Anne and in the prison system's main medical facility, helping to perform diagnostic tests in electroencephalographic laboratories. These procedures were intended to identify neurological conditions such as epilepsy, but also to screen for simulated psychopathology (Eribon, 1991 pp. 41ff.; Macey, 1993 pp. 58–9).[47] During this period he was considering a career in psychiatry, but appears to have had second thoughts when a service user he had befriended was given a pre-frontal lobotomy that condemned him to a 'vegetable existence'. Foucault wondered whether death, or even the worst existential pain, might have been preferable (Macey, 1993 p. 57). Remarkably, it had taken him some time to question the institutional practices he observed and was being inducted into performing.

It seems that experience alone was insufficient to unsettle the aspirant professional, and that a new interpretative framework was needed before critical reflection could bear fruit. In a late interview Foucault describes his discovery of Nietzsche in 1953 as a turning point. *Untimely Meditations* sparked a 'revelation' that provoked him to leave his job in the asylum, and change his life (Martin *et al.*, 1988 pp. 11–13). Foucault's first publication, an extended introduction to a translation of the paper 'Dream and Existence', written by the Heideggerian psychotherapist Ludwig Binswanger, appeared shortly after this, and he would repay Nietzsche later by playing a prominent part in the 'de-Nazification' of his favoured forebear (Eribon, 1991 p. 44; Rajchman, 1985 p. 115).[48] Comparison between the lives and works of the two philosophers has alerted us to a shared propensity to resort to martial imagery that, at least until his return from California, brought Foucault closer to the polemical Nietzsche.[49] The contrast between Foucault as activist, influenced by his engagements with masculinist radicalism, and as postmodern philosopher asking vital questions about the complexities of power, may be less extreme than that between Nietzsche's corresponding subjectivities, but there is clearly an analytical value in separating these voices out. Once again, the philosophy provides conceptual 'tools' applicable well beyond the specific politics of the day, not least when found to be quite strongly consistent with feminist perspectives (Diamond and Quimby, 1988). As well as containing a wealth of material relevant to a critical politics of 'mental health', Foucault's later genealogical works challenge us to transcend simple binary categories, and the false unity of the 'side' we identify with.

Elements within the psychiatric survivor movement have borrowed constructively from gay liberation, but Halperin cautions that this now seems 'a strangely antiquated formula', not least because there is no place outside power to escape to. He argues that far from signalling a retreat into hopelessness and loss of agency, Foucault's analysis of power has proved invaluable during a more hostile and violent post-AIDS era, when the emphasis has switched from liberation to survival and resistance (Halperin, 1995 pp. 30–2).[50] Could this also apply in relation to the complex politics of 'mental health', where users and survivors face an environment in which proliferating technologies of biomedicine and surveillance await deployment within a political culture apparently lurching towards increasing militarisation, privatisation, normalisation and regulation? Foucault's post-Nietzschean 'toolkit' contains some potentially important resources that can be adapted for the purpose of deconstructing, surviving and resisting just such omnipresent forces, not least those proffering inappropriate 'help'. Once the presence of gender in the texts becomes clear, new uses might emerge for the conceptual resources they contain. In particular, undertaking a critique of power/knowledge within practices of eliciting and listening to stories about emotional life begins to look less like a prophylactic against critical work on men's subjectivities than a prerequisite for it.

Chapter 7

Like a marble guest

The nervous illness of Daniel Paul Schreber

> I would count it a great triumph for my dialectical dexterity if through the present essay . . . I should achieve only the one result, to make the physicians shake their heads in doubt as to whether, after all, there was some truth in my so-called delusions and hallucinations.
>
> (Schreber, 1903/2000)

> it seems crucial to resist the myth of interior origins, understood as naturalised or culturally fixed. Only then, gender coherence might be understood as the regulatory fiction it is – rather than the common point of our liberation.
>
> (Butler, 1990b)

Lacan elaborated his influential notion that psychosis is characterised by a gap between the 'psychotic subject' and the world, and in particular by foreclosure of the name-of-the-father, in a seminar (presented during 1955–6) in which he revisited Freud's influential analysis of the published *Memoirs* of Judge Schreber (Benvenuto and Kennedy, 1986). Given the extent of fascination that this remarkable autobiographical work has aroused, it comes as no surprise to find that Foucault regarded it, and the classic 'case history' texts surrounding it, as epitomising the formation of disciplinary power (Foucault, 1975/1977 pp. 193–4).[1] Because of their content, and because these various narratives of experience reflect cultural developments during a period described as crucial in terms of the construction of public masculinities, they also function as vivid dramatisations of the complex interface between the politics of 'mental health' and gender (Hearn, 1992). In this final historical discussion, then, my primary concern will be to trace these two political strands within a genealogical story about disciplinary appropriations of biographical experience. The ready availability of what Foucault called multiple discontinuous commentaries helpfully enables us to approach this material from different angles, and illustrates the potential value of critical postmodern perspectives that acknowledge ambiguity, paradox, pluralism and contradiction, as well as the materiality of power (Foucault, 1973/1975). I begin this discussion with a brief summary of

events, and refer to Schreber's own book and some of the more critical contributions to the literature for further detail (Schreber, 1903/2000; Schatzman, 1973;
Porter, 1987; Lothane, 1992; Santner, 1996).

Daniel Paul Schreber, a contemporary as well as compatriot of Nietzsche, was
an eminent high court judge who was hospitalised in mid-life because of what
he called his 'nervous illness'. Though he recovered from his first breakdown
he was admitted twice more, and spent a total of thirteen years as a psychiatric
patient before dying in an asylum. His privileged class background would
undoubtedly have helped him organise the publication of Memoirs of My Nervous
Illness (1903/2000), based on notes made during incarceration, but did not protect him from exposure to dehumanising conditions, including solitary confinement in padded cells, and enforced medication and feeding. His stated reasons
for publishing an autobiographical account were to challenge the absolute
confidence of medical opinion that his supernatural experiences were merely
delusions and hallucinations, and to attempt to explain 'the necessity' that compelled him to behave in ways that other people considered odd. He hoped that
the truth of his religious ideas might precipitate an overthrow of existing religious systems, and felt that certain knowledge of survival of the soul beyond
death would come as a blessing to mankind (Schreber, 1903/2000 pp. 15,
248–9). While confined, he also sought to limit the contested sphere of medical
and juridical power by writing a legal essay about the circumstances under
which people considered insane could be detained against their will (Santner,
1996 pp. 80–1). Although many other patients have believed they were making
a contribution to psychiatric knowledge, one of the consequences of publication
for Schreber was that he subsequently became the most quoted patient in the
history of psychiatry (Porter, 1987; Schatzman, 1973). A succession of lumin-
aries such as Bleuler, Jaspers, Freud, Lacan, Jung, Klein and Fairburn, as well
as numerous lesser psychoanalytic commentators, have turned to his book in
pursuit of their will to truth about his agonised mental state, and in order to
make general claims about 'psychosis' and 'paranoia' (Leudar and Thomas,
2000; Sass, 1987).

The judge's second and most devastating period of nervous illness was precipitated by the stress induced by his nomination in June 1893 to the post of
Senatspräsident, or presiding judge, at Germany's Supreme Court of Appeals.
At this time he began to dream that his 'former illness had returned', and one
morning in bed, before fully waking, had the feeling that 'it might be rather
pleasant to be a woman succumbing to intercourse' (Schreber, 1903/2000
p. 46). Over-stretched by his work, and by moving to an unfamiliar town with
little opportunity to socialise, he experienced intense sleeplessness and began
to hear a recurrent cracking noise in the wall. After preparing for a suicide
attempt, during the night before the anniversary of his father's death, he was
admitted to hospital, where he remained unable to sleep, and 'passed the days
in endless melancholy'. When, some three months later, his wife went away
for a much needed break, his condition deteriorated so severely that he no

longer wished to be seen by her.[2] He then experienced a 'mental collapse', involving supernatural communication and incessant voices. From this point Schreber believed that his psychiatrist, Professor Flechsig, was persecuting him and maintaining 'nerve-contact' with him when not present. He became convinced that a 'seer of spirits' must be 'unmanned' – transformed into a woman – once in permanent contact with divine nerves or rays (Schreber, 1903/2000 pp. 46–53). He spent time in two other asylums before eventually being released, nine years later, at the age of sixty, into a domestic and largely female-centred existence. Only five years later, his wife suffered a stroke, and he returned to hospital for the last time.

Before looking at Schreber's notion of 'unmanning', I want to draw attention to some commentaries that attempt to place his experiences of incarceration in a critical context. Perhaps significantly, one of the clearest statements about the potential effects of his mistreatment can be found in a contribution from a historian. Porter points out that for five years Schreber 'lived a day-to-day life of extraordinary isolation, spending days on end in his room, punctuated by more or less solitary walks and recreation'. His doctors appeared to have had no sense that relating to his 'delusions', or even engaging with him closely, might be helpful.[3] As well as experiencing their interventions as arbitrary and mystifying, and fearing they might castrate him, Schreber reports brutal treatment at the hands of attendants, being made to sleep in a padded cell for two and a half years, and (for significant periods) lacking any means of occupying himself. Porter suggests that such conditions may be sufficient to explain many of his 'delusions' (Porter, 1987 pp. 165–6). Despite all of this, aspects of Schreber's descriptions of the world he was experiencing look less bizarre once compared with understandings from other cultural environments; indeed some appear to presage subsequent developments at the margins of Western culture.[4]

More recent accounts portray Flechsig as a neuroanatomist renowned for his work on the myelination of nerve fibres and the localisation of nervous diseases in the brain. His appointment to the directorship of a psychiatric clinic is described as signalling a paradigm shift towards extreme medicalisation: 'In one fell swoop . . . the tradition of the soul ended and the reign of the brain began' (Lothane, 1992, cited in Santner, 1996 p. 70).[5] Flechsig's biological determinism permitted no space for agency, no mediating dimension between symbolic meaning and biochemical process. The latter simply determined and produced the former. Some writers find this quality reproduced in Schreber's 'delusions', especially his belief in a 'writing-down-system' in which all his thoughts, phrases, possessions and contacts were being recorded in a highly mechanical and automatic manner (Santner, 1996, citing Kittler, 1990). That this might reflect the reality of psychiatric scrutiny seems to escape many commentators, even when Foucault's work on panopticism is invoked (e.g. Sass, 1987).[6] Santner interprets Schreber's evocative concept of 'soul murder' as a comment upon Flechsig's neuroanatomical paradigm, and Schreber himself associates Kraeplin's 'denial of everything supernatural' with shallow Enlightenment rationalism (Santner, 1996 pp. 74–5; Schreber, 1903/2000 pp. 82–3).

If the material is turned towards a perspective that foregrounds gender, the timing of his crisis, just as he was about to assume a position of considerable authority, and his subsequent dependence upon his wife for emotional support are immediately striking. A psychiatric report, presented to the court in relation to Schreber's appeal against his tutelage order, made much of his desire to publish the Memoirs.[7] Here was a formerly eminent man, about to transgress the masculinist code of the public domain by indulging in excessive disclosure, revealing intimate details of his inner life, and recounting episodes of extreme vulnerability. Moreover, he was about to expose his anguished subjectivity in relatively raw form, at least partially circumventing the mediating filter of professional interpretation and authorisation, by relegating various official reports to the status of appendices to the Memoirs. One of these gives a vivid description of him as a physically strong man who caused so much disturbance by shouting abuse from his window, day and night, that townspeople gathered to complain.[8] His alternation between experimental feminisation and outbursts of apparently spontaneous bellowing, which he attributed to supernatural interference and attempted to control or manage considerately, also invites discussion in terms of masculinity. Such episodes, of course, need to be understood in relation to his prolonged exposure to extreme disciplinary regimes, not only during incarceration, but also, as will soon become apparent, during his early life. Santner has an interesting discussion of Schreber's renunciation of 'dysfunctional' masculinity in the direction of homosexual desire, feminisation and 'Jewification' in the context of a breakdown of authority in fin-de-siècle Germany, but subsumes this as exemplifying an overarching crisis of the Enlightenment subject (Santner, 1996 pp. 55, 145). However we frame the broader context, it seems clear that the social construction of Schreber's madness should not be interpreted simply for what it tells us about the politics of psychiatry. In order to approach this man's story, and the extraordinary public interest it has generated, we need to theorise the operations of gender.

Various contributions from postmodern feminism have interesting implications for understanding the interface between 'madness' and masculinity. Nicholson, for example, identifies a widespread tendency to think of sex as basic, cross-cultural and given, and thus to conceive of the relationship between biology and socialisation as a kind of 'coat-rack'. She refers to this approach as biological foundationalism, and argues that it obscures the differences between women and between men, and impedes understanding of the processes by which people come to be categorised as one or the other. It also fosters a belief that commonalities of sex lead to commonalities of gender, so that while women (or men) are seen as separated by 'race' and class, there is a tendency to assume that the operations of gender are uniform and unmediated.[9] According to Nicholson no common features emanate from biology (Nicholson, 1999 pp. 55–8). As already noted, Butler reads Foucault's account of normalisation as a process in which Nietzsche's expanded interior world of 'the soul' comes to be inscribed on and through the surfaces and actions of bodies. She envisages the social production of gender fantasy as a corollary process, in which the gendered body is constructed through a series of discursive exclusions and denials, producing a 'false stabilisation' in the interests of heterosexually regulated sexuality. This is contrasted with accounts that imply an expressive model that localises and naturalises gender within an interior psychic space or psychological 'core', thereby precluding analysis of the political constitution of the gendered subject. Butler suggests that gender is wholly performative and, applying Nietzsche's insight into the metaphysics of substance, argues that the words, gestures, acts, and desire' of discourse mask the process of social signification being enacted, precisely by fabricating an impression of essential identity (Butler, 1990b pp. 334–7, 20).

Some striking parallels and tensions are immediately apparent between these formulations on gender and postmodern and other critiques of psychopathology that insist on the social construction of distress, and part of the continuing fascination of Schreber's Memoirs is undoubtedly that they encapsulate these so vividly. Freud's paper in which Schreber's 'paranoia' is interpreted as an instance of repressed homosexual desire, and used to illustrate a totalising theory about the cause of paranoia in general, became the classic psychoanalytic case study of this condition (Freud, 1911/1979).[10] Schatzman reminds us, however that, especially in the context of the first half of the twentieth century, homosexuality, persecution, and what is called paranoia can dovetail hellishly'. Using the work of Niederland, he highlights some apparently close links between the painful and humiliating bodily experiences that Schreber describes as miracles, and his father's pedagogical beliefs and practices.[11] Dr Moritz Schreber, an influential paediatrician who believed that harsh discipline was necessary to counter 'weakness, sensuality, indolence, softness and cowardice', devised an elaborate system of orthopaedic devices and exercises, designed both to correct a child's posture and to protect their future mental health.[12] Freud described this man as 'no insignificant person', yet while attempting to interpret his son's childhood history, neglected the content of some forty publications on child rearing written by him, and directed his attention exclusively towards a postulated psychological core, as did his followers for the next fifty years (Schatzman 1973 pp. 124, 16, 9, 142; Niederland, 1984; Freud, 1911/1979 p. 187).

From the point of view of the politics of self-advocacy, it is important to note that Schreber himself does not mention his father in the memoirs. Schatzman understands this invisibility as a function of the state of 'soul murder', or possession, that exposure to a quite sadistic pedagogy had induced in the son. He argues that although Schreber himself likened this state to hypnosis, and managed to unveil a tormenting God behind the figure of Flechsig, he remained unable to discern the imprint of his father behind this image of God. Moritz

Schreber, like many abusive parents, was careful to disguise the relationship of absolute docility he advocated, describing for instance as 'noble independence' the condition in which children did what their parents wanted, while renouncing the moral possibility of doing otherwise and believing they were following their own desires. Like Foucault's prisoners, these children had to internalise and identify with a prohibitive law. The operations of gender were also disguised in his pedagogy, of course, and although it was aimed at children in general, its language of mastery was clearly well suited to the apparently more challenging task of inculcating 'manly heroic spirit'. 'The rearing of a boy is as a rule considerably more difficult', requiring 'more detailed and more weighty . . . explanatory advice' about 'the danger of lust' (Schatzman, 1973 pp. 20, 32–3, 57–8). Sadly, Dr Schreber's mission to socialise by constraining and shaping biology had a particularly devastating impact upon his own two sons. Some seven years before Daniel Paul's first nervous illness, his elder brother Gustav had committed suicide. The value of pluralistic commentary, in which different critical dimensions and perspectives augment, and may sometimes contradict, individual and collective self-advocacy, is underlined by those contributions that relate this absolutist therapeutic regime to the history of National Socialism (Santner, 1996 pp. xi–xii; Schatzman, 1973; Porter, 1987).

It was certainly Schreber's misfortune to experience unusually sustained and intense exposure to what Santner terms 'fathers who know too much'. If Moritz Schreber's programme was 'designed to produce proper Kantian Enlightenment subjects' who would follow an inner voice of reason, it did so by imposing the intimate violences of disciplinary power, well described as a dark counter-law secreted within an over-arching juridical schema that promised liberties (Santner, 1996 pp. 85–6; Foucault, 1975/1977 p. 222). Santner turns to Butler when discussing Schreber's 'unmanning' as a disruption of the compulsively repetitive gender performance required to sustain the stabilisation of rational masculine subjects. Butler's point, again developed from Nietzsche, is that the performance of normality never achieves comprehensive effect, that there always exists the possibility of inadvertent or deviant performances, and that 'queer' performances are productions of the very law they appear to transgress. Although cultural practices of drag and cross-dressing reveal the imitative structure and contingency of gender, the normative force of performativity also works through exclusion. That which is disqualified from 'being' and strictly foreclosed, 'the unlivable, the nonnarrativisable, the traumatic . . . haunts signification at its abject borders' (Butler, 1993 p. 188, quoted in Santner, 1996 pp. 90–9, 14; see also Butler, 1990). In his account of masculinity as homosocial enactment sustained by constant mutual evaluation, Kimmel notes that much of this kind of disciplinary behaviour is furtive, dependent upon secrecy, shame and the observance of minutely coded gender language (Kimmel, 1994 p. 275). One of the most effective ways in which masculinity masks its performative nature, surely, is by reading and monitoring deviant performances as if they alone were performances – constructing them as gaudily excessive against a backdrop of reasonable conformity.

Schreber's 'madness' was clearly scrutinised in this way, by physicians, by the public prosecutor and by other key participants in the theatre of social exclusion (who happened to be male), all of whom were assumed to be 'acting normally' according to the tenets of hegemonic masculinity. Such performances are clearly associated with the highly polarised speaking positions – entailing an expectation of either disclosure or commentary – allocated to different subjects as they are being constituted in relation to regimes of masculinist and psychiatric power (Church, 1995). Of course, a declaration of madness effectively censors deviant performance by disqualifying 'mad' revelations about hegemonic power, and since normative masculinities tend to value an opaque subject, the legacy of the confessional is a strongly gendered one. As Freud puts it in his problematic discussion of homosexuality and paranoia, when an individual is functioning normally, 'it is consequently impossible to see into the depths of their being' (Freud, 1911/1979 p. 197). Conversely, complete transparency is expected of those experiencing extreme states associated with distress, even as coherent thought and agency are being undermined, not least by psychiatric treatments, and anything said or written is subjected to diagnostic interpretation and censorship. Butler's conclusion, that agency emerges out of improvisational variation upon necessary repetition, may be risky or inapplicable in relation to the regulation of distress or madness, because impulsiveness or dissent may be read as pathology, or because it might revive the spectre of romanticisation, and because recovery may depend upon discovering a sense of agency among the often dissonant structures and routines of 'ordinary' life. As previously noted, in relation to masculinity, gestures of autonomy may amount to paradoxical conformity. Seeing madness as performative in Butler's sense would, however, have the merit of highlighting an element of agency and coherence in Schreber's solitary project of 'unmanning', while revealing the prevailing orthodoxy to be a product of the same hegemonic compulsion that constructed and policed his distress (Butler, 1990).[13]

Despite the difficulty, and taking due account of the speaking positions of commentators, it may be constructive to think about men's madness, in which there almost always remains a degree, however tenuous and vestigial, of relative power as always already including a constitutive performance of gender. This kind of perspective might generate pertinent questions about the intricate interdependence between masculinity and culturally sanctioned norms of sanity and reason, at both analytic and practical levels. For example, Schreber's agitated ambivalence towards the injunction from incessant voices that he must be transformed into a woman informed and shaped his understandable resistance against arbitrary and enforced treatment. His alternation between 'manly' and 'feminine' forms of resistance needs to be considered in relation to contemporary cultural and psychiatric discourses on gender.[14] The subsequent rendering of Schreber's personal experience as an object of analysis can be seen as illustrating a tense and complex historical process, integral to the forma-tion of public patriarchies, in which men came to demarcate and dominate a psychological realm (Hearn, 1992 p. 221).[15] If psychoanalytic case history offered a way of bringing men's subjectivity and trauma more fully into the public domain, this appears to have been achieved, ironically, in order to divert attention from the social production of distress and madness by more powerful men.

In his influential essay, Freud courted controversy by equating Schreber's feminisation fantasy with homosexual desire for Flechsig, identifying an indig-nant repudiation of this as an example of true 'masculine protest'. He then situated the material within 'the familiar ground of the father-complex', and explained Schreber's fantasy as a response to the father's 'most dreaded threat, castration' (Freud, 1911/1979 pp. 177, 191). This latter assertion is again chal-lenged by Schatzman, who argues that Schreber's fear of castration was almost certainly grounded in an awareness that Dr Flechsig had actually practised medical castration, and by Bloch, who argues that what Schreber feared was not castration at all, but infanticide (Schatzman, 1973 pp. 106–7; Bloch, 1989).[16] Schreber also expressed an explicit fear of being handed over to another human being for sexual purposes, and used graphic metaphors for abjec-tion, comparing himself with rotting carrion used as bait in hunting. Once again, it seems likely that psychoanalytic discourse, which spirits the imagery of the phallus and of castration into an abstract symbolic register, might have been masking a history of sexual as well as emotional and physical abuse.[17]

Schreber's story clearly has a bearing upon the use of psychoanalytic ideas in critiques of masculinity. Kimmel bases his theorisation of a homophobic under-pinning of normative masculinity upon the Freudian assumption that men con-tinually need to suppress an originally pre-Oedipal homoerotic desire, recast as a feminine desire for other men. Because this homophobic flight from intimacy is never completely successful, it has to be re-enacted in every homosocial rela-tionship. It is possible to overturn psychoanalytic discourse, however, and argue that the social repression of otherwise ubiquitous homosexual desire produces 'paranoia', as internalised feelings of love turn to hatred, inflaming a sense of persecution when others, who still seem aware of these concealed feelings, appear to know our innermost thoughts (Parker, 1997 p. 85). Kimmel also offers a less sexualised, non-psychoanalytic layer of interpretation in which the father is the first man to evaluate a boy's masculine performance. The father's gaze will 'follow him for the rest of his life', and will later be joined by the eyes of 'millions of other men, living and dead' in a regime of perpetual scrutiny (Kimmel, 1994 pp. 129–31; Butler, 1993). This graphic depiction of panoptic masculinity could be taken as an elaboration and confirmation of the continuing political resonance of Freud's observation that 'the strikingly promi-nent features in the causation of paranoia, especially among males, are social humiliations and slights'. But Freud's treatment of the 'disorder' is problematic, not least because it epitomises medicalisation: he characterises paranoia as a condition where interpretation need not involve any acquaintance with the patient (Freud, 1911/1979 p. 197).[18] Not surprisingly, an objectified and exasperated Schreber declared 'paranoia' to be 'a blow in the face of truth which could hardly be worse' (Schreber, 1903/2000 Addendum C).

Nor was Freud's unwillingness to look and listen restricted to his response to 'paranoid' subjects. Bloch attributes the psychoanalyst's 'delusion' about the 'excellence' of Schreber's father, and the son's love for him, to his troubled relationship with his own father. She concludes that it would be difficult to find a more dramatic illustration of the consequences of his retraction of the seduction theory, or reflection of its dynamics, than this 'phenomenal misreading' of Schreber's Memoirs. Freud struggled with but succumbed to his personal investment in the exoneration of abusive fathers, adapted the Oedipus myth accordingly, and subsequently compared the seduction 'fantasies' of his hysterical patients to 'the imaginary creations of paranoiacs' (Bloch, 1989 pp. 185, 191; Freud 1963 cited by Schatzman, 1973 p. 103).[19] Ironically, it seems that commitment to a model of internalisation and an essential psychological core, rather than social construction and inscription, can impel a radically incomplete understanding of the 'depths' of experience. Bloch seeks to restore the heroic dimension of Freud's reputation by outing him as a survivor of abuse (Bloch, 1989 p. 199; cf. Masson 1984/1992). Perhaps because of an understandable caution about the risks inherent in portraying men as victims, Kimmel perpetuates this Freudian omission of any consideration of men's experiences of abusive fatherhood in his account of homophobic flight. Given his recognition that men often feel a sense of powerlessness within power, that fathers loom large as the first witness of their sons' attempts at masculinity, and that violence is often regarded as a hallmark of manhood, this seems a surprising and potentially important oversight (Kimmel, 1994).

Postmodern appropriations of the imagery of madness that rely on Lacan also perpetuate this kind of omission. As already noted, Lacan developed his account of 'schizophrenia' in a tertiary commentary on Freud's misreading of the Memoirs, in which Schreber's 'psychosis' is said to be marked by a 'primordial foreclosure of the name-of-the-father'. Once again the probable causes of Schreber's agony are concealed beneath a series of structuralist abstractions such as 'an accident in the register of the Other', a 'failure of the metaphor of the father', and 'a hole in the place of phallic signification'. Lacan did, however, criticise psychiatry's dismissal of internal voices as hallucinations, and recognise the importance of paying attention to their significance and constituting function for the subject (Benvenuto and Kennedy, 1986 pp. 153, 145). His insistence (in relation to the concept of a mirror stage) that autonomous selfhood is a fiction dependent upon misrecognition and exclusion also has potentially emancipatory implications, which have been taken up by some feminist and postcolonial theorists (Ahmed, 1998 p. 96, citing Lacan, 1966/1977; Fanon, 1952/1986 p. 161). The notion of progression from a fragmented body image in infancy towards armoured subjecthood, driven by a phantasy of 'orthopaedic' totality, appears startlingly resonant here, as does the image of poor 'mad' Schreber, sitting in front of a mirror in his asylum cell, reimagining his body transformed by 'female nerves of voluptuousness' and completing the effect with ornaments made of 'cheap rags and trinkets'.[20] But Lacan's psycho-analytic mythology once again obscures the likelihood that Schreber was decon-structing physical and emotional rigidity instilled throughout childhood by a relentlessly spine-straightening paternal regime, as well as responding to the retraumatising violations of asylum life and not merely reliving some more or less universal primal ontological drama (Schreber, 1903/2000 pp. 370–2).

Ahmed draws attention to Deleuze and Guattari's postmodern appropriation and romanticisation of women's political struggles, in which they privilege 'becoming-woman' as a key mode of becoming, as a 'means through which masculinity announces its impossibility and is re-inscribed otherwise'. In this manoeuvre the masculine subject reinscribes 'woman' as the key to unlocking the opposition between masculinity and femininity, and hence all other dual-ism, in order to instigate and negotiate a dialogue with himself in which his deconstruction of identity effectively renders her imperceptible (Ahmed, 1995 pp. 76–7).[21] In the same account of becoming-other, Deleuze and Guattari also appropriate the ideas and experiences of Artaud and Schreber, while render-ing the materiality of their distress and madness imperceptible.[22] Although Ahmed's analysis of the disjuncture between the postmodern male phantasy of 'becoming-woman' and womanhood reappropriates this imagery without refer-ring to the stark alterity of madness, it casts interesting light upon Schreber's 'mad' enactment of becoming-woman in the face of the impossible inhumanity of his experiences of hegemonic masculinity.

In contrast with psychoanalytic accounts, Santner stresses the interconnect-edness of social stability and psychological 'health', both of which depend upon the efficacy of the performative magic of symbolic investiture, a process whereby individuals are endowed with a mandate that will inform their public identity. The potential significance of investiture as a socio-biographical phenomenon is underscored here by the awful coincidence that the suicide of Schreber's elder brother had occurred during a crisis that had also been pre-cipitated by his appointment to the judiciary – literally by the assumption of juridical power (Santner, 1996 pp. xii, 40, 63 note 52). Focusing on Schreber's 'investiture crisis', Santner expresses surprise that Freud overlooked the impor-tance of two decisively performative speech acts. The official act of inter-pellation nominating him as *Senatspräsident*, and the subsequent declaration by a resoundingly baritone internal voice that he was a *Luder*, destined to be destroyed by God, both proclaimed dramatic changes in symbolic status.[23] Although Santner associates such crises with paranoia, and draws an analogy between them and the prevalence of 'hysteria' in fin-de-siècle Europe, he declines to make a direct association between investiture crises and public masculinity (see Hearn, 1992). Yet if the development of case history as an instrument of disciplinary power reflected public masculinities' need to regulate deviant performance, the overwhelming interest in Schreber may in part be explained as representing an attempt to account for such a pronounced and high-profile failure of patriarchal interpellation, as well as an opportunity to rehearse the concealment of endemic violence. Though Santner contributes towards an appreciation of the complexity of Schreber's story, his search for the causes of paranoia at the heart of political totalitarianism raises as many questions about medicalisation and the pathologisation of masculinity as does Freud's search for homosexual desire at the heart of paranoia.

At a very low point, near the end of his stay at 'Flechsig's asylum', when dreading sexual abuse, or being taken out and drowned, Schreber describes how, sitting in the hospital garden, he 'felt like a marble guest who had returned from times long past into a strange world' (Schreber, 1903/2000 p. 92). This striking image evokes possession by an august ancestral patriarch, a commandingly statuesque embodiment of inherited masculine authority, who, like Schreber himself, would doubtless feel quite out of place among 'lunatics', yet whom Schreber's transformations appear to have been designed both to appease and to undermine. Although Schreber's story is atypical – high court judges scarcely constitute an oppressed group, and the operations of gender are unusually prominent and transparent in his story, men's distress or madness will always be more or less permeated by particular relationships with paternal and patriarchal authority, and traditionally involve performances of masculinity that 'fail' against a benchmark of bland normality, conspicuous achievement, and socially sanctioned domination, personified in the presiding figures of psychiatry.[24] For this reason, the Schreber literature now constitutes a fascinating resource in relation to the genealogy of disciplinary power as a hegemonic instrument of public masculinity, and again illustrates the need for perspectives that adequately conceptualise men's experiences of powerlessness-within-power, while facilitating careful and effective dialogue between overlapping political concerns. It may also tell us something about the historical formation of hegemonic masculinities. Critical postmodern frameworks accommodate this kind of interpretative exploration by distinguishing between the value and necessity of narratives about overarching patterns of social oppression and aspirations to unveil absolute and universal truths.

Part III

Some contemporary debates

Chapter 8

Politics and experience

Engaging with complex subjectivity

'When your headlights hit a hedgehog and it curls up into a ball as a survival instinct, you don't call that catatonic schizophrenia. Yet when a person feels so helpless and distressed that he curls up inside his own reality because the other one is too painful to contemplate, doctors call that paranoid schizophrenia and say it requires lifelong treatment with drugs'. . . . Taking Mike's analogy further, one may switch off the headlights and let the hedgehog go on her way! Alternatively, we may put all efforts into changing the response of the hedgehog – persuading her to ignore the headlights from which she is protecting herself; or administering drugs to the hedgehog so that she is no longer responsive to bright lights.

(Lawson, 1988, cited in Plumb, 1994)

If we start with the assumption that the problems are ones of gender – and that gender refers to particular relations of power that are socially structured and individually embodied – then we are able to be simultaneously critical of men's collective power and the behaviour and attitudes of individual men and to be male affirmative, to say that feminism will enhance the lives of men, that change is a win-win situation but that it requires giving up forms of privilege, power, and control. . . . Our awareness of men's contradictory experiences of power gives us the tools to simultaneously challenge men's power and speak to men's pain. It is the basis of a politics of compassion.

(Kaufmann, 1994)

I have argued for the relevance of a critical postmodern theoretical framework that challenges the ascendancy of masculinist Enlightenment rationality while giving due weight to voices historically excluded from the public realm, and have opened up a discussion about masculinity and madness in the context of four biographical studies that suggests a relationship between the momentum towards unbounded deconstruction and the dynamics of hegemonic masculinity. I now want to consider the application of postmodern thought to current debates in the field. For all its inclusive rhetoric and apparent celebration of diversity, mainstream postmodern social theory has been charged with appropriating understandings wrought from the myriad experiences of women and of people from non-Western cultures, and because of its questioning of assumptions about authenticity and the possibility of coherent subjecthood, of undermining the very basis upon which assertions of difference appear to depend. Critics argue that a postmodern 'we' has been constituted through acts of exclusion and othering, and 'the Other' vaunted, ironically, in order to demonstrate the ultimate meaninglessness of any identity it might contain. 'We are all Others now' (Sardar, 1998 p. 13; Ahmed, 1998 p. 6). On this basis it might be claimed that pivotal to postmodern announcements of the death of a generalised, implicitly masculine subject has been another pattern of appropriation, that of the imagery and experience of madness. In previous chapters I traced the genealogy of this appropriation back to an anguished Nietzsche's allegory of the madman, and to a younger Foucault's exaltation of the madness of Nietzsche and Artaud as a fundamental contestation of Western culture. These influential contributions still resonate, and imagery of madness and schizophrenia continues to emerge with such regularity in discussions about postmodern deconstruction that I want to begin this chapter in cautionary vein by reviewing some instances where madness has been seen, often by practising psychologists, as allegorising, exaggerating or even remedying a contemporary cultural condition.

I then want to discuss the linkages and tensions between various approaches to the politics of experience developed within postmodern feminism and the psychiatric survivor movement, before embarking upon an extended discussion of the implications of both sets of perspectives for understandings of the interface between masculinities and madness or distress. Whereas unbounded postmodern theory works to consign notions of authorship, and therefore ownership and appropriation, to the conceptual scrapheap of modernity, social postmodernism insists upon locating marginalised voices within the context of intersecting patterns of oppression, and can therefore defend situated knowledge claims and argue about authorship, authenticity and accountability. As previously noted, many men who use psychiatric services are highly vulnerable, some who are vulnerable also become threatening or violent in extremis, while others collapse into distress from positions as unambiguous victimisers. Feminist analyses have highlighted both the devastating 'mental health' effects of the abusiveness and violence of a substantial minority of men, and the disproportionate contribution made by women as nurturers and carers. Because of the breadth of diversity of both 'men' and men's experiences of distress and madness, there is clearly a need to disaggregate categories and locate discussions, taking account of ethnicity, sexuality, age, class and disability, as well as the effects of 'mental health' oppression, and acknowledging the lived complexity of individual men's orientations and speaking positions. In the process of exploring these issues, I hope to demonstrate that critical postmodern social theory might overcome the charges of elitism and appropriation levelled at its mainstream elder cousin. It is, after all, in areas characterised by complexity, contradiction and difficulty that a postmodern willingness to invite multiple readings, live with creative tension, and hold back from hasty closure, seems most likely to prove constructive. But before attempting to apply the theory we need to look more closely at some of the ways in which imagery of madness or distress has been linked with postmodern social fragmentation.

'Schizophrenia' and postmodernism, allegory and appropriation

> Schizophrenia . . . is our very own 'malady', modern man's sickness. The end of history has no other meaning. . . . If the human race survives, future men will . . . see that what we call 'schizophrenia' was one of the forms in which, often through quite ordinary people, the light began to break through the cracks in our all too closed minds. . . . Madness need not be all breakdown. It may also be breakthrough.
>
> (Deleuze and Guattari, 1972/1977)

There are some quite strong parallels between the postmodern privileging of 'woman' as a key figure of becoming, and the extensive use made both by writers from within and commentators about postmodern philosophy, of the concept of schizophrenia (Ahmed, 1998 p. 77). Just as the signifier 'woman' has been colonised by an ostensibly reconfigured postmodern masculine subject, the 'schizophrenic disjuncture' somehow 'ceases to entertain a necessary relationship to . . . morbid content . . . and becomes available for more joyous intensities', signifying a new aesthetic or cultural style (Jameson, 1991 p. 29). The contested language of psychopathology is thereby seamlessly pressed into service as a unifying metaphor in the paradoxical and very unpostmodern task of distilling the essence of a presumed postmodern condition characterised by flux, fragmentation and forgetfulness of history. We are, apparently, all 'schizophrenic' now – or at least should aspire to be.[1]

This strange aspiration was epitomised in Deleuze and Guattari's advocacy of a politics of 'schizoanalysis', which would 'schizophrenise' ostensibly 'normal' men and women 'in order to break the holds of power and institute research into a new collective subjectivity and a revolutionary healing of mankind'. *Anti-Oedipus* was announced as a continuation of the project of writers such as Nietzsche and Artaud. The latter's concept of a 'Body without Organs' was freely adapted, and the newly idealised figure of the 'schizo' likened to Zarathustra. Such a man (*sic*) knows incredible sufferings, but

> produces himself as a free man, irresponsible, solitary, and joyous, finally able to say and do something simple in his own name, without asking permission; a desire lacking nothing, a flux that overcomes barriers and codes, a name that no longer designates any ego whatsoever.

These Nietzschean 'new men of desire' seem to constitute an unbounded post-modern riposte to the new men of reason inspired by Kant's 'audere sape' ('dare to know'), while remaining within the same masculinist paradigm (Deleuze and Guattari, 1972 pp. xxi, 131).[2] What was new in the works of Laing and of Guattari, however, was that they spoke from a position as critical 'mental health' professionals, and framed their respective versions of anti-psychiatry and social revolution in a discourse grounded in psychoanalysis.

Guattari regarded his concept of transversality, an adaptation of the notion of transference to the treatment of groups in an institutional setting, as fundamental to the critique of the psychiatric hospital.[3] Genosko argues that the concept mutated, slowly hatching from its psychoanalytic shell, but despite Foucault's emphatic account of the tradition of treating madness as a form of extended childhood, appears not to realise how problematic it might be in relation to the politics of 'mental health' (Genosko, 2000; Foucault, 1961/1967 pp. 252–3). Guattari drew upon Winnicott's model of a child's separation from its mother when conceptualising 'institutional objects', but described both the power he was attempting to confront, and challenges to it, in masculine terms. Psychoanalysis, 'the best capitalist drug', was 'fixated on the superego, indelibly stamped by daddy's authority', and worked to ensure that 'desire is crushed by the injunctions and prohibitions of that same castrating daddy', so that persecution, repression, resignation and guilt prevail, and 'the best a man can hope for is to take his place in the great chain of daddies, cold and remote, like a superego'. This description of 'familialism' portrays a discourse of male victimhood fostering an intractable passivity even where men assume socially powerful positions. But despite celebrating Foucault's analysis of the constitution of the moral authority of the doctor as 'luminous', Guattari's application of his theory now looks decidedly manipulative and tokenistic. In the hospital setting the master 'must allow him/herself to be displaced', not for clear and pressing reasons of democratic accountability, but in order to minimise the likelihood of functioning as a 'superego' for his patients.[4] Thus a project that sought to theorise desire in social rather than narrowly familial terms and rid revolutionary politics of micro-fascistic power seems to have been deeply implicated in the oppression of the selfsame 'schizos' among whom it sought the avatars of a phosphorescent postmodern enlightenment (Genosko, 2000 pp. 108, 111, 117, 131–2).[5]

In his frequently cited post-Marxist commentary upon postmodernism as the 'cultural logic of late capitalism', Jameson identifies 'a whole new type of emotional ground tone'. His description of a new culture of the image or simulacrum is significantly informed by Lacan's description of schizophrenia as a breakdown in the signifying chain. Schizophrenia, understood as a linguistic malfunction, scrambles language into 'a rubble of distinct and unrelated signifiers', thereby rendering impossible the construction of a unified image of personal identity and of the past, present and future of biographical experience. What is left is a series of intense but unrelated present moments, charged with hallucinatory intensity. Jameson banishes the thought that any leading postmodern artist was 'schizophrenic in the clinical sense', and uses a clinical vignette primarily to illustrate this aesthetic intensity and sense of disjuncture. The linkage he makes with a new cultural zeitgeist could perhaps have positive implications in terms of mainstreaming madness, but there are considerable difficulties both in his use of Lacan and in the assumption that postmodernity entails a 'waning of affect', a claim illustrated with reference to Edvard Munch's painting *The Scream* (Jameson, 1991 pp. 6, 26, 11).

This most reproduced of all images, a male artist's depiction of distress, is regarded as canonical of high modernism, with its themes of alienation and isolation. For Jameson it represents but also deconstructs an 'aesthetic of expression' that assumes an autonomous 'bourgeois ego, or monad', conceived as a container within which things are felt, and from which emotions are projected outwards, often with a sense of release and catharsis. Contemporary theory replaces this kind of depth hermeneutic, with its juxtaposition of inner depths against an outer surface, with a conception of discourse and practices, intertextuality and the play of multiple surfaces. Instead of the alienation of a separate subject, condemned by its understanding of subjectivity as a self-sufficient field to experience fulfilment as imprisonment, postmodernism precipitates a decentring and fragmentation of selves. According to Jameson, concepts such as anxiety and alienation are no longer relevant, and the 'death' of the subject may bring liberation not just from anxiety, but from all feeling rooted in personal biography. 'There is no longer a self present to do the feeling' (Jameson, 1991 pp. 14–17).[6] Not only are these last suggestions extravagant, but by insisting on a projective mechanism in which nature becomes 'the wall of the monad', Jameson appears to disregard Munch's own comments, in which he reports not a cathartic release of personal emotion from an imprisoned self, but that he felt 'tired and ill' and 'sensed a scream passing through nature'. During this period, he tells us, 'I followed the impressions my eye took at heightened moments . . . [and painted] lines and forms seen in quickened mood' (Hodin, 1972 pp. 48–50). Thus, in Jameson's terms, the artist was recording what he 'saw' during states of 'hallucinatory intensity' without much affect, not unlike those said to typify the postmodern condition.[7]

For Sass, a psychotherapist working with people diagnosed as schizophrenic and writing within a biomedical framework about schizophrenia, the condition appears as an extreme manifestation of a 'modern malaise', involving a heightening of consciousness, and alienation from emotion, instinct and the body. Sass contrasts this perspective with prevalent views of madness as 'a deficit' or regressed state, or an impassioned Dionysian escape. He draws attention to a 'truth-taking stare' that establishes a mood of radical alienation by seeming to give crystalline insight into the essence of things without yielding any communicable content.[8] This characteristic posture is described as indicative of the early or premonitory stages of psychotic breakdown, and formative of later symptomatology, but also as analogous to a contradiction basic to post-Kantian thought, in which the constitutive power of consciousness is accorded primacy while consciousness simultaneously becomes an object of study. In this context, Sass reads the postmodernism of Derrida as a form of hypermodernism, and concludes that a life lived according to its claims would resemble schizophrenia. His descriptions of both the Dionysian image of madness cultivated by anti-psychiatry, and the hyper-reflexive form he identifies, resonate strikingly with familiar discourses about masculinity. In the former the madman becomes a 'wildman', while in the latter, he turns away from the body and emotional life. The notion of becoming 'a sort of God-machine' – which because it combines ideas of omnipotence and passivity is regarded as 'perhaps the most emblematic delusion' of schizophrenia – evokes not only Foucault's panopticism, but Haraway's depiction of patriarchal Enlightenment epistemology as a 'god-trick' (Sass, 1992 pp. 10, 44–5, 325–6; Haraway, 1991; Foucault, 1975/1977).

Another psychologist, Gergen, looks at the analogy between the construction of relational and ecological postmodern selves and something like schizophrenia from a position critical of individualising discourses about 'mental illness'. Despite a keen sense of the culpability of the mental health professions for generating a burgeoning 'vocabulary of human deficit' and establishing modernist and mechanist conceptions of humanity in order to legitimate their interventions, Gergen nevertheless identifies a new sensibility or pattern of self-consciousness as a syndrome which he calls 'multiphrenia'. Under postmodern conditions of social saturation, characterised by reflexive questioning, irony and linguistic play, we 'exist in a state of continuous construction and reconstruction', and become populated not just by an increasing array of latent selves and voices, but by 'the character of others' (Gergen, 1991 pp. 13–16, 71–3, 7). Whereas for Laing, the politics of experience was largely a question of navigating a path from alienation towards authenticity, for Gergen, postmodernism 'invites a heteroglossia of being'. Although 'the concept of an "authentic self" with knowable characteristics recedes from view', a new sense of polyvocal and relational selfhood opens up new possibilities for transformational dialogue (Laing, 1967; Gergen, 1991 pp. 7, 247, 180; 1999).[9] Critical postmodern perspectives constrain this momentum towards relativism and dispersal by talking about continuing and cumulative selfhood.

Writing in a feminist context, Flax bases her case against insufficient postmodern critiques of the gendered notion of a masterful, mentalist and de-eroticised 'unitary' self on her clinical experience as a psychoanalyst working with women whose painfully fragmented experience is said to mask 'repressed material' widely shared by women in Western culture. She argues that Winnicott's conception of transitional space – in which the boundaries between self and other, inner and outer, reality and illusion, are first negotiated during infancy, and remain susceptible to therapeutic renegotiation – is an important contribution towards post-Enlightenment thinking, and uses it to develop the concept of a 'third space' in which we construct culture, and in which social selves negotiate the processes and practices of justice and citizenship. In particular Flax advocates retaining the conception of a 'core' self – without which such processes would be inconceivable (Flax, 1987, 1992b). Although she recommends consciousness-raising as a way of reconstructing memory as differentiated yet collective experience, and turns feminist therapy against postmodern theorists who reduce oppression to an effect of the binary logic of language, her uncritical use of medicalising discourse appears inconsistent with the postmodern feminist perspective she is developing.[10] 'Re-membered selves' may be a necessary prerequisite for action, but substantial questions arise about uses of therapeutic discourse, not least in the context of a diagnosis (borderline personality disorder) predominantly applied to women, most of whom have been sexually abused by men (Flax, 1990 p. 116, 1987 p. 98; Shaw and Proctor, 2004).

The foregoing examples demonstrate the need to consider the relationship between postmodern theorist-practitioners and the power/knowledge nexus of the 'psy-disciplines' they work within, alongside the operations of gender and other dimensions of power. Although main- and malestream postmodern accounts have evidently appropriated the terms 'woman' and 'madness' for their own theoretical purposes, and have tended to sidestep engagement with either feminism or the politics of the madhouse, postmodern explorations of selfhood, identity and knowledge can clearly help undermine modernist and masculinist accounts of an idealised monadic self and normative reason, thereby potentially transforming the terms of relationship between consensual 'normality' and its various Others (Foucault, 1961/1971 pp. xii–xiii). Such transformation will have limited impact, however, unless it includes and learns from those who have direct experience of exclusion, oppression and emotional injury.

Identity, self-advocacy and the uses of experience

> The most damaging thing about psychiatry is that it negates the value of individual voices and experiences.
>
> (Crepaz-Keay, 2004)

> the characteristics of late modern secular society, in which individuals are buffeted and controlled by global configurations of disciplinary and capitalist power of extraordinary proportions, and are at the same time nakedly individuated . . . together add up to an incitement to *ressentiment* that might have stunned even the finest philosopher of its occasions and logics. Starkly accountable yet dramatically impotent, the late modern liberal subject quite literally seethes with *ressentiment*.
>
> (Brown, 1995)

Since the relationship between politics and personal experience has been an important concern for both feminists and psychiatric survivors, I now want to compare some of the situated understandings of this core issue that have emerged from these two broad political domains. Not least because many prominent survivor activists and theorists have been women, there has been a considerable degree of convergence between the two movements. Kate Millet, perhaps the most high-profile figure to have contributed in both arenas, has described psychiatry as 'one of the meanest systems of oppression ever developed . . . a system of social control of unprecedented thoroughness and pervasiveness' (Millet, 1992, cited in Plumb, 1993 p. 184). Women's greater vulnerability to some of the more contested forms of medicalisation constitutes an obvious area of common interest.[11] There have been many alliances between women as users and workers within the system, some feminist writers on women's mental health issues find much common ground with contemporary service-users and survivors, and some male survivor activists acknowledge a debt to feminism (Barnes and Maple, 1992 p. 141; Barnes and Bowl, 2001 pp. 76–80; Kalinowski and Penny, 1998; Shaw and Proctor, 2004; Lawson, 1991).[12]

Both movements have a keen interest in the interface between public and private realms, in the colonisation of bodies by power/knowledge systems, and in issues around medicalisation and consent. Plumb has compared the experience of violence at the hands of people who were 'supposed to care' in the psychiatric system with domestic violence (Plumb, 1993 p. 173). One of the most consistent messages emanating from the survivor movement has been that recipients of psychiatry have not been listened to, have been treated like objects, categorised on the basis of limited information, and assumed to have no useful knowledge, even about experiences of distress or madness (Campbell, 1990, 1992; Lindow, 1993, 1999; Wallcraft, 1996; Chamberlin, 1977/1988). If these concerns echo those of feminism about the objectification of women, the political response has also often been similar, with an emphasis upon recognising the sensitivity and importance of language and listening to previously silenced voices.[13] Chamberlin adapted the feminist theory and practice of consciousness-raising to ex-patients' mutual support networks in the USA, where reclaiming the validity of experiences and perceptions could be framed as a political rather than a therapeutic process. Drawing on experience from other liberation movements, ex-patients found that separate organisation facilitated the process of self-definition and self-determination (Chamberlin, 1977/1988, 1990). For men, participation in psychiatric survivor groups can raise awareness of gender issues, much as reported by Connell in relation to environmental activism, but also in more immediate and direct ways since the very process of breaking down, and sharing emotional support, can open men up to new conceptions of masculinity (Connell, 1995; Champ, 1999 p. 122).

Plumb has summarised the debate about self-advocacy that took place at the inception of the Survivors Speak Out network in the UK (Plumb, 1993). Although this represented a particular phase in the development of an established movement with much older roots, and although other strands have become more prominent of late, issues about the political nature and uses of personal experience remain pivotal in a field dealing with the individualising effects of normalising power. As already noted, the silencing experienced by psychiatric patients, for whom the disorientating impact of personal crisis is compounded by the effects of being designated 'mentally ill', of pervasive preju- dice, and of invasive forms of treatment, give the concept of self-advocacy par- ticular potency as a political remedy in this context. Crepaz-Keay writes, for instance, that 'the effects drugs can have on memory, on concentration, even the mechanics of standing and speaking, make it very difficult to contribute with confidence' (Crepaz-Keay, 1996 p. 185). Many personal accounts of experi- ences within the psychiatric system remind us why the term 'survivor' was chosen (Greally, 1971; Chamberlin, 1977/1988; Millet, 1990; Plumb, 1993; Pembroke, 1994/1996; OpenMind 1994; Read and Reynolds, 1996). The adop- tion by recipients of psychiatry of a discourse developed within feminist politics around the needs of survivors of rape, incest and sexual assault may appear con- tentious because violence against women and abuse of young girls by men have such profound 'mental health' implications. Feminist and psychiatric survivor concerns overlap significantly in this most sensitive of areas, however. Early 'break-out' groups included provision for male survivors of incest; feminists campaigning against psychiatric medicalisation organised a women's Speak Out protest at the 1986 meeting of the American Psychiatric Association against the inclusion in the DSM-III of a new diagnosis of masochistic (or self- defeating) personality disorder (Armstrong, 1996; Kutchins and Kirk, 1997/ 1999).[14] Furthermore, a feminist commentary on this earlier political use of survivor discourse identifies it as comparable with the discourse of the mad, as discussed by Foucault (Alcoff and Gray, 1993).

Alcoff and Gray draw attention to Foucault's insight into the critical impor- tance of speech and conditions of speaking as a site of political power, and his account of how the 'confessional mode' of speech, involving a strong incitement to disclose, can serve the interests of domination. They argue that survivor speech is transgressive where it challenges conventional speaking arrangements in which women and children are denied the space to speak authoritatively, where their ability to interpret and contradict is curtailed, and where it disrupts dominant discourse by introducing terms such as 'husband rapist'. As a political tactic, the use of personal disclosure, autobiographical narrative and emotional expression in 'speaking out' is fraught with dangers, however. These include the dangers of psychologising the victim and diverting attention from the behaviour of perpetrators, of setting up a false binary separation between 'raw experience' and theoretical understanding, and appearing to legitimate intervention by dispassionate mediators and experts, and of media commodification.[15] Survivor speech is said to be comparable with the discourse of the mad because of these risks and costs, not least because such claims have often been met 'with charges of delusion, hysteria and madness'.[16] There is also a danger that a political or therapeutic impetus towards disclosure can become coercive within survivor movements. It is essential therefore for individuals and groups using this tactic to maintain autonomy over the conditions of speaking, and to obstruct the ability of 'experts' to 'police our statements' (Alcoff and Gray, 1993 pp. 269–70, 279–84).

Psychiatric survivors have explicitly recognised and addressed such dangers, locating the process of speaking out within a context of historical and social understandings of oppression, critiquing cultural prejudice and the medicalisation of distress, and acknowledging a diversity of perceptions and approaches within the movement (Plumb, 1993). Although many published accounts of personal experience focus on and contribute towards a cumulative political critique of psychiatric power, and are thus consistent with the tenets of critical autobiography, tensions have sometimes arisen around the issue of disclosure in this distinctive and complex political arena. Church's poststructuralist-influenced autobiographical deconstruction of her own and others' professional power is no less interesting for describing events within a particular local environment.[17] She applies the feminist notion of 'unsettling relations' to the creatively disruptive impact of the much more direct, personal and emotional style of 'survivor speech' upon the ostensibly more rational public discourse of professionals and institutions. The quite close parallels with gender issues here suggest that further elaboration might be illuminating in relation to the considerable sensitivity of personal disclosure in this setting, not least in relation to the difficulty and danger involved for survivors in expressing anger at the mental health system (Church, 1995 pp. 4, 73, 90, 105).[18] A prominent Canadian psychiatric survivor activist, whose personal experiences have been in print since the late 1960s, has talked about giving his 'ripping my clothes off speech' to hundreds of professional and survivor audiences. I recall survivor colleagues in the 1980s expressing disquiet about the degree of personal exposure happening on public stages in the UK during some campaigning 'road shows'. Bringing the private and personal into public discourse became so prevalent as a strategy for transforming institutional practice that Church even identifies it as the 'mark of a survivor', but as she also notes, such tactics can backfire (Church, 1995 pp. 66, 82). They may, for instance, have exacerbated the tendency noted by Plumb for external commentators to focus on experiential accounts while ignoring psychiatric survivors' history of political analysis and collective struggle (Plumb, 1993 p. 182).

A recent discussion of empowering services for women effectively augments Church's account of professional power by pointing out that women service providers who have been the objects of oppression may have internalised negative images and beliefs, and that these may in turn be amplified during professional acculturation (Kalinowski and Penny, 1998 p. 138). This is helpful in relation to those tensions between feminism and psychiatric survivor politics that arise from the professional allegiance of many feminist commentators, and the invisibility of psychiatric survivor concerns in some feminist writing and practice. Feminist psychiatric survivors have criticised the involvement of feminist psychotherapists in defining the point at which distress becomes 'mental illness' and thus beyond their remit, in the process of compulsory admission, and in practices such as case presentations that perpetuate professional power (Plumb, 1993 pp. 170–1; McNamara 1996). Chamberlin argues that in *Women and Madness*, Chesler appropriated the stories of women patients for her own theorising, accepted the psychiatric mythology of 'genetic and chemical bases of mental illness', and separated women into those who are 'genuinely mad' and those hospitalised for 'conditioned female behaviour' (Chamberlin, 1994 pp. 284–5). The impasse between these two influential radical activists may paradoxically have been fuelled by the closeness of their concerns and the proximity of their ambitions.[19]

Kalinowski and Penny point towards a resolution of such tensions. Using the work of Chamberlin and other American survivor activists, they argue that the complex interactions between misogyny and mentalism, as well as other forms of oppression, must be addressed as a necessary precondition for healing, empowerment and recovery (Kalinowski and Penny, 1998 p. 150). The difficulty of these issues, and, I suspect, a reluctance to theorise and work with contradiction, may perhaps explain, but certainly doesn't justify, the almost complete silence that has emanated from pro-feminist men on the subject of men as recipients of psychiatry since the publication of *Women and Madness* (1972). Notwithstanding psychiatric survivors' overwhelming historical claim to redress for the effects of a fairly comprehensive legacy of silencing, no absolute prerogative can be accorded to voices articulating direct experience. Feminist commentators, and others writing from socially marginal positions, with no personal experience of psychiatry, arguably already speak, to some extent, as indirect objects of its normalising gaze, and may choose to regard that gaze as a secondary instrument of hegemonic (white, middle-class, heterosexist) male power. Because of the legacy of patriarchal violence and oppression that generates most 'mental health' crises, and inescapably colours the politics surrounding them, there is a need to develop approaches that facilitate safe, affirmative and nuanced discussions of the personal dimensions of interlocking patterns of power and discrimination (Ramazanoglu, 1989).[20]

Postmodern feminist writings on politics and experience encourage a careful process of reflexivity, in which we acknowledge our own positions and interests, the constructed nature of our subjectivity, and the contradictions inherent both in selfhood and in the political process. We are invited to step back and listen to different voices or selves, both within and around ourselves, that think and speak from unfamiliar angles. Emphasis is placed on the historical contingency and complexity of patterns of difference and privilege. Political radicalism's pursuit of innocent truths, uncontaminated by relations of domination, is challenged. This kind of approach has been applied to debates across sensitive areas of social policy, such as domestic violence and child welfare (Flax, 1990b, 1992; Featherstone and Trinder, 1997).[21] In similar vein, Brown improvises on a familiar theme from Foucault, and cautions that, unlike their masculinist and modernist counterparts, postmodern feminist political spaces cannot remain pristine havens of non-distorted communication operating behind policed boundaries. Instead they will be characterised by incessant reconfiguration, by partiality of understanding and expression, by cultural chasms that may not be susceptible to resolution, and by recognition that language evokes and suggests rather than simply transmitting meanings (Brown, 1995 p. 50). I take such arguments to be equally, and perhaps even more, applicable, to the spaces in which the politics of distress and madness unfolds, where boundaries are porous and events and phenomena particularly complex and, as social theorists say, overdetermined.[22] Such environments inevitably demand a degree of negotiation and compromise, and the construction of what Flax calls discursive communities, that foster empathy and an appreciation of and desire for difference (Flax, 1992).

Despite the considerable difficulty posed by the concept of impairment, it has been suggested that the user/survivor movement should adopt a disability inclusion model geared towards gaining full citizenship rights, as a unifying political discourse (Sayce, 2000). Concerns have long been expressed, however, about subsuming survivor politics within the broad disability movement.[23] One of the main differences between the politics of disability and the 'politics of the madhouse' is the intensity of overlap between the concerns of the latter and those of the politics of gender, 'race' and sexuality, because of the extent to which distress and madness continually and forcefully direct our attention towards the human costs of other forms of social oppression. This pressure exposes the limitations already inherent in relying upon a minority model of identity-based liberation politics, including forfeiture of common ground and opportunities for reciprocal learning, at the expense of more holistic and pluralistic understandings. It also multiplies potential sites of interruption, discontinuity and tension, and renders psychiatric survivor politics somewhat vulnerable to the charge of being a secondary concern, and thus in effect to further marginalisation among competing liberation narratives. Part of the appeal of a modified 'social model' of distress might be the hope that it would draw together insights that arise from the collectively expressed commonality of psychiatric survivors' experiences. Clearly, however, one of the basic principles informing a social model would be the need to recognise the diversity of contexts in which distress arises. Alliances between black service users, families, workers and community members, for example, have played a vital role in the democratisation of crisis support (Barnes and Bowl, 2001). The case for black and ethnic minority user/survivor-run groups has been made within a disability movement setting, and white psychiatric survivors have attempted to support black survivors by recognising the need for them to organise separately, and working alongside them where appropriate (GLAD, 2003; Sassoon and Lindow, 1995).[24]

There are interesting parallels and some tensions between postmodern feminist discussions of the concept of 'experience' and debates within the survivor movement about self-advocacy. Postmodern feminists have criticised feminist standpoint theory for moving beyond taking women's voices seriously to a point where they are treated as 'unproblematic conduits to "the truth"', and where positions of subordination are romanticised 'as authentic repositories of alternative perspectives' (Featherstone and Trinder, 1997; Burman et al., 1996 p. 4). Postmodern approaches acknowledge that subjectivity is riven with contradiction, that 'each individual is the subject and object of competing and contradictory discourses', and that meaning is relational and contested, and can only be 'fixed' in relation to specific contexts. We possess no ultimate essence or truth beyond that enacted in the various subject positions we occupy (Fawcett and Featherstone, 1994 pp. 42, 45). Scott reminds us that 'what counts as experience is neither self-evident nor straightforward; it is always contested, always therefore political'. Her critique focuses on a tendency within feminism to refer to experience in a way that establishes the prior existence of individuals, thereby naturalising falsely universal categories such as man, woman, black, white, heterosexual or homosexual. Appeals to experience as transparently authentic, incontestable and foundational, as the origin of explanation rather than that which we need to explain, precludes enquiry into the ways in which selves, subjects, subject-positions and identities are produced, in which agency becomes possible, in which dimensions such as race, sexuality and gender intersect, and in which political processes organise and interpret experience (Scott, 1992 pp. 31, 37–8; Hallberg, 1989/1992).

Brown responds to these problems of complexity by calling for a feminist politics that is less orientated towards subjectivity, identity and morality. Postmodernity will leave us vulnerable to domination by technical reason unless we can develop 'democratic processes for formulating collective judgements' based on 'arguing from a vision about the common ("what I want for us") rather than from identity ("who I am"), and from explicitly postulated norms and potential common values rather than from false essentialism or unreconstructed private interest'. Post-identity political positions and conversations might transform a politics of difference into one orientated towards diversity and commonality, towards the world (and its 'structures of dominance within diffused and disorienting orders of power') rather than the self, thereby making available more potent political analyses than can be generated by focusing on the experiential content of fragmented existences alone (Brown, 1995 pp. 50–1).[25] She then undertakes a critique of the politicisation of injury, using Nietzsche's concept of ressentiment (resentment), which raises some sensitive questions about the processes entailed in mobilising a collective discourse around 'a complex and diverse "we" in contexts where intense personal anguish must be negotiated'.[26]

Ressentiment refers to 'the moralising revenge of the powerless, "the triumph of the weak as weak"', and Brown's discussion considers some problems that might arise from an ethicising politics orientated around 'entrenching, restating, dramatising, and inscribing . . . pain in politics', and from the 'psychological and political practice of revenge'. She argues that where politicised identity is premised on pain for its very existence, and installs pain as the foundation of its political claim, it risks perpetuating pain, losing the ability or will to see beyond its own hurting, and becoming attached to its own exclusion. Instead of revenge, such pain may simply long for 'the chance to be heard into a certain release, recognised into self-overcoming, incited into possibilities of triumphing over, and hence losing itself'. The challenge is then to develop a political culture that can sustain such a project without being taken over by it – that 'guards against abetting the steady slide of political into therapeutic discourse, even as we acknowledge the elements of suffering and healing we might be negotiating'. Hence the value of supplanting ontological claims expressed in the language of 'I am' by more explicitly political ones in the language of 'I want this for us', in order to participate in a 'necessarily agonistic theatre for forging a collective future' (Brown, 1995 pp. 66, 74–6).

Though this account explores feminist terrain adjacent to, and in some ways overlapping with, that covered by psychiatric survivor politics, the latter is of course inescapably concerned with personal anguish, and we should not expect to find an exact convergence of interests or responses. Distress or madness, and psychiatric treatment, generate a distinctive set of conditions, issues and dilemmas, and when considering these, critical postmodernism needs, at the very least, to take account of the situated analyses and knowledges of theorists with direct experience (Wilson and Beresford, 2002). This is, after all, a field in which psychiatric discourse has systematically devalued such expertise as 'anecdotal', and dismissed those who resist medicalisation as lacking 'insight' (Perkins and Moodley, 1993). Biomedical psychiatry tends to generate considerable pressure to identify with 'illness', and mask the commonplace reality of recovery.[27] In a context where distressed or mad selves scarcely need further decentring or fragmentation, focusing on commonality of need might seem a particularly constructive move, for personal as well as political reasons.

Within the formulation of self-advocacy developed by Survivors Speak Out, the authenticity, rather than representativeness, of each voice speaking from direct experience is asserted against pervasive silencing, in a context where the fragility and socially constructed nature of selfhood form the raw material of political awareness, and where convoluted biographical experience compounds an often already layered identity (Plumb, 1993).[28] Given a mutually supportive environment, processes of collective authentication can transmute marginalised forms of experience into new kinds of authoritative discourse. In this context I take 'authenticity' to refer to situated claims to interpretative authority, not least where personal stories are being reclaimed from the terrain of case history, rather than to the discovery of newly definitive identities.[29] The sharing of personal testimony has undoubtedly played an important part in building cultures of resistance, generating reservoirs of collective memory, raising awareness, and developing political agendas. Plummer wonders, however, whether a curious sameness evident in the stories of 'abuse survivors' reflects a lingering and unacknowledged influence of modernist discourses about finding a single key to the truth of our lives in certain core experiences. He suggests that, increasingly, the world may not be seen in such straightforwardly transparent and linear terms (Plummer, 1995). I shall be arguing that the need to address the complexity of men's experiences as psychiatric survivors, and perhaps survivors of abuse, but also, unavoidably, as members of a relatively privileged group, suggests the need for more nuanced forms of storytelling that are not solely about recuperating oppressed selves and voices. The postmodern feminist argument, noted above, that experience should be treated not as an explanatory key to pre-existing identities, but as something in need of explanation, is pertinent here (Scott, 1992). Given that contemporary Western culture remains so saturated by therapeutic and medicalising discourse, and that prejudice and discrimination remain prevalent, close attention to the conditions of 'speaking out' is likely to remain a priority for the foreseeable future (Wallcraft and Michaelson, 2001).

Mad Pride's strategy of reclaiming language, celebrating what is positive about the experience of madness, and abandoning 'involvement' in favour of direct action, represents a move away from focusing on pain, but opens up other challenges (Curtis et al., 2000). Postmodern and poststructuralist theorists argue that dependence upon a minority model of liberation politics inevitably results in a conceptual and strategic crisis, because the unitary conception of (female, black, gay and lesbian, or disabled) identity it constructs in order to present a united front has its own normative and disciplinary effects, and leaves many minorities-among-minorities, let alone undecideable strangers, under-represented (Nicholson and Seidman, 1995 p. 17).[30] The notorious slipperiness of madness as a concept, and the degree of irony entailed in any policing of madness as a unitary identity category, may of course help in this respect.[31] Because the survivor movement has been confronting issues around the intersection of simultaneous oppressions, it is quite well placed to learn from the 'necessary errors' of previous movements (Sassoon and Lindow, 1995; Foner, 1995). Although the value of reclaiming 'madness' and of emphasising the distinctiveness of the various kinds of extreme experience (and the realities of radical disempowerment and discrimination that typically accompany psychiatric treatment) described by the term is clear enough, there are also, I think, some persuasive arguments against simply attempting to highlight and then reverse the binary order, in the manner of modernist identity and liberation politics.[32] I now want to summon these in order to suggest a degree of postmodern 'both/and' flexibility.

Masculinities and distress

postmodernism's focus on instability, multiplicity, and contingency, as well as its subsequent celebration of difference, provides an extraordinary basis for interrogating the cultural scripts of normative masculinity.

(Gutterman, 2001)

> Men can clearly be Other if they are Black or gay or both or if they occupy some other Other-ed positioning. To focus on the Other in this way can itself be a form of resistance to dominant formations of men.
>
> (Hearn, 1998)

> In my view it is . . . the ability to take in and honour the pain men suffer that provides the surest foundation for the ability to oppose the pain that men inflict.
>
> (Brod, 1998)

An alternative position stresses a continuum of mental and emotional distress and wellbeing precisely in order to challenge psychiatry's policing of a binary divide between those who 'suffer mental illness' and those who don't, and between the 'psychoses' of the 'dangerous mad' and the 'neuroses' of the 'worried well' (Wilson and Beresford, 2002 p. 154). The propensity to engage in such dividing practices appears to be strongly gendered in Western culture, where an ability to tolerate ambiguity, to enter into the perspectives of others, to accept change and fluidity, and acknowledge non-rational aspects of consciousness, has often been characterised as 'flabby, feminine, and soft' (Bordo, 1990b p. 148; Hollway, 1989; Frosh, 1997). Furthermore, as 'weavers of the fabric of hegemony', psychiatrists participate as 'organising intellectuals' in the regulation and management of the gender regimes that define and enforce 'normal' masculine practice (Donaldson, 1993 p. 646; Hearn, 1987; Busfield, 1996). One corollary of this has been a tendency to assume that women's pain, frequently experienced as crushing depression or extreme anxiety, and dismissively defined as 'neurosis' or 'hysteria', is less real and important than pain expressed in more dramatic and publicly bizarre ways (Barnes and Maple, 1992).

Feminist accounts of women's distress and madness that interpret the political meaning of 'symptomatology', and find historically specific ideological constructions of femininity inscribed on the bodies of 'sufferers', have emphasised a 'continuum between female disorder and "normal" feminine practice' (Bordo, 1990 p. 16). From this perspective then, 'madness' might perhaps be seen to work, for men, as a more euphemistic term than 'distress', insofar as it masks vulnerability with defiance and humour (even occasionally involving ironic references to dangerousness), thereby compounding a tendency widely regarded as a hallmark of masculinity.[33] However understandable it might be for recipients of psychiatry to use the protection of euphemism (in either direction), it remains important to consider the operations of masculinity here, even in relation to the most vulnerable of men. The question arises then, as to whether and in what ways various kinds of distress or madness experienced by men, and various kinds of cultural and professional responses to such experiences, can be seen as echoing, amplifying or subverting normative masculine practice.[34]

If the deconstruction of Enlightenment assumptions about rational selfhood risks undermining expressions of experience and agency among subordinated groups, submerging the subject in discourse and insisting on plural identities seems likely to exacerbate a tendency among dominant groups to evade individual or collective responsibility. Where, we might ask, would such moves leave notions such as integrity (with its appeal to wholeness) and commitment (restricting the freedom to change) that appear so central to processes of relationship? Some writers express concern that focusing on multiple masculinities diverts attention from men as a gender, as well as from the positioning and experiences of women, and consider various issues that arise when men, as members of an 'oppressor class or group', embark upon autocritique (Hearn, 1996, 1994 p. 60). I have some difficulty with unitary conceptions of men as a gender-class, but agree about the importance of retaining a vision of the common in relation to men. There is clearly a need to conceptualise overarching patterns of social oppression, while appreciating how these are reproduced and inter-related in men's practices within widely different contexts.[35] Some writers feel that postmodern theory, with its focus on multiplicity and celebration of difference, provides an extraordinary opportunity for critiquing masculinity (Gutterman, 2001). Stressing the plurality, inconsistency and discursive construction of hegemony, and the complex, contradictory, even chaotic discursive resources from which hegemonic identities are continually reconstituted, enables us to understand how complicity and resistance can co-exist in the same individuals (Wetherell and Edley, 1999). Acknowledging different parts of ourselves can make men more open to feminist and anti-racist claims. It is also argued that (at least some) men have much to gain from engaging with change, not least in terms of emotional development and improved relationships with other men, as well as with women (Hearn, 1994 pp. 60–3; Collinson and Hearn, 1994/2001; Pease, 1999 p. 102, citing Hollway, 1989).

Men who become users/survivors of psychiatry are undoubtedly, in Hearn's terms, 'Other-ed', but are far from being a homogeneous group. As already argued, 'we' need to develop conceptual frameworks that enable us to consider both the considerable vulnerability, and relative power (in relation to similarly positioned women), of the very diverse groups of men who experience distress and madness, and become recipients of psychiatry. The considerable sensitivity of discussions about the implications of founding political claims and premising politicised identities upon pain is compounded here, given a problematic tendency in some quarters to portray men exclusively as victims of political processes, and to foreground men's pain rather than men's power (Brown, 1995; Collinson and Hearn, 1994/2001; Kaufman, 1994). This tendency is compounded by discourses that construct a sense of 'crisis' in male mental health as evidence of a wider crisis of masculinity, that reduce sexual politics to psychology, or that seek to pathologise violence (Coyle and Morgan-Sykes, 1998; McMahon, 1993; Dobash and Dobash, 1992). Although these discourses are not driven by (and may work against) the interests and concerns of most male psychiatric survivors, they certainly complicate a political context that arguably demands a degree of awareness of speaking positions and an acknowledgement of difference and contradiction similar to those called for in discussions of the lived experiences and oppression of disabled men or black men.

Miller and Bell helpfully introduce a critical analysis of men into 'mental health' discourse. They point to the comprehensive failure of psychiatric services (organised in accordance with hegemonic male values) to acknowledge the impact of inequalities on both women's and men's mental health, and to move beyond the assumption that women are 'mad', and men 'bad'. I am concerned, however, that, not least in the opening statement of their central theme, that 'men are at one and the same time both damaged and damage-doing', they themselves effectively perpetuate this last assumption.[36] Since no mention is made of the psychiatric survivor movement, or of concerns about the risks and costs associated with being stereotyped as dangerous, this is at best unsubtle. Miller and Bell write as psychologists working with violent men, and their focus on men who are both vulnerable and violent undoubtedly identifies a key node in the topography of men's 'mental health' that they set out to map. Participants in their workshops speak of violence and brutality in the home and school as normative and unremarkable (Miller and Bell, 1996). Because of an over-reliance on the unitary category 'men', however, they give no sense of the many men who, despite experiencing severe emotional injury and long-term discrimination as recipients of psychiatric services, lead caring and constructive lives, and, masculinity notwithstanding, manage to do remarkably little harm. In 'mental health' contexts, where prejudice often compounds the devaluing impact of psychopathology, it is vital, surely, to encourage positive images of users/survivors. Care needs to be taken, therefore, to protect men who are highly vulnerable, perhaps to the point of only having a precarious foothold on life, from inappropriately generalised negative stereotyping as men, in effect from reverse 'Othering'. The notion of a psychology of 'male entitlement', favoured by Miller and Bell, risks discursively fixing negative imagery at an intrapersonal level, while providing a theoretical alibi for men who want to evade responsibility for their actions.[37] Before returning to the question of violence in the next chapter, I want to look more closely at the connections between men's distress and madness and prevailing discourses about gender.

Predominant among the assumptions about gender embedded within modernist patriarchal psychiatry's constructions of 'mental disorder' has been a consistent association between rationality, agency and masculinity – and a corresponding categorisation of women as passive, emotional and irrational. Busfield comments that this key attribution both reflects the qualities of power per se, and works to regulate and perpetuate differences in power (Busfield, 1996). If we understand men's madness and distress as a Dionysian eruption of repressed emotion and over-civilised instinct, men who 'open up' in this way may seem, at first sight, to be placing themselves outside and against the prevailing orthodoxy of their gender. This seems to be the implication of Seidler's recommendation of Foucault's Madness and Civilisation (1961/1971) as a valuable source on the history of exclusion of the imaginal realm and of unreason

(Seidler, 1994 p. xii). Mad men of this kind, such as Artaud, who also develop a critique of the power of psychiatry's Enlightenment science, and its pervasive influence on the shaping of selfhood, would appear to be resisting dominant formations of men in a potentially quite powerful way. It would be simplistic, however, to suggest that, for unreconstructed men, Dionysian outpourings of emotion constitute an intrinsically counter-cultural practice. Another ubiqui-tous set of discourses about men, after all, proclaim, paradoxically, that 'we' are also creatures driven by overpowering instinct, that male sexual dominance, the phallic imperative that drives history, is impelled by a primordial and trans-historical biological drive (Segal, 1990/1997 pp. 207–9).[38] Moreover, other models, or perhaps forms, of madness, such as those described by Sass as amounting to a hyper-reflexive exaggeration of consciousness, in which idiosyn-cratic and incommunicable illumination becomes a refuge from emotion and the body, appear to echo or amplify familiar facets of hegemonic masculinity from another direction (Sass, 1992). This kind of intense yet fragile intro-spection is unlikely to produce the kind of gendered reflexivity that has been identified as essential for personal and political change in men, without sensi-tive and appropriate support and encouragement (Whitehead and Barrett, 2001 p. 352).

Lived reality tends to be a lot more complex than such mappings suggest, of course, and critical postmodern perspectives would approach men's distress and madness by listening to particular stories, and looking at its painful produc-tion within particular social environments from a variety of often contradictory and chaotic emotional, material and cultural resources. Such is the consensus linking dominant patriarchal discourses and normative rationality, however, that no critique of psychiatry, as it affects men, can reasonably proceed without reference to feminist and pro-feminist analyses of this overarching cultural con-figuration. Petersen, for example, who cites Young's account of the exclusion-ary fiction of impartiality, concludes that this pervasive masculinist ideal has performed a regulative function (Petersen, 1998 p. 89; Young, 1990). Hearn's development of feminist understandings of the power of 'public men' and the public domain, over women and the private domain, may prove important in helping us think about the relationship between various groups of men and a psychiatric system deeply implicated in the publicisation of the social world. Hearn locates men and conceptualises public patriarchies in relation to a politi-cal economy of reproduction, and argues that differentiation between men, and the resultant oppression by dominant groups of men of other groups of men, is instrumental in the continued oppression of women.[39] The historical formation of a gendered public/private division, in which passion, desire and the body are confined to the invisibility of the private domain while reason, knowledge and the mind enjoy the visibility of an 'adult' public world is, therefore, once again, located within a discourse about men's power (Hearn, 1992 pp. 30ff., 80–1). Hearn's analysis can usefully be read alongside Foucault's account of the historical construction of a new reign of reason based upon a 'parental complex', in which the authority of the physician was modelled on the intimate law of the family patriarch (Foucault, 1961/1971 p. 272).

The medical profession, traditionally a male bastion, has arguably played a pivotal role in the historical transition towards public patriarchies by assuming responsibility for the categorisation and regulation of gendered states, by policing social exclusion, and (along with psychoanalysis) by promoting 'men's domination of the psychological and psychodynamic arenas' (Hearn, 1992 pp. 219, 15; Witz, 1992).[40] Biopsychiatry, in particular, has been aptly described as caricaturing male values (Breggin, 1993 p. 410). That psychiatry has functioned historically as an instrument of hegemonic masculinity, helping the dominant grouping of men from which it has overwhelmingly recruited to carve out and maintain steeply hierarchical social divisions, is abundantly clear in relation to a significant legacy of mistreatment of men from subordinated groups. The formality, detachment and objectification demanded by public masculinity and enshrined in psychiatry's criteria of rationality, as well as in its procedures and practices, have often compounded the social chasm between male professionals and users/survivors, to the point where 'mental health' and other oppressions become inseparably and devastatingly combined.

The story of how homosexuality was pathologised, and its removal from the *Diagnostic and Statistical Manual* in 1973 following concerted campaigning by lesbian and gay activists, initially from outside, and then also from within the profession, confirms the political nature of the process of classifying mental disorders. Interestingly, the identification of male homosexuality as a 'sexual deviation' was particularly influenced by psychoanalytic psychiatrists' belief that it was caused by families with a cold rejecting father and overprotective mother. Activists pursuing a rights agenda insisted that questions about infantile psychosexual development were irrelevant, but also had to challenge psychiatric attempts to 'cure' homosexuality using a range of crude physical interventions such as electroshock and aversion therapy, that led directly to the death of at least one person (Kutchins and Kirk, 1997/1999; Golding, 1997; Tatchell, 2000; Smith et al., 2004).[41] Declassification has not ended mistreatment, of course. In the UK as many as a third of gay men still report lack of empathy, discrimination, harassment and sometimes violence within the mental health system, yet many also experience difficulties in talking to other gay men about experiences of distress (MIND 2003).

Psychiatry has an equally problematic record in relation to black and ethnic minority men, amounting at times to an active allegiance with oppression. In 1851, for instance, an American psychiatrist borrowed the Latin word *drapetes* (meaning 'runaway slave') in order to devise a new category of mental disorder. Drapetomania, or flight-from-home-madness, medicalised the condition of absconding slaves – a condition that could be prevented by the simple expedient of 'whipping the devil out of them' (Kutchins and Kirk, 1997/1999 p. 210). In contemporary Western societies, young black men are particularly vulnerable to a diagnosis of schizophrenia and to compulsory admission into a mental health system that relies excessively on medication and fails to provide early support, advocacy or aftercare (Sainsbury Centre, 2002). Racist assumptions still inform both philosophy and practice, and globalisation threatens to impose a 'mental illness' model wherever non-Western traditions survive (Bracken, 1993; Sashidharan and Francis, 1999; Fernando, 2004). Black men may experience particular difficulty coming out as psychiatric survivors, for fear of further mistreatment within the system, or because of a need to appear strong within their own communities (Faulkner and Sayce, 1997 p. 9). These factors may contribute to a tendency for black men to be less willing than black women to make linkages between political oppression and psychic pain, and to engage in recovery and self-help movements as well as activism (hooks, 1995 pp. 140–3).

Hegemonic masculinity has maintained its monopoly claim over dispassionate and disembodied reason by firmly associating all uncertain and disorderly aspects of existence with those designated as Others, by ensuring that men become desensitised, and that expressions of male vulnerability are thoroughly purged and sequestered. Hence the censorship in men of most emotions other than anger, the repression of receptive forms of male sexuality, and the institutionalisation of men who are physically disabled or deemed insane, might all be understood as instances of the same exclusionary dynamic (Young, 1990; Segal, 1990/1997). The value of this, often unconscious, strategy for maintaining what Connell refers to (in the singular) as an increasingly visible, co-ordinated and global gender order is readily apparent. But Connell also argues that the scale of contemporary violence suggests crisis tendencies in this overarching order (Connell, 1995 pp. 200, 84). Both world wars, for example, destabilised gender ideology, and brought men's 'mental health' into the cultural limelight.

Kutchins and Kirk remind us that American psychiatrists have always played an important role in war, and trace medical involvement in the diagnosis and treatment of soldiers' emotional injuries from an eighteenth-century diagnosis of 'nostalgia' developed by Swiss physicians. In the First World War, mounting concern about the depletion of Germany's forces and about the cost of shell-shocked casualties prompted a shift from neurological understandings towards concepts such as 'greed neurosis' and 'pension struggle hysteria' that implied malingering. The use of electroshock was duly introduced as a frightening alternative to returning to the trenches (Kutchins and Kirk, 1997/1999 pp. 103–4). In Britain, class privilege ensured that Siegfried Sassoon received a diagnosis of neurasthenia, and was given psychoanalytic treatment. During the process of recovery he distanced himself from other 'more or less dotty' officers, and simultaneously affirmed his sanity and masculinity by recanting his objection to the war, and returning to his station as officer and gentleman. By contrast, a twenty-four-year-old private who had become mute after fighting in the worst campaigns of the war was 'treated' with electroshocks, 'hot plates' in his mouth, and cigarette burns on the tip of the tongue, in order to force him to speak. Elaborating upon Goffman's comparison between the powerlessness of soldiers and the position of women, Showalter notes that 'shell shock' provided a suitably masculine-sounding alternative to the effeminate associations of 'hysteria', and that when military psychiatrists dismissed men as cowards, there was often an implication of effeminacy or homosexuality (Showalter, 1987 pp. 172–88). During the Second World War, we learn from a prominent psychiatrist Dr William Sargant that 'millions of pounds in pensions were . . . saved, simply because it was at last realised that immediate and heavy "front line" sedation was generally more effective in the prevention of chronic neuroses, and so-called "malingering" reactions'. Sargant also recalled patients in mental institutions in the 1930s being kept in states of chronic intoxication with 'truly enormous doses' of the same bromides (Sargant, 1958 cited by Medawar, 1992 pp. 49–50).

Setting this implicit comparison in the context of a large-scale historical narrative about hegemonic masculinity enables us to reframe explorations of the extent to which experiences of collective trauma are related to, and comparable with, individual crises that rupture ordinary social worlds. Connell's invitation to map crisis tendencies in the gender order is taken up, more or less explicitly, by several pro-feminist commentators who point to the possibility that such crises present opportunities not just for retrenchment but also for constructive change. Kaufman, for instance, argues that recent progress in the direction of gender equality has rendered the pain associated with practices of masculinity more visible, and that a recognition of contradictory experiences of power can open up an effective politics of compassion that is both critical and male-affirmative (Kaufman, 1994; Brod, 1998). Frosh discusses men's responses to a crisis in traditional paternal authority under postmodern conditions, quite closely echoing Hearn's analysis of the historic transformation towards public patriarchy (Frosh, 1997b pp. 48–52).

A characteristic male response to crisis conditions has been to fall back on emotional inexpressiveness, in order to consolidate power and conceal vulnerability (Sattel, 1976/1989). Reich derived his familiar metaphor of emotional armouring from the predominantly masculine tradition of warfare. The realisation that it appears to have taken the exaggerated terrors of industrialised trench warfare to bring men's 'mental health' to centre stage in Western culture, and that 'shell shock' persisted long after hostilities ceased (when it was subsequently discussed largely by women), appears to confirm the pervasiveness and tenacity of this ingrained cultural tactic. Care needs to be taken, however, to avoid the essentialism and over-generalisation implicit in phrases such as 'the inexpressive male'. Silence can sometimes be an appropriate and constructive response to traumatic circumstances. There are also times when distress or madness, compounded by the effects of psychiatric interventions, induces an involuntary and problematic withdrawal from human contact. Pro-feminist commentators should recognise that, under such circumstances, social relations move into a different register. Many of the men who become users and survivors of psychiatric services are subject to two or more intersecting regimes of power (such as those formed around 'race', class, sexuality and physical disability, as well as psychiatry), and can therefore be said to belong to both oppressed and oppressing groups.

When discussing this it may be important to note the potential disjuncture between the impact of 'oppression' in colloquial discourse, where it can become a red button term eliciting visceral responses that tap into personal and collective reservoirs of cumulative pain, and its life as a theoretical concept. Difficulties negotiating this terrain may also be compounded by a tendency to conflate oppression and anguish, and to overlook the indeterminacy involved in operations of power.[42] Although the association between oppression and personal pain or emotional injury is well established, some men (as well as women) from materially comfortable backgrounds experience severe and disabling distress or madness, while many whose lives are marked by manifest oppression do not. Mike Lawson's hedgehog allegory vividly expresses the case for some kind of social model, but if we are to understand the impact of masculinity, yet another layer of interpretation is perhaps needed. For many men, culturally sanctioned masculine inexpressiveness not only exacerbates emotional injury by impairing the ability to ask for and benefit from emotional support – particularly from male peers – but also proves hopelessly insufficient as a means of protection in a hostile world. For some other men, unfortunately, the cosy hedgehog will be unconvincing as a totem animal. Clearly we need to locate men's pain in relation to entrenched patterns of violence and abuse against women, and men's continuing domination of public institutions. Careful use of large-scale historical counter-narratives should enable us to depict the evolving social context within which men's distress and madness are produced.

Postmodern feminist critics of standpoint theory caution against collapsing complexity and producing simple moral antagonisms between monolithic identity categories, so that men or psychiatrists are portrayed as utterly complicit and all-powerful, and women or survivors/service-users as intrinsically innocent and helpless (Fawcett and Featherstone, 1994; Featherstone and Trinder, 1997). Perspectives that assume an invariant and unidirectional flow of power and oppression are arguably both unduly pessimistic and inadequate as a basis for negotiating the ineluctable contingencies and convolutions of biographical and social experience (Foucault, 1976/1978; Liddle, 1993).[43] Dominant sexist discourses continually reproduce meanings that predispose men and women to misrecognise themselves, and each other (Hollway, 1984/1998).[44] Tensions arising because of the relative positionings of men and women within the 'mental health' system will not always be reducible to misrecognition or to dissonance between the sexist expectations of some men and the reality of their powerlessness, however. The challenge for services and self-help or self-advocacy groups is to remain flexible enough in terms of philosophy and practice to be able to respond with clarity, and in a supportive manner, to circumstances that may confound expectations, and for which there can be no 'correct' analysis or painless remedy.

In *Women and Madness*, Chesler commented on the ineffective and effectively punished 'masculine protest' of women, and the 'feminine' passivity of
many men diagnosed as schizophrenic (Chesler, 1972 pp. 52–5). As previously
argued, 'schizophrenia', a condition said by Lacan to be characterised by a
catastrophe of the signifier, a collapse in the phallocentric ordering of the
world through language, has been energetically adopted by mainstream theorists
of postmodernity, and should also interest commentators on masculinity. Judge
Schreber's is not the only story in which madness appears consequent upon a
breakdown and unravelling of hegemonic masculinity. Connell draws attention
to the discussion of 'David' in Laing's classic study of 'schizophrenic and schizoid
persons' *The Divided Self* (Laing, 1959/1965). David, a young male student who
seems to have been diagnosed as 'borderline' because of his unusual clothes and
manner of speaking, had been playing a range of female parts in front of a mirror
since his mother died when he was ten years old. From his point of view,
his unusual public manner protected him against an engulfing femininity.
Describing him as driven towards psychosis by the unresolvable contradiction
between, in effect, attempting to be his dead mother or becoming a man,
Connell argues that if masculinity did not involve fear and hatred of femininity,
and thus of the 'woman inside him', this agonising dilemma would not have
arisen (Connell, 1987, p. 214, 1995 p. 19). Connell also notes Laing's failure
to pick up on the relevance of his work to understandings of gender, but overlooks the operations of disciplinary power here (Connell, 1994).[45]

Setting out to recuperate the 'schizophrenic credit' – those qualities of
heightened sensitivity and empathy that can be acquired through experiencing
the outer limits of sanity, but which become distorted during 'maximum
derangement' – Chadwick gives a vivid autobiographical account of his energetic
rejection of a formerly conventional 'macho' identity. He likens his personal
journey – from being a schoolboy with no father, whose idea of being a man
was to be 'physically powerful, highly sexed, and sexist', through 'stormy days
of cross-race and cross-gender transition', eventually emerging as a 'peaceful
feminine man of placid lifestyle' – to Dante's journey through hell. A funda-
mentalist masculinity that derided the 'music', grace and style embodied by
women, black people and homosexuals, reinforced by homophobic school bullies
and then by 'community paranoia' and prejudice, is understood to have played
a critical part in inducing the self-loathing that precipitated 'persecutory
delusions' and ultimately a suicide attempt that led to a positive experience of
hospitalisation (Chadwick, 1997 pp. 30, 34–7). Many of the themes in
Chadwick's book are consistent with the postmodern framework he subsequently recommends (Chadwick, 2002). During his auto-deconstructive trajectory, he rejects the notion of a core Self in favour of 'severalising' the self. His
writings explore multiple accounts in order to elucidate the complexity of
psychosis, and the 'socially uncategorisable' phenomenon of 'borderliners',
people of great sensitivity and fluidity whose identity is in process, among
whom he still counts himself. Postmodern theorists might also be expected to

be receptive to the kinds of sexual ambiguity and dissent he champions, and to respect his holistic mixing of models.

Chadwick's subjective phenomenological writing is counterbalanced, however, by the truth-testing modernist realism and male-coded rationalism of another voice – that of an empirical psychologist who deploys batteries of tests in order to separate psychopathology from spiritual inspiration. While this orientation may have served as an effective bulwark against terrors past, such training, and an adherence to medical-model discourse, might be seen by some as a recipe for internalised oppression. Chadwick does see reality as a story, however, and identifies as an artist, even when immersed in experientially informed 'science-like' experimentation. Pro-feminist readers might worry that in his concluding comments, on the need for dignity and empowerment for people who experience spiritual overwhelm and 'psychosis', Chadwick seems to lose sight of his 'mad' insights into his own social co-ordinates and the pivotal role of masculinity at both personal and social levels.[46] Such critics should perhaps consider whether their own political vision has been sufficiently multifocal to allow them to appreciate the circumstances of those engaged in the kind of protracted and precarious struggle towards recovery that Chadwick describes. Unless a seemingly normative cultural amnesia about men's power is challenged, however, narratives of men's pain can function to reinforce a belief that men's liberation from the undoubted harm inflicted in the cause of masculinity is a sufficient political concern.

Thanks to the cumulative political campaigns and self-advocacy of feminists and psychiatric survivors, we now know that for some people, voice hearing is associated with a history of sexual abuse (Romme and Escher, 1993; Coleman, 1999). Coleman's autobiographical account of 'the making of a schizophrenic' can be read as another instructive sequel to Schreber's memoirs, insofar as, more than eighty years on, professionals were still trying to repair what they saw as faulty biology, rather than listen to an abuse history, masked behind tormenting voices. After a decade of painfully ineffective treatment, during which he became 'little better than a zombie who viewed life through a legalised drug-induced smog', Coleman found a way out of the system with the help of friends, 'navigators' and the hearing voices network. A protective politicised community empowered him to speak out about highly sensitive personal experience, and produce a wide-ranging critique of medicalisation and the psychiatric system (Coleman, 1999 pp. 12–14, 1998). Like Chadwick, he has contributed significantly to knowledge about and revaluation of psychosis, encouraged positive thinking in a field long mired in clinical pessimism, and developed practical guidelines for helping people to survive and recover. Coleman even includes a democratised 'case study' report on how a colleague worked with someone called 'David', a man troubled by a 'Satan' voice that urged him to have oral sex with the men around him. His work makes clear the inadequacy of treating such voices as meaningless symptoms of metabolic disturbance.

Dominant discourses of masculinity would seem to account for some striking continuities in the ways in which men experience personal pain, but many questions remain to be answered, in various social and cultural contexts, about the relationship between hegemonic masculinities and distress. Some 'Othered' men's distress or madness can be understood as emotional injury consequent upon exclusion from a hegemonic gender order. Some may even amount to an act of conscientious objection to the process of interpellation – a 'call-up' that imposes pain and alienation as a condition of recruitment to positions of masculinist power. While such pain and powerlessness must clearly be acknowledged, it is vital that such understandings aren't allowed to obscure awareness of 'our' often closely interconnected and countervailing power, especially in relation to women. There is a need to challenge treatment regimes that function as a disciplinary attempt to reinstate this relative power, by shoehorning men back into the patriarchal fold, and punishing dissent.

The tradition of mutual support and qualities of heightened sensitivity, empathy, compassion and tolerance often found among survivor communities creates a space in which men can begin to embrace more caring, expressive and egalitarian – not to mention less 'logocentric' – forms of masculinity. Pro-feminist men may have much to learn from political survivors, whose situated knowledge comes from close acquaintance with the impact of different oppressions. While it is important not to romanticise the torments (or ecstatic insights) of solitary madness, it seems that the experience of being in crisis can sometimes become an alchemical process during which the protective but distorting rigidity of masculinity is transmuted, and hegemonic habits abandoned. Successful transformation of crisis into opportunity of this kind seems likely to depend upon access to the right kind of supportive community, one grounded in a sufficiently open-minded and open-hearted critical sensitivity. How much better it would be, though, if we could build communities in which men's sensitivity and empathy were valued from the outset, and the violence and oppression that generate most distress and madness were no longer endemic.

A moment of recognition

Just as I was settling into my seat and beginning to doze off, I recognised someone entering at the opposite end of the rather full train carriage. Our eyes met, and as 'Allan' began to make his way along the swaying corridor towards me, I realised he was looking agitated, in fact extremely angry. I'd known him well enough, and for long enough, not to be particularly worried by this, but could have done without any drama that morning. He flopped heavily into the seat next to me and, staring into space, continued to radiate a somewhat menacing aura. Then he punched the back of the seat in front of him, hard enough to make it shake. This was not good. I asked him what was going on, but he ignored me, and punched the seat again. Although I felt confident that he wouldn't want to hurt anyone, my fellow passengers were not to know this, and of course, couldn't be expected to know about the long sequence of difficulties that had pulled him into such an abyss of depression and 'paranoia'.

Something had to be done. I withdrew into myself, and staring at the back of the seat in front of me, silently summoned and radiated my own anger, with as much ferocity as I could muster. The effect was dramatic. Allan's rage evaporated immediately, he deflated visibly. His expression softened and, turning towards me, he looked puzzled for a moment, then relaxed and began to talk very quietly. It was as though an internalised barrier dividing normality from abnormality, sanity from madness, had somehow visibly dissolved.

Although this kind of recognition may happen spontaneously in non-hierarchical mutual-aid environments, I'd heard from a friend (who is a survivor and therapist) that mirroring someone's distressed state for them has been developed as a therapeutic intervention, and I thought it worth trying as an anti-havoc tactic.* But was my action a step too far towards proto-professionalisation, an incursion of discourse into everyday life? Was my 'acting' inadmissible deceit or tactical necessity? I plead self-preservation and haven't repeated the offence, but if I'd been driven to a point where I seemed about to cause mayhem, or even consternation, in public, I would rather someone had resorted to this kind of benign trickery than calling in the cavalry.

* In Process Orientated Psychotherapy, a therapist might, in exceptional circumstances, act the part of someone in a similar 'extreme state' to the person in crisis, in order to avert harm (Mindell, 1988). Particular issues arise where such methods are used in professional settings, of course.

Chapter 9

Masculinities and risk
Negotiating the politics of complexity

> it was taken for granted that my desire to be myself in the decision making process about myself was in actual fact nothing more than lack of insight on my part. The frightened self (which felt controlled by the external voices I heard) . . . gave way to the angry frightened self that the psychiatric system perceived as aggression and part of the deterioration of my illness. This led to the continuation of the conflict that in turn led to the absence of recovery. The focus of professionals in understanding feelings as part of the illness process also means that they perceive '*my self*' as damaged and in need of repair.
>
> (Coleman, 1999)

> once diagnosed mentally ill one is faced with the profoundly held association in the public mind between madness and danger. Images of the 'mad axeman' stare back from the pages of newspapers . . . MIND has heard from relatives of people diagnosed mentally ill that they are terrified the individual may become violent – on the grounds that 'it's part of the illness, isn't it?' – even when there is absolutely no evidence of any inclination towards violence.
>
> (Sayce, 1995)

At the time of writing, an unprecedentedly broad alliance of mental health professionals, voluntary organisations and service-users/survivors has been campaigning against draconian proposals for increased coercion set out in the UK government's draft mental health bill. These proposals seem set to provide for the compulsory treatment of people living in their own homes with prescribed drugs that may have serious adverse effects, and for the preventive incarceration of individuals solely on the basis of a diagnostic category newly formulated by politicians and civil servants.[1] Although the proportion of homicides committed by people deemed to have a mental disorder relevant to the offence declined significantly between 1957 and 1995 (by an average of 3 per cent annually), high-profile campaigns by pressure groups such as SANE, aided and abetted by media representations erroneously linking 'schizophrenia' and voice-hearing with violence, have presented community care as a grossly irresponsible failure. This has fuelled the pervasive and damaging stereotyping of psychiatric patients, especially those who happen to be young black men, as dangerous, yet male psychiatric patients are very much more likely to take their own lives than to kill someone else, particularly a stranger (Taylor and Gunn, 1999; Beresford and Croft, 2001; Fernando et al., 1998; Crepaz-Keay, 1996; Leudar and Thomas, 2000). Challenging such prejudice is an essential prerequisite to ensuring that political, policy and service responses to the needs of a small minority of male service-users who really are threatening as well as vulnerable are both considered and appropriate.[2] Yet the political clamour surrounding a small number of high-profile tragedies in which psychiatric patients have either killed, or spectacularly ended their own lives, has been accompanied by a resounding silence on the significance of violence as a cause rather than consequence of distress (Rogers and Pilgrim, 2003). Moreover, the number of psychiatric patient deaths associated with neuroleptic drugs – possibly as many as one a week in the UK, or four times the rate of 'mad' homicides – and the greater exposure of black patients to higher doses of potentially harmful medication has attracted far less interest and concern (Sayce, 1995; Littlewood and Lipsedge, 1982/1997 pp. 259–60).

A concomitant reluctance to explore the linkages between masculinity and violence in this context undoubtedly reflects an unwillingness to negotiate complex political terrain. Since issues around violence can become highly sensitive within the politics of 'mental health' as well as within feminism, this is clearly a key area where potential tensions between discourses – political stories addressing various aspects of the same social worlds from different positions and perspectives – demand careful attention. The practice of politics within (and between) discursive communities may warrant specific exploration. One of the implications common to both self-advocacy and pro-feminist politics is that how we speak matters as much as what we say. It may be helpful, for instance, to attend to the ways in which subjectivity is implicated in how we 'do' the politics of gender and 'mental health', in terms of institutional practices as well as in the conduct of advocacy and self-advocacy (Church, 1995). Once again, critical postmodern approaches which emphasise a willingness to accept and work with the creative tension between plural frameworks and explanations might prove invaluable. Despite our best efforts to transpose politics into a human key, however, temporary chaos may ensue as 'the necessarily agonistic theatre of discursively forging an alternative future' unfolds (Brown, 1995 p. 76). When it does, in this context perhaps more than any other, continuity of emotional support and human value needs to be underwritten within the political process.

There may, of course, be political aporia here: contradictions that are genuinely intractable, where a pragmatic separation of concerns will remain the best option. But if this is the case, such a choice should be made following careful deliberation rather than avoidance. These preliminary observations apply equally to the ways in which we read, theorise and debate these issues, not least since the 'mental health' arena aspires to be a prejudice-free zone, in which respect accorded to the humanity of all participants, whatever they may currently be thinking and saying. This, after all, is complex terrain, where the weight of circumstance bears heavily upon questions about disclosure and concealment: where stories of intense pain need to be listened to, and may be withheld for good reason, or prove impossible to tell, but also where stories of power-within-powerlessness may be declaimed in an idiom of prerogative and dominance.

In this chapter I consider a variety of perspectives on 'dangerousness' and risk, and discuss the predominantly male phenomena of homicide and suicide. I am interested in the way in which patterns of convergence or disjuncture between different discourses affect how we manage to think and speak, or more commonly not to think and speak, about the relationship between masculinities, distress or madness, and 'risk'. Various commentators, including some writing from within the survivor movement, provide summaries of an extensive litera-ture on the latter. Although I comment cautiously on some findings (and include generous endnotes), as a postmodern critic of medicalisation I have both political and philosophical difficulty entering a literature couched almost exclusively in positivist and bio-medical terms. Since papers presenting the results of empirical studies tend to privilege diagnostic categories while masking the social context and subjective meaning of extreme acts, and making the operations of gender difficult to trace, my emphasis on the latter might be seen as compensating for the bias of dominant discourse. In the following account I juxtapose a range of contributions from social theorists, psychiatric survivors, psychiatrists and psychologists, feminist and pro-feminist writers, and commentators on 'race' and ethnicity, whose interests converge around this problematic area of policy and practice.

Locating risk and 'dangerousness'

> while society continues to see our crises as signs of mental illness and thus fundamentally dangerous and incommunicable, our journeys through distress may continue to be unnecessarily lonely and violent.
>
> (Campbell, 1995)

> If we are serious about public safety, then it has to be all public safety, and we have to review all the ways people are at risk. There must be no 'sacred cows' like alcohol, masculinity, or the car, and no scapegoats like people with a mental health label.
>
> (Simpson, 1999)

After more than three decades, feminist concerns are now beginning to be incorporated into mainstream mental health policy (Department of Health, 2003b). Various writers urge men to engage reflexively and self-critically with a patriarchal gender order, and emphasise attention to men's violence against

e for emancipatory practice (Pease, 2002; Hearn, 1998).
discourses developed around this imperative be assumed
challenging a simultaneous trend in mental health policy
liance upon coercion and control, forms of psychiatric
lisproportionately, in terms of frequency at least, at male
atric services? Given the sensitivity about stereotyping
already, _ _ and given that among the diverse population of men who
become psychiatric patients a small minority have been extremely violent
while others will be 'normally' misogynistic, and that women face the additional
risk of re-victimisation within the system, this is a complex question (Pilgrim,
1997 pp. 60–1).

A comparative reading of the domestic violence and critical mental health
literatures reveals two apparently contrasting sets of discourses about violence.
The literature on men's violences against women has promoted a gendered,
inclusive and agentic model of violence, stressing the importance of definitions
wide enough to encompass pushing and breaking things, the violences of 'talk
and text', and the visual violence of pornography. The purpose of this is to
counter violent men's denial and minimisation of the impact of their actions,
and to foreground accountability (Hearn, 1996 p. 104).[3] An explicit theoretical
focus on men as the main 'doers of violence' draws attention to the ubiquitous
connections between violence and masculinity, and to the function of violence
as a resource for demonstrating manhood. Professional discourses about a cycle
of violence are regarded as problematic because they are readily appropriated
to excuse men's violence (Hearn, 1998 pp. 35–7). Agencies are criticised for
failing to intervene urgently, or consistently, in situations traditionally conceptualised as private, particularly in ethnic minority settings (Hanmer, 1996).
Postmodern feminists critique a tendency to rely on fixed and essentialist
gender categories, arguing that violence is diverse, context-specific and constructed in discourse, and that a nuanced view of men provides a more effective
basis for practice as well as focusing blame on those most culpable (Featherstone
and Trinder, 1997).

The critical mental health literature also approaches the issue of violence
from an advocacy perspective, but in this case motivated by a need to defend
the interests of a group misleadingly and harmfully characterised as intrinsically
dangerous. Here we find an emphasis on the need to take full account of any
systemic provocation, to distinguish between various kinds and levels of violence,
and to understand and interrupt cycles of fear and violence (Sayce, 1995; Huka,
1996; Sainsbury Centre, 2002). Professionals are taken to task both for minimising violent incidents and for over-predicting 'dangerousness' (Parker and
McCullogh, 1999; Fernando et al., 1998).[4] Agencies are criticised for the
manner of their intrusion into the private domain, and are often cast as the perpetrators of violence, particularly where institutionalised racism is also involved.
Ethnic minority experience is thus highlighted as epitomising an almost diametrically opposite objection. Where these two sets of critical discourses agree

about the problematic nature of clinical discourse, particularly when isolated from sexual politics and social analysis, it may also be for rather different reasons. The violence literature critiques a tendency for therapeutic understandings of men's violence to minimise responsibility and let men off the hook (Dobash and Dobash, 1992). Foucauldian critiques of psychopathology, by contrast, often emphasise the ensnaring disciplinary nature of power/knowledge regimes. Crucially, however, these two broad agendas converge where they agree that male violence, per se, should not be treated as indicative of psychopathology. It is precisely the gendered assumption of a unified rational self that positions violence as exceptional rather than implicit in patriarchal social relations (Hearn, 1998). This same exclusion brackets violence and madness, so that public discussion is shaped by a dominant discourse that detaches 'insane' violence from the moral domain by representing it as impelled by voices or as characteristic of conditions such as 'schizophrenia' (Leudar and Thomas, 2000).

In 'mental health' environments, the kinds of contradictions outlined above may manifest, for instance, in tensions between the need to maintain a realistic pro-feminist suspicion of unknown men (because of the violence and abusiveness of a substantial minority of men, and the deviousness that often accompanies it) and an imperative to believe at least in the symbolic truth of what users and survivors of psychiatry are saying (because of the historic dismissal of any possibility of value or meaning in anything that 'mad' people say). Once psychiatric institutions are analysed in terms of the extent to which they function as public patriarchies, considerable light can be cast upon the selective and regressive operations of disciplinary power. As 'weavers of the fabric of hegemony', 'organising intellectuals' implicated in the maintenance of gender regimes that define 'normal' masculine practice, psychiatrists should perhaps be subject to as much attention in discussions around gender and violence, as the male service-users/survivors whose very existence often seems to be problematised (Donaldson, 1993 p. 646; Beresford and Hopton, 2001).[5] This function has clearly shaped the violences and violations experienced by survivors within the psychiatric system.

Looking back on his earlier work on the asylum, Foucault comments that he perhaps over-emphasised techniques of domination at the expense of what he calls 'technologies of the self' (Rabinow, 1994/2000 p. 177).[6] He argues that the 'psychiatrisation of criminal danger' coincided with developments in the criminal justice system that privileged questions about the nature of the criminal, and reconceptualised punishment as a means of reforming the individual. In his genealogy of psychiatry, Foucault attributes the new discipline's claim to legitimacy as a distinctive branch of medicine to this willingness to engage in public hygiene of the social body, especially by identifying and confronting social danger (Kritzman, 1988). Thus, although patriarchal and disciplinary modes of power are not co-terminous, the juridico-moral concept of the dangerous individual arose out of a particular configuration of social developments characteristic of emergent modernity, crystallising a markedly gendered dynamic of suspicion and silence that came to define the psychiatric enterprise.

Though by no means all such cases involved male criminals, Foucault opens his account of 'the dangerous individual' with reference to a contemporary drama that might be taken to epitomise what has subsequently been described as masculine inexpressiveness. A young man accused (in 1975) of serial rape and attempted rape 'jammed the machinery of justice' by refusing to say anything in court in response to questions about who he was. The presiding judge attempted to elicit a confessional discourse of memories and intimate disclosures in order to evaluate the case properly, but the young man refused even to defend himself. Foucault presents him simply as resisting authority and refusing to play the game of juridical power.[7] He then goes on to consider the early development of a 'pathology of the monstrous', based upon the 'great criminal events' of the early nineteenth century, that seemed to arise out of an excess of passion or rage, but were neither preceded, accompanied nor followed by recognisable signs of madness. A new category of 'homicidal monomania' was devised to characterise a form of insanity that was invisible before the point of eruption, so that only a trained eye would be able to detect premonitory indications. Because this construct inscribed the possibility of 'dangerousness' into the social body, it also served the interests of an emerging discipline by strengthening the case for establishing therapeutic confinement (Kritzman, 1988 pp. 130–5). Along with Pinel's 'moral insanity', homicidal monomania has been identified as a precursor to psychopathy, a condition said to share many core features with white male subjectivity (Parker et al., 1995; Stowell-Smith and McKeown, 1999).[8] The resonance of Foucault's genealogy with recent debates is striking, and invites questions about the production of 'dangerous individuals' under postmodern conditions of economic and cultural turbulence.

Surveying the social landscape of the contemporary West, Bauman identifies a renewed paradigm of exclusion associated with a post-correctional age. Focusing upon a Californian 'state of the art' supermax prison, automated to the extent that inmates have virtually no face-to-face contact with anyone, he argues that any superficial resemblance to the Panopticon is misleading. Unlike panoptical institutions, which were essentially workhouses for a new industrial era, these 'laboratories' of globalised society are designed solely to explore the limits of confinement and incarceration (Bauman, 2000, 1997). The mirror-clad Bonaventure Hotel in downtown Los Angeles is said to evoke a 'technological sublime' and epitomise Jameson's 'schizophrenic disjuncture' of postmodernity, but Gregory's description of this condition as 'a moment of explosive arrest . . . in which the possibilities of the present are thrown into frozen relief' is more graphically manifested in another, similarly anonymous building, in that same city, which turns out to be another prison (Gregory, 1994 pp. 154–7; Jameson 1991). The eight-storey 'Twin Towers' jail, reportedly functions as the largest mental institution in the USA. Concealed behind its equally opaque façade, a disorientating labyrinth of steel-reinforced sliding doors and soundproof security glass, likened by visitors to an aquarium, catacomb or funeral parlour, serves as the first 'care facility' for many homeless people and war veterans. Higher floors are designated for more 'unstable' prisoners, on progressively higher levels of medication (Campbell, 2003).[9] Processes that pathologise and criminalise marginalised groups have thus become inextricable in the sterile micro-practices of an incipient postmodern gulag.

Elaborating upon Foucault's concept of governmentality, understood as 'a calculated supervision and maximisation of the forces of society', Rose also identifies an exclusionary logic, reconfiguring urban space in advanced liberal societies by isolating and insulating an archipelago of secured zones – consumerist 'enclaves of contentment' – from unprotected zones and marginalised spaces (Rose, 1989/1999 p. 5, 2000 p. 331). A new penology appears much less concerned with issues of responsibility or diagnosis than with identifying, classifying and managing social groupings according to criteria of dangerousness (Feeley and Simon, 1992). In this context, control professionals are increasingly engaged in, and charged with responsibility for, 'risk thinking' – with 'management of the marginalia' and surveillance of the usual suspects, their gaze and their encounters with clients, formatted by the demands of risk management. Agencies are required to ascertain who can be managed within open circuits of control and who must be excluded. A group of intractably risky and 'monstrous' individuals (sex offenders, paedophiles, drug dealers, serial killers, the incorrigibly antisocial) re-emerge to face a variety of paralegal forms of confinement and more or less permanent sequestration (Rose, 2000 pp. 332–4). At this point, critics of disciplinary power and medicalisation may find themselves agreeing, albeit for different reasons and in different terms, with those psychiatrists who, unlike their Victorian forebears, stress that individuals classified as having a psychopathic personality disorder are not recognisably 'mentally ill'.

Applying this analysis specifically to the operations of contemporary psychiatry, Rose comments on a shift from a vocabulary concerned with the dangerousness of certain types of individuals to one in which risk has become the organising term. Whereas dangerousness applied to a minority of the psychiatric patient population, the new vocabulary of risk applies much more widely, relating to a widespread cultural impetus to discipline uncertainty and, in particular, to discipline and standardise the clinical gaze and govern professional activity. An obligation to assess, evaluate and minimise risk under 'the shadow of the law' now takes precedence, so that diagnosis becomes technical, administrative and 'quotidian', concerned with the management of the everyday, an 'interminable task of inscription' (Rose, 1998 pp. 185, 190).[10] There has been a rapid rise in compulsory admissions under the Mental Health Act (by 45 per cent between 1991 and 1995), and increasing pressure has driven clinicians to turn towards a quantification of risk, not least in an attempt to curb a consistent over-prediction of dangerousness.[11] In a supposedly post-decarceration period the predominant rationale for confinement has become one of public security. Discourses of probabilistic risk assessment make it increasingly difficult to articulate reciprocal obligations, to strengthen recipients' rights and guarantee protection from prejudice and violence in 'the community'. Rose observes that if anything unifies the various figures gathered together by new designations of the monstrous, it is their predatory nature. Such people are portrayed as radically different, anomalous and exceptional. They embody gross pathology, even evil, and constitute a menacing spectre threatening our 'seductive fantasies of ideal communities' without risk, 'where individuals and families are free to live an untroubled life . . . understood as [the] pursuit of contentment and lifestyle maximisation' (Rose, 1998 p. 191). At which point this powerful analysis of the governance of everyday life through crime and madness, and the consequent production of vengeful 'good conscience', appears to emanate from a position of radical libertarian innocence. There is no sense of the realities of violence disproportionately faced by disadvantaged communities, and because Rose says little here about the complicating operations of gender, 'race' or class, little sense of the forces that converge around the construction of discourses about 'monstrous' and predatory individuals.

Masculinity, psychiatry and risk debates

Before attempting to address this problematic omission I want to summarise some recent discussions of risk within the psychiatric system in relation to intersections between the politics of gender and of 'mental health'. Although the 'mental health' field inescapably involves risky situations, it is perhaps important to distinguish between pervasive, diffuse, inappropriately managerial, and exclusionary 'risk thinking', and focused risk assessment, such as that which is motivated by a need (and duty) to care for people who appear actively suicidal or threatening. Even within these specific circumstances, however, the importance of developing a pluralistic and contextualised understanding of power relations cannot be overstated. Survivor-informed recommendations for good practice include taking into account the effects of institutional provocation – such as discriminatory practices or a simple failure to listen to service-users – and always assessing any risks to a service-user while considering whether a risk is posed to others (Langan and Lindow, 2000).

Potential hazards to patients within the hospital environment include sexual abuse, institutional racism, iatrogenic injury and what Campbell calls 'therapeutic aggression'. Poor ward environments and lack of care amplify distress, and Sayce draws attention to an urgent need to identify environmental triggers to anger (Campbell, 1995; Sayce, 1995).[12] Many black men have expressed the not unreasonable fear that involvement with psychiatry could lead to their death (Sainsbury Centre, 2002; Francis, 2004). Returning patients into situations where there is 'unfinished business' can add further risk (Prins, 1999 p. 104). The uniform application of a 'risk gaze', associated with defensive practice, unrealistic expectations of risk elimination, and increased use of compulsion, particularly in the absence of accessible services, are widely regarded as likely to undermine safety by driving more people to avoid services (Morgan, 2000; Beresford and Croft, 2001).[13] While there are various summaries of the often flawed studies investigating linkages between particular manifestations of distress and violence, and continuing attempts to hone predictive instruments, Beresford notes that despite government rhetoric about evidence-based approaches, policy has been driven by fear of scandal (Beresford and Hopton, 2001).[14] Langan concludes that although social workers should keep abreast of findings, they will have to continue to live with uncertainty (Langan, 1999).

Survivors have written about the depth of anger, intensity of fear, and feelings of shame and humiliation experienced as an inpatient. In the epigraph at the head of this chapter, Coleman talks about an 'angry frightened self' produced by psychiatrists' unwillingness to listen, and interpreted by them as lack of 'insight' and aggression (Coleman, 1999 p. 58). Simpson recalls long-suppressed 'white hot anger' about the mental health system, that he was eventually able to process in a survivor co-counselling group (Simpson, 1996). Campbell argues that, despite media sensationalism, most violence within the system is 'more humdrum and insidious', and often amounts to 'the last communication' (Campbell, 1995 p. 19).[15] The conclusion reported by a number of studies of violent incidents in ward environments, that women patients are equally if not more 'assaultive' in this context, suggests that we should be looking at how the objectifying and monological procedures of masculinist psychiatry contribute to this kind of reactive anger and violence. It may also have served to deflect attention away from the contribution of masculinity to the greater involvement of male service-users in more serious violence, and in violence in community settings, however.[16] Women survivors and service-users, who commonly report harassment, sexual exploitation and violence in ward settings, and according to one survey only 3 per cent of whom want to be on mixed wards, are important stakeholders in 'risk' debates (Darton et al., 1994, cited in Sayce, 1995). A strong association between 'psychiatric patient violence', drug and alcohol abuse, antisocial acts, and criminality, fostered by the growth of a masculinist culture of violence in disadvantaged areas, has arguably fuelled the prejudice directed against service recipients experiencing 'psychosis alone' in recent years (Pilgrim and Rogers, 1993/1999, pp. 56–7; Rogers and Pilgrim, 2003; Swanson et al., 1990; Walker and Seifert, 1994; Crichton, 1995).[17] Yet little attention has been paid to understanding the continuum between spontaneous acts of violence associated with mental anguish, and more calculated, habitual and instrumental forms of violence, or to the ways in which masculinity is mediated through class and 'race' in cultural environments devastated by poverty and oppression.

In their review of the relationship between gender and dangerousness, Pilgrim and Rogers point out, for instance, that in the case of 'schizophrenia', men tend to be diagnosed younger, when physically strong, and that women's problems are more likely to be dealt with at the 'soft' end of psychiatry (Pilgrim and Rogers, 1993/1999 pp. 56–8). Pilgrim suggests that men disproportionately experience psychiatric oppression because of a generalised expectation of dangerousness (Pilgrim, 1997).[18] The violences of some men who become psychiatric patients also need to be considered in pro-feminist terms, however. An American study of 169 people diagnosed as having a serious mental illness and living in the community found that 70 per cent of violent acts were committed by men, and that women were the victims in 60 per cent of cases, but crucially it also commented that very little supported housing was available which would have enabled individuals to live independently (Estroff et al., 1994).[19] While recurrent findings that the small minority of mentally distressed people who do attack someone else are markedly less likely to assault strangers than people known to them may allay public fears about 'mad axemen', they inevitably raise another set of questions about gender, 'caring' and family relationships (Department of Health, 2001). Such questions are highly sensitive and complex, of course, because of the possibility that distressed individuals or family members (or indeed both or neither) might act abusively. In a context driven by the need to formulate defensive arguments against politically driven proposals for draconian social control measures, issues around masculinity and violence might, of course, be seen as divisive. They could also be selectively appropriated by 'politically correct' post-liberal politicians, or by psychiatrists in support of medicalisation and governmentality, understood as regulatory power directed at marginalised and oppressed populations.

Although men are, unfortunately, dramatically over-represented in the contested statistics for homicides committed by people deemed to be suffering from a mental disorder, and wives, girlfriends or mothers are over-represented among their victims, discussions have rarely considered the contribution of hegemonic forms of masculinity to the construction of misogynistic distress (Boyd, 1994; Department of Health, 2001 p. 11; Morrall, 2000).[20] The ostensibly definitive 'Falling Shadow' report (into circumstances leading to the fatal stabbing by Andrew Robinson of a female occupational therapist in a hospital in 1993), for example, overlooked some implications of the crude and occasionally lurid misogyny that surfaced around earlier events in this man's life (Blom-Cooper et al., 1995).[21] Arguably, the pessimistic account of schizophrenia that enlists all manner of events, thoughts and reactions as evidence of a relentlessly deteriorating disease process requiring indefinite maintenance on heavy-duty medication closed down some potentially fruitful avenues of enquiry into what was actually going on for this young man, as well as some potential avenues of social accountability, while reinforcing stigma by associating 'mental illness' and violence.

Had his distress and rage been conceptualised in relation to normative masculinity, this would have suggested the possibility of negotiating with him about what it might mean to be a man, and how 'we' come to learn about this, and drawn attention to a range of cultural influences in his life. It is just possible that careful attention, especially at an early stage, to the personal meaning of his experiences, might have averted the tragedy that major tranquillisers, sadly, failed to prevent. I am struck, for example, by the report's lack of interest in whether and how services helped him deal with the sexual difficulties that so obviously tormented him.[22] Despite commenting on the potentially serious threat Robinson posed to women, the report discusses management of risk and principles of care without recommending single-sex accommodation and, for example, seems untroubled that he was able to embark upon a relationship with a woman he met in a hospital, who subsequently had his child.[23] There is a need to acknowledge the intimate co-existence of violence and vulnerability in such men, within a context of complex power relations. Constructing this story as being about a man with a marked propensity towards misogynistic violence who also experienced mental distress, rather than about a 'schizophrenic', might have generated a less discriminatory set of proposals – about citizenship, civil liberties and community protection.

Comments from survivors indicate an understandable ambivalence about violent individuals detained in hospital settings. A situated knowledge of the kinds of cumulative emotional injury and devaluation that can enrage desperately vulnerable people has prompted some to express sympathy, and a degree of solidarity with those incarcerated at the sharp end of the psychiatric system.[24] Beresford points out, however, that while many survivors experience psychiatry as an oppressive, overpowering and stigmatising institution, it often affords unwarranted protection for perpetrators and 'law-breakers' who seek a mental illness diagnosis in order to mitigate responsibility for the effects of their actions (Beresford and Hopton, 2001). The political repercussions of the social control function of psychiatry are epitomised in secure institutions where narratives of madness, criminality and dangerousness intersect tensely with those of gender and 'race'. The English Special Hospitals reverberate with histories of gross psychiatric oppression, particularly in relation to black 'schizophrenic' inmates, but also juxtapose male sex offenders and women patients who are extremely vulnerable to re-victimisation because of sexual abuse histories and extreme self-harm.[25] Warner nevertheless uses Foucault and Butler to critique advocacy structures in this setting for their dependence upon a binary victim–abuser story that undermines women's right to self-determination, to make 'poor choices' and to be 'bad', by continually producing them as 'good' and passive. This is important in the context of the operation of these institutions not just as places of exclusion but as 'technologies of production, of individualisation of the gendered subject' (Warner, 1996 pp. 111–12, 105). How then does socially instituted gender asymmetry work in relation to the mostly 'mad and bad' men in these hospitals, who are usually storied only as abusers? Should 'we' not be deconstructing any use of totalising and immobilising gender categories (as well as diagnostic categories) that reproduces these highly problematic groups of men as inherently monstrous and essentially dangerous?

Insofar as feminist, pro-feminist and critical mental health discourses rely upon an invariant logic of domination and subordination, the complexities of these extreme and pivotal disciplinary environments are likely to remain politically unthinkable. When 'we' seek to dissociate ourselves in absolute and fundamental terms from the 'villains' and perpetrators in our midst, we should perhaps ask whether we are reproducing the dividing practices of dominant culture. It is, after all, axiomatic that such practices headline individual dangerousness in order to scapegoat 'others', and distract attention from the dangerousness of a social system predicated upon domination.[26] Postmodern perspectives put in question any simple or universal answers to such troubling questions, as do genealogies of the logic of exclusion such as Mariani's account of American bio-behavioural research into 'antisocial behaviour' (childhood behavioural disorders and Antisocial Personality Disorder (APD) or psychopathy) and the associated development of biologically invasive social control techniques. The infamous 'Violence Initiative', based upon dubious assumptions about a genetic predisposition towards violence, was designed to detect early warning signs and direct medical interventions (including psychosurgery) at the predominantly black children regarded as being 'at risk' of turning to crime or delinquency.[27] Mariani identifies nineteenth-century moral management – which she sees as attempting to contain gender-class traitors by classifying psychopathy as the negative pole of bourgeois masculinity – as the precursor to contemporary bio-criminology, and its interest in a wide variety of rogue males. Exponents of this discipline deploy scare tactics and promulgate preposterous statistics on the numerical strength of an invisible enemy presence, and although Hare and Mednick's psychopathy checklist – now 'the industry standard worldwide' – identifies traits consistent with patriarchal capitalist mores, they are at pains to dismiss social explanations (Mariani, 1995).[28] Meanwhile, a large proportion of the distressed people rejected by psychiatric services, who arguably constitute today's 'undeserving poor', are young and often homeless single men, with a tendency towards 'reckless and disturbed behaviour', and a diagnosis of personality disorder (Repper and Perkins, 1995 pp. 495–6). The spectre of preventive detention looming over such men suggests that no adequate attempt will be made to reconfigure services in order to address their admittedly complex needs.[29]

Brown's analysis of the gendering of state power augments the bleak cartography developed by Rose by theorising the contribution of masculine hegemony to the paradigm of exclusion that still underpins and bisects the diversity and contingency of postmodern regimes of control. Using Foucault's late work, she foregrounds the contradictory nature of a protean and multifaceted masculinist state. Identifying a 'prerogative modality' of state power, Brown cites Weber's theory that marauding male 'warrior leagues', and correspondingly defensive male household authority, constituted a gendered and sexual underpinning to the political formations from which the state emerged. From this perspective, violence, violation and 'dangerousness' appear endemic both to the fabric of state institutions that have the power to protect and that are 'often all that stands between women and rape, women and starvation, women and brutal mates', and to 'the community' which masculinist state power regulates. Because agencies of the state actively colonise, by configuring, administering and producing both subjects and the issues that concern them, Brown emphatically warns about surrendering control of codification, but concludes that state power can be exploited and subverted because of its multiple and unsystematic composition (Brown, 1995 pp. 174, 178–91, 196). Parallels have been drawn between dilemmas faced by lesbian and gay communities wanting to secure funding, services and anti-discrimination measures from governments that are also regarded as oppressive, and those faced by psychiatric survivors opposing forced treatment but demanding decent and democratic services and protection from prejudice (Sayce, 2000 p. 128). Brown's perspective foregrounds the presence of masculinist institutional power, while signalling the need to account for men's violences across the familiar debates and ethical dilemmas surrounding citizenship, agency, capacity to consent, enforced treatment, risk, surveillance and the incarceration of 'monstrous individuals'. Men's contributions to debates about risk and violence need to be based upon an acknowledgement of our various, and often contradictory, orientations and positionings in relation to hegemonic discourse.

Racism and 'dangerousness'

When we turn the material and look at the racialised nature of masculinist state power, all of these concerns, debates and dilemmas are intensified, and the operation of discourses about individual dangerousness and the dangerousness of supposedly protective institutions becomes dramatically apparent. Black and ethnic minority recipients of psychiatric services, and young black men in particular, have repeatedly been shown to be disproportionately vulnerable to coercive and oppressive treatment within the psychiatric system, leading to vicious circles of control, anger and 'non-compliance' (Fernando, 1991; Sayce, 1995; Prins, 1999; Fernando et al., 1998; Sainsbury Centre, 2002; Bhui, 2002). Mama points out that enslavement and colonisation were not only about material exploitation and subordination, but also 'transformed and subjected Africans to the imaginings and caprices of imperial culture and psychology' (Mama, 1995 p. 17). In response to this legacy, another set of counter-discourses about violence has emerged. Marriott, who is among many contemporary commentators to draw on the work of Fanon, writes that 'anger has long been a chosen vocation for black men desperate to retain their separatedness'.

He also cites James Baldwin's telling observation that the idea that black experience is somehow incommunicable is unwittingly mirrored in black forms of anger (Marriott, 2000 pp. viii–ix; Fanon, 1952/1986; Baldwin 1964).

In 1968, two black American psychodynamic psychiatrists published a book called *Black Rage*, in which they described the realistic and appropriate depression and grief that results from turning the hatred of racism in on the self. This was an unpopular reality to 'sufferers' who preferred to see themselves in a more heroic posture. As this grief lifted, suppressed hatred would be redirected outwards in an attack whose fury would be proportionate to the depth of grief experienced. Although Grier and Cobbs wrote from a generically male perspective, they did specifically discuss black masculinity, in terms of a never-ending battle to acquire the prerogatives and privileges (of money, the power to 'control and direct other men', and to understand and alter one's life) accorded to their white counterparts. The legacy of slavery had necessitated the suppression of 'manly' aggression and assertion. Central to Grier and Cobbs's argument was their differentiation between a 'black norm' – the 'normal complement of psychological devices' acquired by black men in order to survive racism – and the 'illness' that remains after this has been subtracted, and is 'a proper subject for therapeutic endeavour' (Grier and Cobbs, 1968 p. 179). Because the 'black norm' entails a suspicion bordering upon paranoia, and because 'the mental disorder into which black people most frequently fall is paranoid psychosis', the boundaries of madness may not be clear, however. There are obvious parallels here with Chesler's contentious differentiation between those hospitalised women who are suffering from the effects of mistreatment and oppression and those who really are 'mentally ill' (Chamberlin, 1994).

More recently, the theme of black rage has been taken up by hooks, who stresses the importance of understanding rage as 'a potentially healing response to oppression and exploitation'. She argues that neither the movement for racial uplift nor contemporary 'narratives of pleasure and cool' adequately address the psychic wounds of racist aggression. Failure to address these wounds leads directly to a psychology of victimhood, in which learned helplessness, despair and uncontrollable rage abound in the psyches of black people. While black women's fiction and the writings of black feminists have repeatedly demanded an interrogation of personal histories in order to break silences and heal wounds, the black male response to any focus on individual trauma and psychological recovery has, with the exception of black gay men, generally been negative. Despite reservations about Grier and Cobbs's Eurocentric and patriarchal assumptions, hooks regrets that their contribution has not been embraced and developed, and that current mental health work rarely makes the link with political injustice in order to combine emotional healing with politicisation and social activism (hooks, 1995 pp. 12, 137).

Her observations on media representations of black rage as useless, meaningless and destructive are pertinent in relation to the recent prominence of media portrayals of young 'schizophrenic' African-Caribbean men as 'big, black and dangerous'. A central argument in Fanon's *Black Skin, White Masks* is that an imago or fantasy of the black man has been constructed in order to allow a certain purging or purifying of European culture. This purging necessitates 'a vicious pantomime of unvarying reification and compulsive fascination, of whites looking at themselves through images of black desolation' (Marriott, 2000 pp. 67, xiv). Thus the genealogy of imagery of the black madman includes a mythology of violent, aggressive, and 'animalistic' black sexuality, 'fabricated and fictioned by the all-powerful white master to allay his fears and anxieties, as well as providing a means to justify the brutalisation of the colonised'. Fanon analysed the internalisation of this oppression, and its contribution to intracommunal violence (Mercer and Julien, 1988 pp. 134, 115; Staples, 1982). Black feminists have emphasised, however, that social conditions should not be used to exonerate black men's sexism and exploitation of women, and Majors has called on black males to reject the false promise of recuperating patriarchal privilege (Segal, 1990/1997 pp. 186–7, citing hooks, 1989; Majors, 2001).

Fernando approaches dangerousness in a 'mental health' context with reference to discourses about black rage, and cites Amos Wilson's understanding of black adolescent men's violence in the context of the criminogenic effects of white American society. He argues that the psychiatrisation of 'rage, alienation, and (what is seen as) bizarre behaviour' is comparable with the psychiatrisation of escaped slaves, and that the construction of schizophrenia (a description of 'mad' people who could not be understood, as alien) at a time when Europeans' fear of unknown 'dark' forces was focused upon the 'alien' cultures of colonised black peoples made it the 'natural' diagnosis to use in the medicalisation of black protest, despair and anger (Fernando et al., 1998 pp. 66–8, 80, citing Wilson, 1991). These twin narratives of the mad and black alien have converged tragically in the lives of many young black men. The random fatal stabbing of Jonathan Zito by Christopher Clunis at a London underground station in December 1992, though highly atypical, came to be seen as emblematic of the dangerousness of 'schizophrenics' who were supposedly being 'freed to kill' in alarming numbers (Sayce, 2000; Crepaz-Keay, 1996). This tragic event remains significant since the inquiry set up to investigate it, and the moral panic that was precipitated around it, heralded a progressive expansion of the coercive reach of the psychiatric system. Since much has been written about this elsewhere I want to focus briefly upon the contribution of black commentators who have challenged the dominant discourse about containment and control of risky individuals that quickly enveloped mainstream public understanding of this case and others like it.

Wilson unsurprisingly argues that young black men have been victims of failures in the system – in particular of a lack of communication, a lack of access to appropriate services, and an unwillingness to relate to black recipients in a non-stereotyping manner – and that 'had something been done earlier to meet Christopher Clunis' most basic needs for housing and employment, the whole situation could have been prevented' (Wilson, in Fernando et al., 1998 pp. 196–7). A review of the inquiry report produced for the Race Equality Unit draws attention to Clunis's attempts to negotiate a review of the exceedingly high doses of chlorpromazine he was being given, and criticises the complacency of the inquiry team in relation to the bankruptcy of a 'total drugs policy'. The inquiry's criticism of a nurse for his reluctance to assist in returning Clunis to a drug regime he described as a 'chemical straitjacket' and felt was potentially dangerous, demonstrates the simplistic nature of calls for transparent inter-disciplinary co-operation (based upon modernist assumptions about the neutrality of diagnostic information) and for coercive outreach to guarantee 'compliance'. One element in the institutional racism identified by Harris is an assumption that black men need to be treated with heavy dosages of medication or ECT rather than being offered psychotherapy or counselling. He found no evidence of due concern for two key losses in Clunis's life, the loss of a 'girlfriend' and, crucially perhaps, in the following year, the death of his mother (Harris, 1994 pp. 17–21).[30] Once again it was black psychiatrists, countering the hegemonic objectification of their discipline, who raised issues around black men's subjectivity. Feelings of rage are commonly reported in association with grief, especially where the process of grieving is in some way interrupted, as it was for Clunis. Given that he was experiencing institutional racism from the people who were meant to be helping him, and no doubt encountering racism elsewhere (he reportedly heard voices taunting him with racist insults) it is perhaps not so remarkable that events took a tragic turn. hooks has written about a sequence of racist incidents that left her feeling so enraged that she wanted to stab the white man who happened to be sitting next to her. Her 'killing rage' turned to grief, and she wept – which is, of course a much less socially accepted option for men, and perhaps particularly for black men (hooks, 1995 p. 11). When interviewed by the inquiry panel Clunis recalled needing help, but not knowing how to ask for it (Ritchie, 1994).

Critics of postmodern perspectives might expect those engaged in resisting pervasive and often virulent oppression to jettison attention to diversity and complexity as impractical luxuries, in favour of an orchestrating vocabulary of solidarity. A shift in the opposite direction has been described, however, in which the saliency of 'black' as a unifying signifier has been gradually eroded as issues of globalisation and diaspora become prominent, and 'rainbow coalitions' emerge as an alternative to ethnic absolutisms (Hall, 1992; Rattansi, 1995). Various postcolonial commentators have discussed the need to take the paradigm of articulation seriously, to interrogate and transcend claims that assert the primacy of a particular axis of differentiation over all others (Brah, 1996 p. 246; Mercer and Julien, 1988 p. 102). Mama has critiqued the unitary subject and notions of an 'essential African core' in black psychology (Mama, 1995). In contemporary discussions of mental health service provision the work of Brah has been cited to emphasise that difference should not be assumed simply to reflect pre-given ethnic or cultural traits amenable to standardised responses, and that the politics of gender and 'race' are inseparable. Black and ethnic minority service-users want 'an appropriate and dignified service' that feels safe and affirming (Sainsbury Centre, 2002 pp. 63–5; Bhui, 2002 p. 43).[31] This is likely to entail helping individuals break a cycle of oppression and distress involving both mentalism and racism, and deal with internalised racism (Trivedi, 2002). At the time of writing, another inquiry report into the death of a black male patient has identified institutional racism in the NHS, reminding us that this is a continuing story.[32]

Risk and suicide

> If suicide rates indicate a social disturbance in the relation of the individual to the group – a breakdown of social integration and regulation, the remedy must be social.
>
> (Seidman, 1994/2004, summarising Durkheim, 1897/1952)

The other main area of risk strongly associated with men is, of course, the risk of suicide. Although much more common than homicide, and somewhat less culturally charged, this is another politically complex area, not least since the headline 'social facts' about increasing rates of suicides by young men have been central to claims that there is a 'crisis of masculinity' in the West (Coyle and Morgan-Sykes, 1998). Interestingly, Durkheim's *Suicide* was one of many monographs on the subject published during the nineteenth century, often documenting a rise in suicides as evidence of a moral crisis of European civilisation. As previously noted, this was also quite widely framed as a crisis of masculinity, and in statistics on suicide Durkheim found 'definite proof' of 'the unhappy moral conflict actually dividing the sexes'. His work showed that this ultimate desperate assertion of individuality is paradoxically and intimately immersed in the operations of the social order (Giddens, 1978; Durkheim, 1897/1952 p. 386). During the twenty years to 2000, suicide rates in the UK fell for women and older men, but rose markedly for younger men, so that suicide became the commonest cause of death in men under thirty-five.[33] Another striking pattern that emerges is the extent to which unemployment, social deprivation and exclusion increase the likelihood of suicide (Pritchard, 1992; Department of Health, 2002). The rapid increase in young suicides in the UK coincided with the ascendancy of neo-liberal political economy during the 1980s. Clare reports that male suicides have risen strikingly across age groups and in most countries over the past thirty years while female rates have remained stable, and that the predominance of young male suicides is a new phenomenon.[34] Locating these trends within a crisis discourse about the 'waning Y' chromosome, he advocates a reassertion of the normatively 'protective' figure of 'old man', who eschews feminine influence but reorientates himself towards family and personal relationships (Clare, 2001 pp. 82–4, 221).

A rather different picture has been provided by Canetto, who notes that in many Western countries women have higher rates of suicidal ideation and behaviour while men have higher mortality from suicide. Calling this the gender paradox in suicide, she reviews empirical studies noting considerable local variation, and considers whether cultural assumptions facilitate differences in suicidal behaviour, and lead to an under-reporting of 'non-fatal suicidal acts' in men, and an under-recording of female suicides (Canetto, 1992–3; Canetto and Sakinofsky, 1998).[35] Other reviewers have questioned both the constructions of meaning upon which statistics depend and the interpretations being placed upon them, but noted that in recent years male rates of self-harm have been rising, and the gender gap in attempted suicide diminishing (Payne and Lart, 2004). A large study of young men in the UK finds levels of depression similar to those already reported by young women, but identifies a range of distinct issues, especially around obstacles to obtaining help and support (Katz et al., 1999).[36] Stack summarises possible explanations for the disproportionately high suicide rates in men, including much higher rates of alcohol abuse, a cultural emphasis on being impulsive, decisive and 'strong', the greater visibility of failure in the 'primary adult male role', and (in some countries) greater access to firearms. Women tend to be protected by better coping skills and support networks, an ability to recognise 'warning signs' (such as depression) and a willingness to ask for help (Stack, 2000 p. 146). The gender gap in suicide figures may also reflect differences in methods of self-harm.[37] Notwithstanding these complexities, rising levels of male suicide undoubtedly represent a disturbing trend, justifying policy interventions, hopefully based upon nuanced understandings of the operations of power rather than discursive attempts to reposition men as the new victims vis-à-vis women.

One approach to the phenomenon has been to suggest that since Durkheim linked suicide with the rapid social transformations of early modernity, and in particular with processes of social integration, his theorisation may be even more applicable to the more profound instability generated by current sociocultural upheavals. Because men have difficulty with feelings of ambivalence and uncertainty, with remaining socially connected, and with expressing 'negative' emotions such as anxiety, uncertainty, weakness or sadness in a culture of 'winners', some facets of postmodern individualism may affect them ('us') more adversely than women (Moller-Leimkuhler, 2003). Social comparison has been identified as an important issue for some men, especially in relation to 'breadwinner suicides', and Scourfield notes that suicide may result from a perceived loss of honour when the patriarchal dividend fails to deliver the privileges of masculinity (Scourfield, 2004; Connell, 1995). Durkheim's positivistic interest in distinguishing social normality from social pathology, and the affinity between his functionalism and the widely contested sex role theory, make his perspective quite problematic, but his ideas are still favoured, for instance by some contemporary exponents of communitarianism (Giddens, 1978; Whitehead, 2002; Erben, 2004). When observing that men were more susceptible to what he called 'conjugal anomie' as a result of divorce, however, he did attribute this to the unequal involvement of men and women in social life, and to the 'obviously opposed' interests of husband and wife in marriage (Durkheim, 1897/1952 pp. 384–6). Pritchard invoked the concept of anomie when describing unemployed men as 'deprived of a role', and felt that psychiatry should become involved in alerting employment agencies to the psychosocial stresses of unemployment (Pritchard, 1992 p. 755).[38] The difficulty with this approach is that it obscures the 'obviously opposed' interests that determine distribution of means, as well as the workings of postmodern power/knowledge regimes that manage subjectivity in contexts of entrenched inequality, accompanied by a steady erosion of social welfare.

Another important limitation of much current research is that it treats 'men' and 'women' as unitary categories, and consequently de-emphasises both the considerable diversity of masculinities, and the range of circumstances in which men's suicides are occurring. Social policy debates often exacerbate this limitation by portraying men in polarised terms, as either victims or perpetrators. Noting that a minority of men kill themselves in order to punish a woman partner, and that violent men commonly use suicide threats or attempts in the context of divorce or custody battles, Scourfield challenges the expectation that men who take their own lives are necessarily or simply victims (Scourfield, 2004). Clare observes that 'suicide is a very aggressive act, even if it is not intended to be so'. There can be a close relationship between suicide and homicide, insofar as overwhelming homicidal feelings may be checked, or concealed, by suicide, or because suicidal intentions may unleash a homicide (Clare, 2001 citing Hendin, 1999).[39] This link between some suicides and aggression is also reflected in the particularly high suicide rate among male prisoners convicted of violence against the person (Erben, 2004). Bracken notes that Durkheim's finding – that suicide rates fell during the civil wars of his day – also applied in most European countries during the two world wars (Bracken, 2002). Although increased social cohesion would no doubt contribute to this effect, the removal of most men from 'ordinary life' into military service, and a collective experience of mayhem, is also susceptible to less comfortable gendered readings.[40] While acknowledging the intense ambiguity of many suicidal acts, it is important in the context of men who use psychiatric services to emphasise the profound, and often carefully masked, vulnerability of many men who are driven to this extremity, as well as some issues particular to service-users.[41] There is also a need to engage with debates in criminology, since a high risk of suicide among prisoners and released prisoners means that custodial sentences amount to a death penalty for a significant number (Wilson, 2005). Aggregate studies and general theorisations about 'men' inevitably convey little sense of the desperate social environments, personal contingencies or ontological implosions that make escape by means of violent self-destruction appear a more bearable option than struggling on.[42]

Young men's distress

I want to conclude this section by looking, in a way that conveys a sense of the lived experience involved, at two studies that focus on young men who are widely identified as both particularly vulnerable and 'hard to reach' by professionals and researchers. A large survey of young men in the UK found that one in three of those who had attempted suicide would 'smash something up' if they were very worried or upset, while many would pick a fight or get involved in 'antisocial acts'. Another third would simply keep their feelings to themselves. One of the most significant factors differentiating the 'suicidal' group was an extensive experience of violence in their lives, and this was coupled with a greater likelihood of having a father who would expect them to 'fight their own battles'. These young men, who are in a very real sense the victims of male-on-male violence, are described as living in an 'emotional landscape limited by the myths of masculinity'.[43] Less than one in five of the overall (self-selected) sample said they would go to their father for emotional support, and the report's authors comment that 'it was striking that so many told us that "nobody ever asks me about how I really feel"'. 'Sky rocket narratives' about cultural achievement were scarce here, with only about a third of the depressed and suicidal respondents saying they felt they wanted, or could cope with, a job and a family. Another potentially important, though perhaps not surprising, finding was that those boys and young men who were struggling with a sense of worthlessness, victimhood or isolation were considerably less supportive of the prospect of women's equality, and more inclined to feel that men were losing their rights (Katz et al., 1999, p. 12). Accounts such as this show how vulnerability and violence can be intimately linked in the context of subordinated or marginalised masculinities, and implicitly undermine simple binary assumptions about good and evil, guilt and innocence, perpetrators and victims, purity and contamination, agency and structure.

McQueen and Henwood (2002) adopt an explicitly postmodern theoretical perspective in their fine-grain analysis of how cultural constructions of gender available within particular social contexts shape the ways in which young men talk about their emotional lives and experiences. They regard the 'turn to text' as especially relevant in a setting where therapeutic engagement relies upon the medium of language, and draw upon discussions by Frosh of the fragmentation or dislocation of contemporary Western identities, based increasingly upon consumption rather than production (Frosh, 1991, 1997). Constant cultural change, not least a decentring and problematising of male experience in response to feminist advances, is likely to pose difficulties for men whose self-concepts are embedded within traditions of machismo or masculine rationality. Adolescent boys beginning to define themselves as adult men may find it particularly difficult to exist within, or find alternatives to, traditional but fragmenting forms of masculinity. The discourse analytic study looks at how young men enter the mental health system, and at how the cultural ideas and concepts available to them influence the way they talk about their experiences. It is argued that the decontextualisation of teenage boys' distress, coupled with an assumption that language is descriptive rather than constitutive of the experience of distress, impair professionals' ability to work effectively with them.[44]

One of the two participants discussed, a young man with a history of being bullied, intimidated and socially isolated from male peers, expresses stoicism, and attempts to salvage agency rather than talking about feeling anxious or worried. This is understood in the context of physical struggles for power, and a class-specific homophobic discourse in which admitting emotional distress would undermine masculine identity. The authors emphasise the distinction between this contextual understanding of his statements that 'I just blocked it out' and 'I got used to it', and therapeutic discourses then might read these as repression of a definitive emotional state or dissociation from emotions. Another young man with a history of violence initially arising out of the need for self-defence minimises this and attempts to diminish his responsibility by presenting himself in the childlike position of being 'naughty'. The study attempts to develop a non-pathologising and socially informed approach to understanding male subjectivities and mental health by focusing on subject positions within narratives, and on the importance of overcoming tensions between contradictory positionings rather than using psychoanalytic or cognitive frameworks. Viewed from this perspective, aggressive behaviour, for instance, would be recognised as one of the few powerful subject positions left for young men with limited life chances, whose accounts of experience are constrained by dominant discourses of a masculine–feminine polarity (McQueen and Henwood, 2002).

Conclusion

Discussions of both suicide and homicide crystallise some potentially productive tensions between the politics of 'mental health' and a series of other overlapping political concerns, especially those of feminism. Because these topics are difficult and culturally charged, I would again emphasise the value of developing theoretical perspectives capable of addressing a 'reconceived ethics' of complexity, grounded in an appreciation of multiple and locally embodied differences, and of attending to the practice of political dialogue (Price and Shildrick, 1998 pp. 225–36). Postmodern perspectives on the immanence of power and surveillance within networks of everyday existence, on the reinvigoration of the impetus to incarcerate, on the constitutive force of language, and on the complexity and instability of identity, are all pertinent to any theorisation of risk and masculinities. If homicide represents the lethal apex of a culture of pervasive violence, and suicide epitomises the precariousness of hierarchical (hegemonic and subordinated) masculinities at an individual performative level, then interventions aimed at reducing the incidence of violence or self-harm need to be informed by a critical understanding of dominant discourses about masculinity that foster harmful and self-destructive beliefs and practices. Such interventions, whether originating within 'mental health' agendas or not, should also be informed by a critical understanding of discourses, practices and power relations within the 'mental health' arena, taking account of the potential dangerousness of psychiatry and the extreme vulnerability of many men who are users/survivors of psychiatric services.

A complicated bereavement?

In the circles I moved in we regarded therapy, the kind dealing with personal growth not pathology, as a valued part of everyday life, indeed almost a political imperative for men. The therapist I was seeing was a man whose background and perspective were compatible with my own, who was reasonably client-centred (he saw himself as an advocate for my unconscious processes) and was affordable.* I found the continual process of discovery compelling, even at times enjoyable, and felt that working on my 'own stuff' helped me in my work with other people.

On 19 May 1989, I went for what turned out to be a very 'heavy' session. What came up was a 'horrendous image of a cancerous breast'. I felt revulsion and rage, and was plunged into gut-wrenching sobbing, a full grieving reaction that came out of a clear blue sky and continued through the next day. This made little sense, since I'd just visited my mother, and according to my diary, found her 'fit and active'. The summer passed fairly uneventfully, but on 23 November she rang me to say that she'd had some tests on a lump in her breast. They'd given her some large tablets to take, but had not told her whether it was malignant and she hadn't asked. She'd not thought much about it, or wanted to tell me before her six-monthly check-up. This meant, of course, that my otherwise inexplicable grieving had coincided, fairly closely, with her discovery of the lump. As things turned out, it also preceded her death, and my 'real' bereavement, by just over two years.

A decade later, on 14 July 2000, my partner and I decided to stop off at Llangollen on the way home from a holiday on Anglesey. Walking on to

* He had a sliding scale and belonged to an organisation that made provision for people unable to pay. Therapy and counselling services vary considerably, so good independent information is important.

the ancient bridge, which I remembered from several family holidays almost forty years before, I looked up at the towering hills, and then noticed a local bus coming towards us. I'd adored buses as a boy and, seeing the name Bryn Melyn Motor Services painted on its side, I was suddenly transported into another time. Tears welled up powerfully inside me, and I let them flow. Noticing that almost everyone on the bridge had become transfixed by the remarkable sight of a man crying in public, I turned away to face the roaring green body of the river, and, with my partner marshalling the audience, topped it up a bit. Afterwards I felt much better, and carried on driving home. This was nine years after my mother's death.

Between these uncharacteristic outpourings, the epicentre of my bereavement was an extraordinary and transformative moment. I've felt a strong need to protect a sacred space around the memories associated with it, for a number of reasons. One is that I'm now afflicted by 'N-door syndrome' (where n is about 20), a condition that develops after repeated exposure, on entering yet another room, to formal demands for yet another summary of a quite traumatic story. (I don't recall anyone apologising for intruding in this way, incidentally.) Another is that the sheer complexity and richness of what unfolded defy description, let alone encapsulation. I've been telling people that I experienced a 'complicated' bereavement, but have since learned that precisely this term has been used to medicalise mourning deemed abnormal because of its duration or timing (Foote and Frank, 1999). I offer these peripheral stories, therefore, against the will to interpretation and to unsettle expectations that 'knowledge' is a healing balm.

Chapter 10

Reconstructing men's lives

Power/knowledge, personal recovery and social transformation

> no-one can be masculine through and through without constantly, and in the end rather obviously, doing violence to many of the most basic human attributes; the capacity for sensitivity to oneself and others, the expression of fear, the admission of weakness, the wisdom of co-operation, the satisfaction of servicing, the pleasures of passivity, the need to be needed – all quint-essentially 'feminine'.
>
> (Segal, 1993)

> By taking part in self-conscious and critically reflective practice that challenges dominant discourses and constructs alternatives, and by adopting non-patriarchal speaking positions, we (men) can begin to reconstitute our sense of who we are and who we might, both individually and collectively, become.
>
> (Pease, 1999)

Given the self-evident importance in 'mental health' environments of retaining a compassionate and affirmative attitude towards vulnerable men and maintaining an optimistic sense of the possibilities for change in men's lives, a quite widespread tendency to pathologise masculinity, within both mainstream and critical discourse, constitutes another area of potential difficulty in the complex political matrix surrounding contemporary responses to men's distress. Since our understandings of and orientations towards masculinity will inevitably inform, and may decisively shape, any work 'we' might do as men, on our selves or with each other, I begin this chapter by reviewing some relevant histories and debates. As already noted, various feminist and critical psy-professionals have contributed influential analyses of the gendered and racialised nature of social violence within masculinist culture. Notwithstanding an understandable suspicion of therapeutic over-generosity towards physically abusive men, such accounts have often drawn upon the conceptual resources and discursive force of psychopathology, psychoanalysis and psychology in order to critique characteristic manifestations of masculine hegemony, such as the 'madness' of racism or 'homophobia'. Although the rhetorical appeal of such a strategy may be understandable, attempts to appropriate and redirect disciplinary power in the service of social transformation can appear, at best, questionable when set against histories of psychiatric oppression. The following discussion invites reconsideration of the pervasive influence of power-knowledge systems, and the interchange between 'clinical' and political discourse, in the context of potential exchanges between pro-feminism and 'the politics of the madhouse', and recognition that there may well be areas here where tensions between different interests and discourses defy formulaic resolution. In the context of what Bauman calls the pluralism of authority, purposive action that can no longer be substantiated monologically necessarily becomes subject to ethical dialogue (Bauman in Beilharz, 2001, p. 186).

Alongside and underpinning immediate forms of crisis support, there is an evident need for various cultural spaces where individual and collective memory and identity can be re-evaluated. Despite a range of concerns associated with what has been called the therapeutic turn, and despite the very real difficulties of recommending such a strategy in the context of the 'mental health' field, where oppressive scrutiny and appropriation of biography have been commonplace, I am inclined to believe that working with male subjectivity can be both counter-cultural and potentially helpful for individual men. In order to test this proposition I want to explore an apparent contradiction between pro-feminist claims that psychoanalytic thinking is a valuable source of critical deconstructive insight into the formation of masculinities, and appropriate psychotherapy an important site for the personal-political transformation of men, and another set of concerns about the politics of disclosure, about therapeutic discourses and practices, and regimes of surveillance and control, that arise within environments dominated by psychiatry and psychology. Because the former arguments constitute such an emphatic strand within critical studies of masculinity, because men have traditionally been reluctant to seek help during the early stages of distress, because some critics of psychiatry cautiously advocate psychotherapy, and because some alternative and survivor-led projects make use of broadly therapeutic methods and discourses, I devote considerable attention to these issues, and once again recommend the postmodern possibilities of ambivalence and patience in the face of incommensurable positions.[1]

In the final section I discuss the interdependence of personal and social change, and consider critical life-story work, a form of identity work rooted in social postmodern understandings of selfhood, and drawing on critical auto/ biography as a potential resource for working with male subjectivity without medicalising or individualising men's distress, and for promoting emotional wellbeing both among men and within communities affected by men's sexist assumptions and practices. Although most of the material discussed in this chapter relates more closely to crisis prevention or recovery than to emergency support, my hope is that these explorations may also have some bearing upon the questions raised by the tall dark male stranger at the crisis house door, alluded to in Chapter 1 above.

Pathologising masculinity

> Psychoanalysis on the one hand has enriched almost every current of radical
> thought in the twentieth century, from Marxism, surrealism, and existential-
> ism to anti-colonialism, feminism, and gay liberation. On the other hand, it
> has evolved into a medical technology of surveillance and conformity,
> acting as a gender police and a bulwark of conservative gender ideology.
>
> (Connell, 1994)

Although some social psychiatry has upheld hegemonic values, Frantz Fanon
brought a sharply defined critical edge to his 'sociodiagnostic psychiatry', and
wielded it against the 'madness' of racism. Bhabha comments on the intricate
irony of turning the European psychoanalytic tradition to face the history of
the Negro, which it had never contemplated – an irony represented on the
dust jacket of *Black Skin, White Masks* by the figure of a black man wearing
a white coat signifying the authoritative speaking position of the doctor.
Even though Fanon directed his critical gaze towards what he described as the
'Manichaean delirium' of colonial and racist consciousness, rather than explicitly at white hegemonic masculinity, his influential oppositional discourse
crystallises some issues at stake in this debate. Bhabha points out that Fanon
was neither raising the question of the universal rights of 'colonial man' in
liberal-humanist terms, nor historicizing colonial experience in terms of a
Marxisant master–slave dialectic. Instead he suggested that a reading of Lacan's
Other might be more relevant, and proceeded to identify the colonial subject
variously 'inscribed in the texts of history, literature, science, and myth', and
to evoke the colonial condition through image and fantasy (Bhabha, in
Fanon, 1952/1986 pp. xii–xiii; Bhabha, 1994 p. 32). Fanon affirmed the importance of renouncing what he referred to as 'hate complexes' (such as the scapegoat complex), but rejected theories positing latent conditions which traumatic
circumstances merely make manifest.[2] For Bhabha, his distinctive achievement,
however, was to see 'the phobic image of the Negro, the native, the colonised,
deeply woven into the psychic pattern of the West'. This insight enabled a
deeper reflection on relations between coloniser and colonised, and brought
'hope of a difficult, even dangerous, freedom' (Bhabha, 1994 pp. 63, 52).
    Bhabha develops an intricate poststructuralist improvisation on Fanon's
theme, using Lacan to stress the importance of language in the construction of
identity. In particular Fanon deals with the doubling of identity: the difference
between personal identity as an 'intimation of reality' or being, and a psychoanalytic process of identification through which a 'socially and psychically
authenticated' human subject emerges. Identification is about the problematic
process of access to an image of totality that must remain both 'an illusion of
presence' and 'a sign of . . . absence or loss'. Out of this liminal tension
Fanon, echoing Freud's famous question about women, asks 'What does a *black*

man want?' His answer, that he wants the confrontation with otherness that 'an unconscious disavowal of the negating, splitting moment of desire' in the colonial subject denies, makes the personal political by exposing racism to inter-rogation by 'a politics of narcissism' (Bhabha, 1994 pp. 51–2, 63–4). Fanon declares not only that colonialism makes the Negro 'a phobogenic object', but that 'the negrophobic man is a repressed homosexual' (Fanon, 1952/1986 p. 156; see also Segal, 1990/1977 p. 177). Rather than cementing an internalisa-tion and privatisation of experience, Hall argues that it is precisely Fanon's con-ception of otherness as an internal compulsion that allows cultural identity to be seen as a point of identification made within discourses of history, refracted though memory, fantasy, narrative and myth, as a positioning rather than a fixed essence (Hall, 1990). The mapping of power relations involved in the con-struction of this account is complex. Fanon, a black male psychiatrist, illustrates his notion of negrophobia using a psychiatric case history taken from a young white female inpatient, and reporting the results of a word association test carried out on his patients (confirming the prevalence of racist stereotypes); he also writes about the precariousness of his position as a black doctor in 1950s France, where he concluded that he was 'hated, despised, detested, not by the neighbour across the street or my cousin on my mother's side, but by an entire race' (Fanon, 1952/1986 p. 118; Macey, 2000 pp. 136–7).[3]

The closely analogous term 'homophobia' also emanated from within the 'psy-complex', first appearing in psychological writings in the late 1960s and gaining wider currency after 1973, when it was used in a popular book by the psychoanalyst George Weinberg. Weinberg defined it as describing 'an irrational persistent fear or dread of homosexuals', or 'an irrational fear or intolerance of homosexuality' (Weinberg, 1973; Kitzinger, 1997 p. 211). Doubtless because this term has subsequently become embedded within the conceptual currency of public discourse, there has been much more debate about its political impli-cations and, at least within critical 'mental health' circles, about the implica-tions of its provenance. Given that Kimmel concludes that homophobia is 'the central organising principle of our cultural definition of manhood', and that it propels exaggerated masculine behaviours including the gendered rage of racism, this is a debate that puts in question the terms in which we discuss and challenge hegemonic forms of masculinity (Kimmel, 1994).

Some defences of the term 'homophobia' within lesbian and gay politics have quite serious, albeit unintended, repercussions for users/survivors of psychiatry. Hopkins, for example, notes that, for some, the phobia suffix codes anti-gay and anti-lesbian acts as irrational and uncontrollable individual aberrations that belong to a clinical realm in which moral responsibility and political critique seem inapplicable, and within which 'homophobes' may enlist inappropriate sympathy. His own analysis becomes particularly problematical where he sug-gests that 'heterosexism' should apply to institutional prejudice so that 'homo-phobia' can be reserved for 'physical violence and strong verbal, economic, and financial abuse of gays'. Only the notion of phobia, it seems, will suffice to describe virulent and sadistic acts of violence, which may also appear 'semi-psychotic' and amount to 'evidence of a radical kind of evil'. Hopkins appears to sense the difficulty with this, and attempts to avert the problem by arguing that homophobia does not parallel claustrophobia or agoraphobia because it has been developed within political rather than psychiatric discourse. Though the 'repression hypothesis' (that homophobia is driven by a need to conceal and compensate for unacknowledged homosexuality) often seems appropriate, prejudice is a product of binary gender systems, and will only cease when these are supplanted (Hopkins, 1996 p. 99).[4] For Halperin, however, the pervasive and multiform nature of homophobia exemplifies Foucault's late formulation of power. Its discourses are constructed from an infinite number of interchangeable assertions that are impervious to rational disqualification, and form part of a general and systematic strategy of delegitimation. Yet despite arguing that Foucault's anti-psychoanalytic approach enables homophobia to be treated as a political rather than a psychological problem, and that its causes are to be found in (what Bersani calls) 'a political anxiety' about subversive social change rather than within psychic life, Halperin leaves the term itself unquestioned (Halperin, 1995 pp. 32–3, 121–2, citing Bersani, 1995).

Writing from within the traditions of critical psychology and radical feminism, Kitzinger reaches a different conclusion. Because psychology systematically replaces political explanations (dealing with structural, economic and institutional oppression) with personal ones (focusing on 'the dark workings of the psyche, the mysterious functioning of the subconscious'), the term is challenged for imputing sickness to individuals who deviate, albeit in an illiberal direction, from society's expectations. That the notion of homophobia reinforces the power of psychology to label people as 'sick' or 'mentally healthy' is confirmed by the development not only of scales to measure and diagnose homophobia, but of a related category 'internalised homophobia', which perpetuates the pathologisation of homosexuality.[5] Kitzinger argues that a psychology of prejudice that depends upon programmes to change individuals (and proposes remedies involving education, psychotherapy or different forms of child rearing) diverts attention away from structural oppression and collective political action, and is analogous, for instance, to attempts by psychologists to attribute unemployment to 'state benefit neurosis' (Kitzinger, 1997 pp. 210–12). Foucauldian perspectives complement such suspicion about attempts to harness the power of governmentality and normative psychology, with their traditions of moral pedagogy, moral treatment (of those deemed insane), remoralisation and now responsibilisation, to progressive political projects (Rose, 1998).

It is possible to agree with Hopkins that the vehemence of extreme violence, which is almost always a male phenomenon, requires particular explanatory attention, without accepting that the language of phobia is appropriate for the task. Insofar as the notion of phobia implies abnormality, this is clearly inapplicable if the repudiation of homosexuality is fundamental to the construction of hegemonic masculinity, yet part of the appeal of the term is that it strategically undermines the insistent masculinist coupling of normative violence and bravery. The sight of an older man breaking into a profuse cold sweat when the subject of sexuality came up for discussion in a group also reminds me that at an individual level the experience in question can sometimes resemble other forms of fear and anxiety widely referred to as phobias.[6] From the point of view of the politics of 'mental health', however, the last thing that is needed is yet another discourse linking a clinical (or clinical-sounding) term with violence. Use of the phobia suffix has not been invoked in relation to prejudice and violence against women, although this is widely related to a very similar socially constructed psychic process of repudiation, and is typically neither concurrent with, nor driven by, any immediate subjective experience of anguish for the man. Evolving discussions such as this suggest the need for a language about subjectivity and power grounded in an open-ended and pluralist political aware-ness, rather than superficial conformity to prevailing notions of correctness, a language that facilitates processes of speaking and listening across the bound-aries constructed by necessary fictions of identity, between distinct but inter-related communities of interest. Because the user/survivor movement potentially includes so many members of other 'Othered' communities, it is well placed to develop such languages and processes.

There is also a history of concepts migrating in the other direction, from poli-tical into clinical discourse. Bracken points out that many of the people involved in research into post-traumatic stress disorder (PTSD) had a back-ground in feminist, anti-war or human rights struggles, and were looking for scientific legitimation of particular political positions. Noting that PTSD was 'recognised' as a medical condition at about the same time as homosexuality was being 'de-recognised', he observes that psychiatrists (and others) campaign-ing for this saw it as an 'always-already-there object in the world', rather than as a construct being shaped around a specific moral and social agenda (Bracken, 2002 p. 47). Significant numbers of Vietnam veterans arriving in the clinics and wards of hospitals with serious psychological injuries were told that they were suffering from long-term psychiatric disorders that were inducing delu-sional thinking about the war. In one celebrated case, psychiatrists responded to the disturbing testimony of a man who witnessed, but did not participate in, the killing of large numbers of women and children at My-Lai, by diagnos-ing paranoid schizophrenia and declaring that he was 'obviously in full-blown psychosis'. Veterans groups, encouraged by the decisive success of political advocacy in the homosexuality controversy, responded by demanding acknowl-edgement that their experiences of trauma were principally attributable to what had happened in Vietnam, not least in order to claim disability benefits and compensation (Kutchins and Kirk, 1997/1999 pp. 107–10, 116). Interestingly, when the new diagnostic category was finally accepted, it was categorised as a separate disorder, distanced from serious psychiatric conditions, in order to minimise the effects of stigma on veterans who were becoming psychiatric patients (Busfield, 1996 citing Gersons and Carlier, 1992). This contrasts markedly with the former classification of homosexuality as a sexual deviation under the rubric of personality disorders.

Insofar as it focuses on issues of meaningfulness and subjectivity in a context where both are systematically undermined, Bracken considers the clinical and cultural popularity of PTSD in terms of its function as a 'disorder of postmodernity' (Bracken, 2002 p. 187). Lembcke's social constructionist account shows that, as befits a postmodern condition, media and film representations of the traumatised veteran played an important part in its inception. He argues that by the time mental health professionals came to interpret the experiences of Vietnam veterans, a cultural image of the 'unanchored vet' was already well established. 'Flashbacks' in Vietnam war films (where these were usually disturbing mental events rather than simply depictions of memory used as a narrative device) pre-dated the adoption of the term in mental health practice. Here they became a way of reinterpreting and even reimagining both events and the identities of veterans qua veterans, just as in film they had functioned to rewrite American history. A discourse of trauma came to displace political discourses about pacifism and anti-imperialism developed by the veterans' movement, and was used to discredit the anti-war movement. Although 85 per cent of men who went to Vietnam did not see combat and many encountered resistance to military authority, they came under intense pressure to conform to a culturally constructed 'false memory syndrome' that demanded stories about war as a male rite of passage. One ironic effect of this ostensibly sympathetic discourse was to stereotype veterans as unusually violent. Lembcke concludes that the PTSD framing effectively diverted attention from the war itself towards individual victimised veterans, thus undermining understandings of America as the aggressor, and reconfiguring the nation's memory of Vietnam 'as a preparatory step to its revival as a major military power in the 1990's' (Lembcke, 1999 pp. 53–4, 59).

Kutchins and Kirk argue that although much of the initial impetus to establish PTSD came from a need to include the experiences of non-combatants, veterans subsequently failed to differentiate between men who were victims and those who had been perpetrators of atrocities (Kutchins and Kirk, 1997/1999 p. 116). Based on a study of a PTSD unit of a veterans' administration hospital, Karner identifies a 'protocol for "telling"', in which an initial reaffirmation of the quintessentially masculine activity of combat preceded any contradictory sentiments. She found that a masculine stance was maintained in peer groups, and that statements about crying or anxiety were made in private, usually with female psychologists or nurses, or in her interviews. PTSD was constructed as a 'masculine malady' in various ways. In addition to understanding behaviours such as aggression, social isolation and emotional distance, fighting and drinking, and soldierly hyper-vigilance as characteristically masculine, veterans could invoke PTSD itself as proof of manhood since it implied survival of unusually extreme combat experiences. The gathering of veterans in the unit replicated the camaraderie of combat, allowing men to overcome the supposedly emasculating process of becoming a patient and identifying vulnerability. The medicalisation of biography – a narrative reconstruction of identity incorporating a ready-made technical vocabulary of stressors, flashbacks, traumas and hyper-vigilance – provided an interpretative frame for addressing the disjuncture between lived experience and conventionally idealised images of war and manhood. For Karner, however, PTSD served to reinforce toxic notions of masculinity by focusing treatment on elements of hyper-masculinity (such as violence, drinking and thrill seeking) and encouraging a belief that all such 'symptoms' derived from behaviour learned in combat, so that internalised cultural models of normative masculinity were left intact (Karner, 1995).

Recommending a critical postmodern perspective on the false memory debate, Atmore cites Foucault's argument that discourses are sets of themes that can become attached to very different, even contradictory political projects (Atmore, 1997; Foucault, 1980).[7] Nowhere is this more evident than in the application of PTSD to both the wartime traumas of men and the experiences of people, mostly women, who have survived sexual abuse and domestic violence. For Herman, the similarity between psychological syndromes found in these disparate groups provided evidence of a war between the sexes. Her account developed a structural understanding of trauma in terms of power relations rather than intra-psychic processes, but perpetuated the assumption that PTSD was a pre-existing condition awaiting recognition (Herman, 1992; Busfield, 1996; Bracken, 2002)[8]. Feminist campaigns against the victim-blaming diagnosis of 'masochistic (or self-defeating) personality disorder', which had been devised as a means of overcoming difficulties in applying PTSD to victims of abuse, culminated in moves to establish a new diagnostic category of 'delusional dominating personality disorder', specifically directed against the tactics and attributes of masculinist power (Kutchins and Kirk, 1997/1999 pp. 167–75). Although the failure to gain recognition for DDPD clearly reflected the gendered institutional bias of American psychiatry, the adoption of categories to delineate disorders of power poses potential difficulties for both feminists (by exceptionalising and depoliticising abusive behaviour, and appearing to minimise agency) and psychiatric survivors (by reinforcing the linkage between 'mental illness' and violence, and psychiatry and social regulation).

Similar considerations arise with other attempts to fix masculinity as psychopathology, and with the importation of the language of pathology into critical discourse. Thus, for example, a hyper-masculinity inventory has been devised in order to delineate a 'macho personality constellation', with the somewhat tautological promise that this will help us understand criminal behaviour, predict dangerousness and treat male offenders (Zaitchik and Mosher, 1993).[9] Perhaps the clearest instance of problematical pro-feminist work is Jukes's assertion, generalised from his unavoidably confrontational psycho-educational work with violent men, that a 'gendered psychosis', forged during a necessarily traumatic original separation from the primary object (the mother), is the source of a universal male misogyny. This balefully monolithic construct repeats the double calumny of associating psychosis, and implicitly those diagnosed as psychotic, with Stygian rage and an innate propensity for violence, and imputing to 'all men' an orientation of unmitigated hatred and enmity towards women (Jukes, 1993, 1996).[10] Other applications of psychoanalytic thought, such as Fanon on racism, Santner on paranoia and fascism, and Kimmel on masculinity as homophobia, attest to the pervasiveness of narratives linking a repudiation of otherness characteristic of dominant forms of Western masculinity with a critical stage of early development theorised as the Oedipal constellation. While such accounts risk over-estimating the influence of early childhood experience and over-valuing individualistic and therapeutic remedies, their cumulative force does suggest that formative processes shaping male individuation need to be considered, alongside and in the context of the social and cultural dimension.

The politics of therapeutic disclosure

> The obligation to confess is now relayed through so many different points, is so deeply ingrained in us, that we no longer perceive it as the effect of a power that constrains us, on the contrary, it seems to us that truth, lodged in our most secret nature, 'demands' only to surface . . . one has to have an inverted image of power in order to believe that all these voices which have spoken so long in our civilisation – repeating the formidable injunction to tell what one is and what one does . . . are speaking to us of freedom.
>
> (Foucault, 1976/1978)

> Men who may wish to stay in control of conversation may quite accurately perceive that the disclosure of their emotions leads to a reduction in control, with the result that they may not find the prospect of self-revelation an enticing one.
>
> (Spender, 1980)

> with an ideology based on an objectifying trajectory, manifested psychologically in the splitting of intellect from feeling and the repression of the latter, it ceases to be possible to adequately construe the self – to make sense of one's own experience and emotional confusion . . . men's own experience is left uninterpretable because masculinity is based upon its repression – a particularly significant issue in relation to therapy. Self-control, mastery of nature and of our 'nature', is a defining marker of the masculine state.
>
> (Frosh, 1995)

Connell concludes that psychoanalysis, despite its evolution from a debatable method of therapy into a normalising technology of surveillance and control, has also functioned as a 'remarkable tool of research' and contributed significant insights and lines of enquiry into the necessarily conflict-ridden and in some

ways precarious construction of masculinity. Freud's assertion of an 'architecture' of gender, and his exploration of the 'contradictions and fissures'
within male identities, constituted a significant challenge to prevalent cultural
assumptions both about masculine rationality and about an a-priori masculinity
inherent in biology. Although he celebrates the Freudians for making the 'first
serious attempt at scientific research on masculinity', what Connell appears to
value in their work is its discursive fecundity. Psychoanalysis originally involved
'the decoding of personal meanings in an extraordinarily fine-grained way',
requiring 'a strenuous balancing of concern for the person and critique of what
the person says'. Freud's account of psychosexual development centres upon
the Oedipus complex not as a simple sequence of rigid stages but as a continually updated map, a script for the drama of masculine development. Because
this narrative process can unfold along different paths, Connell makes the paradoxical claim that this paradigmatic meta-discourse yields some of the strongest
evidence for the currently popular notion of multiple masculinities. Moreover,
psychoanalysis is social from the outset, insofar as it forces recognition 'that
the social is present in the person . . . and that power invests desire in its very
foundations' (Connell, 1994 p. 16).

Seidler, who maps masculinity in terms of the Enlightenment tradition with
its privileging of rationality and 'objectivity' and its institutionalised Cartesian
splitting between bodies and minds, acknowledges Freud's challenge to utilitar-
ian conceptions of identity, but also advocates therapeutic practice as fundamental to a politics of personal transformation for men. Unless 'we' learn to
face our past histories with honesty and compassion they will continue to
haunt us, but because we have so much invested in maintaining an externalised
and culturally sanctioned work-orientated image of ourselves, the process is
likely to prove 'scary' (Seidler, 1994, 1997 p. 161). Seidler is far from alone in
this; indeed Rowan makes the stronger and curiously reifying claim that only
therapy is capable of exploring 'the nooks and crannies of a man's psychology
in enough detail to leave nothing untouched in the end', and thus of effecting
an initiation 'at every level' (Rowan, 1997 p. 5). In Seidler's account, therapy
is a learning process in which men can come to recognise 'our' conformity to
dominant discourses about emotion and identity, and in which we must forgo
the quest for immediate explanations and solutions in favour of a gradual discovery of feelings. 'We' may learn, for instance, that we have studiously been
avoiding certain difficult feelings, such as those associated with bereavement
(Seidler, 1994, 1997).

Petersen offers a postmodern critique of Seidler's work, arguing that his discussion of the mind–body split actually suggests a rationalistic and cognitive
encounter between a 'pre-social fixed subject and self' and a stable domain of
bodily 'feelings' and 'desires' for which men need to take greater responsibility.
Because culturally constructed dualisms, such as man–woman, mind–body and
reason–emotion, become naturalised in his texts, and retain a universalist and

essentialist quality, and because he presupposes a natural realm beyond relations of power and knowledge, Seidler unwittingly reinforces the dualistic thinking he sets out to challenge. He writes as though men were being shaped by social and historical conditions not of their own making, and assumes a commonality of generic male experience 'unmarked by "race", ethnicity, sexuality, age, physical ability and so on'. Petersen highlights the contribution of post-Darwinian psychology and psychoanalysis towards constructing the notion of an alienated male subject, cut off from his body, his 'true feelings' and significant others, and cites various commentators who argue that a confessional style of writing about masculinity has attributed male domination to a non-relational masculine psychology, rather than to social arrangements or material and political practices (Petersen, 1998 pp. 89–93).[11]

Some of these objections may be overstated, and the latter point, for example, appears to depend upon the very dualistic thinking that Seidler explicitly counters by insisting upon emotion as a source of knowledge. In a later discussion, Seidler also replies to Connell's dismissal of consciousness-raising as a 'therapeutic' distraction from the need for men to come to terms with their experience in critical ways, by invoking 'the personal is political' as a key feminist insight that men have learned from. Addressing the relationship between masculinity, violence and emotional life, Seidler arguably demonstrates the material and political nature of men's discursive and relational practices. In doing so he suggests that the assumption of discourse theorists that experience and identity can be reconstituted in language relies on a modernist paradigm that not only underestimates the tension between discourse and subjectivity but mirrors violent men's insistence on control and denial (Seidler, 1998; see also Henriques et al., 1984/1998 p. 204). I take this as implying that a more psychologically informed approach might usefully augment the tradition that has taken a cognitivist and voluntaristic view of men's apparent difficulty with talking about personal issues, regarding this primarily as a conscious strategy (Spender, 1980 p. 47).

Writing as a psychotherapist who has worked with sexually abused children and their families, Frosh locates his influential discussion of therapeutic work with men specifically within the context of postmodernity and the deconstruction of traditional Western notions of masculinity. Affirming the importance of Seidler's contention about men's historical appropriation of rationality for the marginalisation of both 'femininity' and madness, he argues that psychoanalysis 'is *founded* on the ambiguities of gender – the tension induced by the apparent oppositions of masculinity and femininity, of desire and otherness'. Although 'embroiled in patriarchal conceptions of sexual difference' it provides conceptual and practical tools for the deconstruction of a masculine mastery that appears to be constructed primarily in relation to difference – as something that is 'not not-masculine'. Femininity is also constructed in negative terms, but as productively empty, lacking active consciousness, a contentless receptacle for disowned male projective fantasies. Deconstructing masculinity and femininity therefore entails recognising both as constructed categories with no establishable essence (Frosh, 1994 pp. 10–12, 89–90). Like Connell, Frosh points to a long-standing psychoanalytic interest in interpreting personal linguistic texts (Frosh, 1995). In the process of therapy, clients' talk about themselves and their relationships 'becomes an object to be revolved and examined' (Frosh, 1997 p. 74). Like Seidler, he argues that disrupting masculinist fantasies of superior rationality is a key element in this process, not least since a concealed vulnerability – 'the sense that masculinity is built upon emptiness', and especially upon a disavowal of reciprocal neediness and intimacy – accounts for much of men's violence. In a socially contextualised psychological exposition of why some men abuse, he suggests that the construction of masculinity leads to an over-reliance on sex as a channel for emotion and intimacy, and can generate an unbearable tension between one momentum towards dependency and dissolution, and another towards mastery and control (Frosh, 1995 p. 230, 1994 pp. 113–15).[12]

Feminist advances have decentred male experience, rendering masculine identity uncertain and unstable rather than something that can be assumed. As masculinities come to be regarded as heterogeneous and the image of monolithic phallic authority fragments, many men cling to traditional masculinity, repudiating homosexuality and 'feminisation' even more desperately. In this context a therapeutic stance of 'holding' and creating a supportive environment can facilitate a gradual reframing of selfhood and identity as a way of narrating experience, rather than as a static entity to be defended against fears of annihilation (Frosh, 1995).[13] Whereas some narrative therapists contest the 'expert rationalist model' of therapy by limiting themselves to opening up 'a more vibrant recognition' of the complexity and constitutive nature of people's stories, Frosh argues that many of the conflicts that generate distress operate 'at the edge of language', so that the therapist often needs to engage in a struggle to articulate that which has not yet been spoken – to make meaning known (Frosh, 1997 p. 75). Although he describes this as a pre-postmodern insight, treating such newly shared meaning as a contingent and particular co-creation would be consistent with critical postmodernism, and Frosh, elsewhere, outlines an 'imaginary' in which qualities traditionally coded as 'feminine', from irrationality to 'jouissance', continually emerge from the margins of personal experience, 'prodding away eventually to puncture all assertions of full mastery, knowledge, and control'. Exposure to the possibility of everlasting change leaves 'us' with a series of provisional positions, consistent with the 'little narratives' of postmodernism (Frosh, 1994 pp. 143–4).

Although Frosh critiques psychoanalysis as a gendered project that has sought to colonise the irrational and subjugate it to reason and science, and hopes to transform its discursive practices, his account remains that of a practitioner in a medicalising field. He refers to patients or analysands, and retains diagnostic labels, as when arguing that Dora may have 'stayed a hysteric all her life'

(Frosh, 1994 p. 127). His defence of psychoanalysis against Masson's influential polemic remains in a theoretical register that effectively masks the detail of elitist and oppressive practice, as well as the key issue of abuse within therapeutic situations (Frosh, 1999; Masson, 1984/1992, 1990).[14] As with Seidler, there is little sense of how the heterogeneity of the social informs the development of male subjectivities and differentiates between various experiences of 'masculinity' and 'femininity'. Frosh sometimes, perhaps inevitably, appears inconsistent with his own postmodern direction. He continues to talk, for example, about 'the unconscious', as opposed to unconscious processes, and about 'the irrational', which carries connotations of a failure of logic, an incapacity to reason, rather than the 'non-rational', a less judgemental term inclusive of intuitive and otherwise inspired knowledge. Others have attempted to demonstrate that the limitations of both psychoanalysis and discourse theory can be overcome by combining insights from the former with poststructuralist perspectives on subjectivity and power-knowledge. This would effectively 'unlock the closed circle' of psychoanalysis, and facilitate the development of strategies of resistance encompassing change in both subjects and circumstances (Henriques et al., 1984/1998 pp. 225–6).[15]

Even the ostensibly transformational proposal that a male therapist can help a male patient in a manner analogous to a view of mothering that entails intimate instinctive knowledge and generous responsiveness to destructive feelings, by making the therapeutic situation 'as "soft" as possible', is far from unproblematic. Frosh acknowledges that the assumption on which 'reverie' is based, that an analyst can 'know' someone's unconscious mind simply by being there and noting their own emotional responses to what is being said to them, has potentially oppressive implications.[16] It does, after all, tacitly position the service recipient as infant (Frosh, 1992 pp. 157–9, 1994 pp. 31–5; Bion, 1962). One way of considering just how oppressive and silencing such an assumption about knowledge might become is to return to Foucault's account of the confessional paradigm which, as the epigraph at the head of this section indicates, appears to radically undermine any claims for therapeutic liberation. For Foucault, psychoanalysis crowns the repressive hypothesis (that power works through negation and prohibition) in a paradoxical manner, by productively inciting a confessional impulse and developing expert discourses of interpretation and normalisation that not only construct 'truths' about selfhood but construe these as necessarily opaque to the confessing subject. An entire disciplinary grid has developed around this proliferating medium of constitutive power, so that every confessional act situates the individual as an object of knowledge within a relationship of power, and every story about experience becomes a case (Foucault 1976/1978; Dreyfus and Rabinow, 1982). This scenario, in which empathy facilitates surveillance, may appear unduly bleak, but reminds us to look carefully at the social dimensions of power-knowledge shaping any and every context where psychoanalytic ideas are being applied to problems of masculinity.

Rose has brought Foucault's notion of the confessional to bear in an extended critique of the ways in which contemporary lives have become saturated by a complex and heterogeneous array of political technologies of individuality, identifiable as 'psychotherapeutics'. He argues that this trend is consistent with the regulatory apparatus of post-liberalism, which is characterised by a fragmentation of the social state and marketisation of the public sector. A spectacular expansion of the realm of the psyche has coincided with a paradoxical and pervasive mode of governance that obliges us to become free, autonomous, choosing individuals. Although the relentless expansion of the therapeutic 'allows the play of values and aspirations from widely varying ethico-political positions', its significance lies in the consequent pluralisation of agencies and mechanisms that regulate subjectivity by attaching selves to 'the project of freedom'. A whole matrix of power-knowledge is devoted to applying forms of expertise that promise to enhance autonomy, framing our relation to ourselves within an individualising ethic, and anchoring us ever more firmly to the project of our own identity. Burgeoning therapeutic discourses of self-mastery contribute to a climate of responsibilisation in which the effects of poverty, discrimination, distress or illness can be recast in terms of personal failure, incompetence and lifestyle choice. Rose acknowledges that there are some benefits associated with this ethos, but envisages another kind of freedom: 'an ethics whose vectors do not run from outer to inner, and do not question appearances in the name of their hidden truth . . . that does not seek to problematise, to celebrate, or to govern the soul' (Rose, 1989/1999 pp. 261–2, 272, also 1996, 1999).

In this context he identifies the ethicalising political genre of 'speaking out', in which hidden injury becomes a marker of identity and legitimacy, as a reversal of the traditional problematic of stigma, but also as a therapeutisation of politics (Rose, 1989/1999 p. 269). Once again, Brown addresses similar terrain from a feminist perspective. She argues, for instance, that feminist standpoint theory (and much of modernist feminism) treats consciousness-raising in a manner analogous to psychoanalysis or the confessional, insofar as material excavated there is valued as the hidden truth of women's existence – 'true because hidden, and hidden because women's subordination functions in part through silencing, marginalisation, and privatisation'. Yet it is precisely because women are positioned 'as private – sexual, familial, emotional . . . produced and inscribed in the domain of both domestic and psychic interiors' that the voicing of their experiences takes on a confessional quality. Brown therefore invokes Foucault's caution against assuming that, under such circumstances, truthtelling about experience amounts to liberation, particularly since the status of such truths as 'the secret of our souls' has been established by those seeking to use them to discipline us (Brown, 1995 pp. 41–2). Foucault did, however, move from analysing how productive power operates through 'technologies of the self' to taking a belated interest in the creative potential of such practices (Rabinow, 1994/2000 p. 177).

While recognising some negative repercussions of what she terms 'the therapeutic turn', notably the adaptation of ideas of an insatiable and malleable self
to the demands of capitalist consumer culture, Nicholson has more to say than
Rose about its democratic possibilities. An increased willingness to attend to
'emotion', to 'what I feel', and to 'the relatively non-linguistic', has opened up
spaces of resistance, legitimised idiosyncrasy, and provided an important source
of challenge to forms of social rationality that depend on devaluing others.
Because it has exposed the psychological as well as material effects of oppression
to scrutiny, the individualising or at least anti-communitarian impetus of the
therapeutic turn has greatly extended the range of critique 'and left a powerful and importantly democratic imprint on the shape of our politics'. Early
consciousness-raising groups were able to combine the therapeutic and political
in creative ways because they were also informed by an assumption that distress
was socially shared and historically contingent (Nicholson, 1999 pp. 151, 161).
This difference in emphasis between the positions taken up by Nicholson and
by Rose again appears to reflect a gendered response to issues around subjectivity.[17] As already argued, feminists have long identified men's resistance
to disclosure as a strategy for maintaining power, and pointed out that 'men's
stories, of private, gendered and domestic lives, still need telling' (Spender,
1980; Allen and Laird, 1991 p. 76). If we accept Connell's evaluation of psychoanalysis, one of the key areas opened up to political critique, in part at least as
a result of the therapeutic turn, has been male subjectivity (Connell, 1994;
Jackson, 1990).

    In reply to Rose, it is possible to envisage forms of freedom that are more
social, collective and action-oriented without insisting upon a 'resolutely superficial' ethics that arguably protects a depth–surface binary distinction (Rose,
1989/1999 p. 272). Instead we might talk about postmodern subjectivities in
ways that reconceptualise the relationship between surface, depth and 'truth',
without abandoning the devalued 'feminine' metaphor of depths (and the
socially formed imaginal insights, intuitive processes and mysterious convolutions of memory associated with it), in favour of a rationalistic genealogy of
appearances. Since issues about masculinity and selfhood have to be negotiated
in a cultural climate that positions the privileged generality of men as public
and rational, technologies of the self surely need to be evaluated in terms of
whether or not they challenge this over-arching hegemonic arrangement.
Despite the evident appeal of politically regressive 'masculinity therapy', Frosh
and others clearly demonstrate that critical therapeutic practice with and
among men is, at least in terms of the politics of gender, possible (Connell,
1995; Frosh, 1997; Real, 1997; Rowan, 1997; Law, 1999; Tudor, 1999).[18]
Psychiatric survivors, who remain overwhelmingly excluded from the public
realm by the effects of discrimination, and devalued as embodying absolute
unreason, bring to bear a political sensibility shaped by a collective history
of exposure to subjection through the appropriation and objectification of

biography. Writing about disability, Shakespeare notes that men can be victims and oppressors at the same time, and that hegemonic masculinity both undermines disabled men's subjectivity and contributes towards generating prejudice about disability (Shakespeare, 1999). For men experiencing distress or madness, disempowerment in relation to hegemonic masculinity is likely to be experienced with particular intensity in encounters with psychiatry. It is crucial, therefore, that any proposals for transformational therapeutic work with men address not only questions of differences between men but also the complexities of power relations between men as service recipients and professionals, not least where the latter assume a mantle of expertise in sexual politics.

Beyond the closed circle of individualisation

In an influential early exposition of narrative therapy, White and Epston use Foucault's 'toolkit' in order to challenge the normalising practices of power-knowledge, but understandably look elsewhere when developing ideas about personal agency and authorship.[19] Although they contribute significantly towards debates about the democratisation of therapeutic practice, and propose to critique their own work, I want to focus briefly on some concerns that are likely to be apparent to readers who are users of services. Firstly, the reproduction of a series of personal accounts, albeit in anonymous form – and this method of therapy centres upon the process of 'restorying' experience, with little apparent acknowledgement (and seemingly without the permission) of the people whose success in becoming the 'privileged authors' of their lives is being celebrated – means that the whole document uncomfortably resembles, and is summarised very much like, a series of conventional cases histories.[20] Secondly, the parameters of narrative practice are defined as encouraging polysemy and multiple perspectives, but encapsulated in a way that implies universal applicability and appears strangely forgetful of social, historical and cultural contexts.[21] Thirdly, and despite worrying over the term 'therapy', some of the methods advocated that do reach beyond the closed circle of individualisation, including investigation of family and community archives and historical documentation in order to develop and facilitate the performance and circulation of subjugated knowledges, controversially expand the reach of therapeutics (White and Epston, 1990 p. 83).[22] Other difficulties can occur when the therapeutic process itself becomes politicised. There appears to be a reluctance to recognise the potential collective agency and insight of diverse groups of service-users and clients, and unpack the relationship between political and professional discourses.[23] Henriques et al. argue that narrative approaches tend to under-theorise the subject and overlook the contribution of both practices and relations, and unconscious processes, in constructing subjectivity (Henriques et al., 1984/1998).

Others have nonetheless developed White and Epston's theoretical theme in interesting ways by engaging with feminist critiques of therapy and postmodern feminist discussions of Foucault. Swan, for example, believes that narrative therapy can achieve the elusive end of politicising the personal (Swan, 1999).[24] Allen and Laird argue that men's lives are storied in a sociocultural context in which powerful myths about masculinity inform the 'gender folklore' of families. Men who rigidly accept these myths will be uncomfortable with the implication that they need help, or may have '"emotional" problems'. The therapist therefore sets out, with the client, to construct a coherent story of the problematic situation from his point of view, but will question how he has engaged with it, who has influenced his storying of it as a problem, and what meanings others give to it. In family situations it is noted that 'men tend to have more storying power and claim more verbal space', but also tend to be less comfortable with relationship language. An 'ecology of ideas' about masculinity needs to be disrupted and deconstructed in a collaborative process involving co-interpretation, the co-construction of new meanings, and the co-invention of more workable stories. One of the goals of this social rereading of biography is to help men move from a position of rigid autonomy towards greater connectedness, and face the challenge of relating a changed story about identity to the wider world (Allen and Laird, 1991 p. 91). Addressing the dilemmas of the male therapist, Law argues that a discursive approach can support counter-practices that constitute resistance to hegemonic discourses. Because the tradition of confidentiality is seen as protecting therapeutic processes from scrutiny, and exacerbating a historical failure of men, collectively, to 'self-regulate', moves towards greater transparency and accountability represent an interesting deconstruction of the confessional (Law, 1999).[25]

Law gives an account of working with a man he calls Don, who confessed to an incident in his late teens, some fifteen years previously, in which he had humiliated a girlfriend by forcing her to have sex against her will. Noting Foucault's argument that the confessional talks sexuality into a religious/moral discourse, he sought to transpose this story into an ethical discourse of accountability by naming the man's action as rape, and inviting him to speculate about how the experience of rape may have affected the young woman. After it was acknowledged that the therapeutic relationship was not immune from reproducing gender discourse, it became possible to explore the ways in which the 'gender archive' had informed his client's involvement in practices of domination and shaped his sense of selfhood. In particular, a moral discourse of shame and humiliation identified as integral to processes of regulation and self-regulation within 'male culture' had driven Don into a state of withdrawal and depression, and fuelled anger and resentment towards his therapist. Directing him towards an ethical discourse would enable him to take some responsibility for addressing issues of sexism and sexual violence, rather than languishing in self-punishment or hoping for forgiveness. In this context, Don's agreement that his story should become partially public is seen as a political act against the usual discursive practice of secrecy. Law also argues that the standard shaming practice in which men who rape are permanently constructed and excluded

as monsters allows other men to regard themselves as having no connection
with or responsibility for the effects of such acts. Once the link is understood
as being about participation in hegemonic discursive practices rather than a
question of guilt by association, the connection becomes clear and political
(Law, 1999 pp. 120, 115).[26] This kind of open and accountable professional
practice includes the therapist in a democratising loop, in which political
knowledge is brought to bear upon a reinterpretation of experience, which in
turn contributes to new political understandings.

A more directly political approach to working with men's subjectivity has
been developed from within the traditions of the anti-sexist men's movement
and associated critical studies of masculinity. Removing such work from an
overtly therapeutic milieu does not guarantee immunity from charges of therapeutisation, however. Petersen, for example, refers to Jackson's influential
critical autobiography as an instance of a confessional style of writing about
men that became prevalent in the 1990s (Petersen, 1998). Although *Unmasking
Masculinity* includes some quite detailed descriptions of intimate biographical
moments, Jackson refuses to present 'a unified seamless voice' or search for a
true self, and explicitly orientates his writing towards a critical deconstruction
of what Foucault called the 'will to knowledge'.[27] This entails disrupting an
archaic and quite pervasive silence about the contradictory detail of men's
personal, emotional and domestic 'private' lives (Jackson, 1990 p. 10). As previously noted, Western philosophy has long regarded the personal, the particular and the emotional as devalued 'feminine' concerns that mark women as
irrational and uncomfortably close to nature, while privileging 'male' impartiality, universality, rationality and culture (Lloyd, 1984). The confessional
paradigm in its modernist Enlightenment guise is clearly intended to police
the messiness of private subjectivity, but as Foucault also points out, discursive
strategies and practices conceived as instruments of power can be reclaimed as
points of resistance, sites of reversal, starting points for oppositional strategies
(Foucault, 1976/1978 pp. 100–2). This is arguably what Jackson has done, drawing on feminist life-history work, and resisting an injunction against the 'self-
indulgence' of disclosure which is often more immediately apparent in the
male-defined domain of public discourse than any incitement to confess.

In order to effect this transformation – and notwithstanding the difficulty
inherent in theorising the relationship between multiple selves, the cumulative
continuities of biographical memory, and choices men make about whether to
take up or reject subject positions within masculinising discourses – Jackson
emphasises political agency. He does this by locating the doer behind his own
deeds, and taking care to avoid representing himself as passive and powerless.[28]
Choice and change become possible, he argues, once the commonalities in
men's experience are understood as socially constructed. As more men with a
range of different experiences and backgrounds 'come out of hiding', and map
the terrain of their sedimented life histories by 'making more publicly visible

the specific institutional conditions and relations of their shaping', critical inventories can be compiled that expose covert networks of male power and counter essentialist assumptions about men's supposedly inherent aggressiveness or rationality. Again there is a circular process of critical deconstruction, involving 'a long and tortuous movement towards reconstruction' (Jackson, 1990 pp. 265, 268).

Although Jackson's writing is quite strongly influenced by psychoanalysis – he talks, for instance, about still being affected by 'blockages and avoidances', and sets out to understand his emotional investment in taking up positions within discourses that confer power by examining the historical production of 'unconscious structures' – he also focuses specifically on shifting relations and practices, such as doing more housework. Gradually, the distinctive contribution of critical life-history work enables him to see that thinking in terms of 'unblocking the past', or 'unmasking' himself, implies a fixed unified identity waiting to be uncovered, and he comes to understand autobiography as a transformative process of selective reconstruction guided by anti-patriarchal and anti-capitalist values. Tracing the formation of different voices (in contexts such as the family and the school, and in relation to themes such as sexuality, sport and boyhood literature) can help dissolve rigidly defended boundaries between private and public identities, and reintegrate reason and emotion in men's lives. His insight, that undoubtedly has resonances here, is that using critical methods to investigate the social construction of masculinity (and for him, social class) allows men to move away from seeing personal problems and failings in terms of individual weakness or neurosis, towards a more political perspective from which such experiences can be reframed as 'socially shaped conflicts and struggles', and constructively shared with other men (Jackson, 1990 pp. 3, 253, 265–9).

A similar approach has been developed by Pease, in the context of participatory research based on postmodern feminism and a postmodern reworking of feminist standpoint theory.[29] He argues that conceiving of masculinities as discursive frameworks within which men learn to position themselves as male opens up possibilities for self-critical engagement with privilege in ways that humanist notions of innate masculinity do not. Such engagement can be fostered by combining collective memory work with participatory research methods based on anti-patriarchal consciousness-raising, reconceptualised as a collective process concerned with destabilising identity rather than the discovery of true selves, and with the production of alternative discourses that question men's dominant positioning in the gender order without attempting to establish a definitive critique (Weedon, 1997). Once again, a therapeutic strand is discernible in the intention to explore 'the emotional and psychological basis of our relationships with women and other men'. In this formulation a group of co-researchers work on their chosen theme by writing down memories (using a third-person voice to avoid rationalisation) and collectively analysing the material. Although common elements are identified and responses to cultural imperatives discerned in order to arrive at critical understandings, a postmodern willingness to live with a degree of contradiction is acknowledged as relevant to the dilemmas faced by men attempting to formulate pro-feminist subjectivities and practices.[30] In the process, Pease summarises issues that arise when pro-feminist men act as allies to feminists and gay men (Pease, 2000 pp. 147, 150).

Considered from a critical 'mental health' perspective, social life-story research has the merit of opening up possibilities for working with men's subjectivities and individual difficulties in ways that are non-medicalising, personally transformative and politically awakening. There are clear parallels with the principles of self-advocacy, understood as a politically embedded and collective as well as individual process, in which people from marginalised groups develop and articulate shared perspectives (Plumb, 1993). Both traditions involve men in processes of sharing emotional support while reinterpreting biographical experiences in social terms, and analysing social worlds in the light of reformulated experiential knowledge, and there is fairly obvious common ground. Effective challenges to men's violences and abuses against women, children and other men clearly need to be integrated into policy frameworks for promoting wellbeing or positive 'mental health'. During episodes of 'breaking down' and being there for each other in times of crisis, men who experience madness or distress implicitly reject some of the key ground rules of masculinity, particularly where trust, intimacy and physical warmth are shared between pairs or groups of men, and where equal opportunities perspectives are actively developed and supported. Men who have been through this kind of process often emerge more emotionally open and compassionate. When asked whether he minded another man who was in the depths of a horrific bereavement phoning him in the middle of the night, a close friend of mine replied 'Of course not – he were grabbin' at cobwebs.'

Where self-advocacy galvanises users'/survivors' expertise-by-experience about ways in which psychiatry and psychology colonise biographical experience and produce individuals as patients in order to overturn the medicalisation of identity, critical life-story work with men entails a more explicit dual focus on the contradictory relationships that all men from marginalised and subordinated groups have with hegemonic masculinity. Although both perspectives critique structures of power, the former privileges the recovery of oppressed voices or selves, while the latter starts from a position of asking men to identify 'our' histories of negotiation with, and investment in, dominant stories about masculinity, to deconstruct privileged voices or selves and to construct new narratives about ourselves as men. One reason for the lack of progress towards developing anti-sexist activism within communities of 'Othered' men has been the difficulty of developing new kinds of stories that encourage men to articulate and negotiate dual or contradictory positionings, particularly perhaps where, as with some uses of survivor discourse, politicised identities have been constructed in ethicalising terms around male versions of a paradigm of victim-hood (Brown, 1995).[31] In 'mental health' contexts, moving beyond individua-listic misconceptions of self-advocacy in order to look at how men's lived experiences impact upon women in both public and private realms, and chal-lenge ways in which men who are users/survivors (or have experienced distress or madness) might be identifying or colluding with hegemonic gender discourse, requires due sensitivity and local knowledge.

Any importation of life-story work with men into 'mental health' settings, where Foucault's critique of the incitement to confess takes on particular signi-ficance, inevitably brings questions about therapeutisation into sharp focus. It should not be difficult for professionals already engaged in reflexive practice to consider critiques of normalisation, medicalisation and political power-knowledge alongside and in relation to gender issues. I make no apology for re-emphasising the caveat that issues of professional power and differences in power between men need to be carefully addressed. The construction of mascu-linities, power relations between men and women, the politics of disclosure, and getting the balance right between the need for constructive challenge and personal affirmation are all likely to look quite different when mediated by 'race' and ethnicity, class, sexuality, disability or experiences of psychiatry. Many questions inevitably arise about specific needs and issues that are particu-lar to, or become accentuated within, 'mental health' environments.[32] In terms of which men want to take part, and how individual men feel about moving beyond discussing experiences of masculinity in relation to relatively safe or familiar topics (such as employment, sport, schooling and politics and, in self-advocacy environments, psychiatry), towards more intimate arenas (such as the family, adolescence, sex or sexuality) that are likely to have been the site of very difficult experiences, life-story work should learn from self-advocacy, and proceed on the basis of informed consent and self-determination. Although many men are likely to find such discussions helpful and interesting, others will not feel up to it, and should not of course be pressured into participating. Although Pease comes from a critical social work background, an advantage of life-story research is that it can take place in settings unconnected with psy-chiatry, such as community education, community groups, writer's groups, local publishing projects and pro-feminist men's groups or conferences (Jackson, 1990; Pease, 2002).

Although psychiatric survivors have good reason to challenge normalising therapy, provision of counselling has long been a political demand, and positive experiences have been reported with culturally appropriate and holistic therapy. I have noted that feminist and pro-feminist commentators have tended to take a relatively optimistic view of the therapeutic turn. Men's attitudes towards therapy and counselling, and towards the use of therapeutic discourse within self-help and crisis support environments, are still likely to be influenced by gender socialisation that strongly discourages disclosure of vulnerability. Within this pattern, however, some men who are psychiatric survivors have valued co-counselling for its toolkit of practical self-help therapeutic/survival skills based on working in pairs and taking turns to listen and express 'distress', for its relatively democratic support networks, and for linking personal liberation to social change. Although their accounts seem, at first sight, radically counter-cultural, we should perhaps exercise a Foucauldian suspicion about treating such networks as already liberated spaces existing outside power and beyond critique (Mental Health Foundation, 2001).[33] Paths towards survival and recovery will inevitably reflect cultural diversity and historical contingency, and may bear little resemblance to formal notions of therapy. Visitors to crisis houses often specifically prefer the informality of 'someone to talk to' (Faulkner et al., 2002).[34] The potential value of community development work has been recognised in relation to the emotional wellbeing ('mental health') of women and people from ethnic minorities, and should also be mentioned in relation to the heterogeneous and marginalised groups of men who use, or in some cases either don't manage or want to use, mental health services.

Inconclusion

For people experiencing crisis, immediate survival needs take precedence, and the speed and sensitivity of responses remains a paramount concern. Faced with acute wards that have become 'more custodial and drug dominated', the survivor movement continues to challenge dominant medicalising discourse that interprets any crisis as an onset of 'mental illness'. User-led community-orientated crisis houses are developing approaches that reframe crises as potential turning points from which recovery is possible (Campbell, 1998; Faulkner et al., 2002). The individual experiences of men who really have been in crisis might usefully inform political reflection and collective action towards recon-structing masculinities, a transformative process that could have consider-able potential benefits at both personal and cultural levels. Survivor activists, researchers, theorists and writers are well placed to build on existing work that points in this direction, and to negotiate what can often be highly sensitive as well as contradictory issues for individual men. At the time of writing, with an even more coercive legislative framework on the immediate horizon, driven largely by ill-conceived responses to the challenge posed by a small minority of men who are both distressed and threatening or violent, mutual crisis support is likely to go underground, with survivors providing refuge against the threat of sectioning and compulsory treatment in the community (Faulkner et al., 2002). In this context, well-informed discussion is needed about the position of 'men' as users and providers of services, advocacy and crisis support in relation to critical deconstructive understandings of masculinity and reconstructive initia-tives promoting cultural change in the direction of 'saner', safer, more holistic and politically reflexive masculinities.

The postmodern democratic impulse – to attend to diversity, accept ambigu-ity and contradiction, and forgo totalising explanatory frameworks, evident in the decolonising agendas of post-psychiatry, transcultural psychiatry, critical psychology, postmodern social work and similar paradigms for critical professional practice – will hopefully mitigate the impact of increased coercion, and improve the chances of services dealing with these concerns in a good-humoured and non-prescriptive spirit (Bracken and Thomas, 2001; Swartz, 1996; Pozatek, 1994; Timimi, 2005). In particular, treating accounts of experience as narrative fictions, stories that are always open to reconstruction and reinterpretation, rather than as repositories of data encoding universal 'truths' about pathology, could remove much of the tension around disclosure, and release a significant barrier that masculinist therapeutic discourse places around men's already guarded subjectivities. One of the themes that emerges clearly from the critical biographies, especially from the story of Antonin Artaud, is the importance of looking at recovery as a social and cultural, rather than predominantly psychological or medical process, and the importance of gender and masculinity in shaping the personal and social horizons envisaged by professionals and service-users/survivors. An absence of emotionally sustainable and nurturing communities among men, and the inability or unwillingness of many men to engage in mutual relationship, not only hurts women and children but effectively undermines such men's recovery.

Postmodern feminist critiques of reliance upon universalising and essentialist identity categories such as 'women' and 'men' are particularly helpful in this context. In environments where some men are extremely vulnerable, to the point of having only a fairly tenuous hold on life, it is vital that critiques of collective masculine power are handled carefully. While it is important to understand the continuing prevalence and effects of the violence and abuse enacted by a substantial minority of men against women and children, and the persistence of oppression and discrimination faced by women, care must be taken not to superimpose a second 'vocabulary of deficit' about men, over the already extensive vocabularies of deficit in place about 'the mentally ill', and other stigmatised groups (Gergen, 1991).[35] I have drawn attention to a broad agreement that pathologising violence works against the interests of both women and service-users/survivors, have questioned a tendency to appropriate the language of psychopathology for emancipatory ends, and am less interested in debates about adjusting diagnostic categories to encompass men's pain than in ongoing survivor critiques of medicalisation – which, as I understand it, challenge the hegemony of the medical model without precluding well-informed, and preferably self-managed, use of medication. Because men's distress can manifest in chauvinistic forms that produce hatred and rage, albeit sometimes combined with extreme vulnerability, there is clearly a need to challenge any importation into the 'mental health' field of hegemonic masculinist discourses, such as those claiming a 'crisis' or feminisation of masculinity, invoking crude biological essentialism, or demanding retaliatory men's rights.

Although many male writers have managed to combine postmodern aspirations with an inability to notice gender, our engagements with the construction of theory itself, and its translation into political or professional practice, are inevitably gendered. For me, one of the most striking themes to emerge from the critical biographical chapters is the inevitability that 'we' men address our fathers, as images of or lenses through which we see and respond to patriarchal power. How, we might ask, have public men come to construct a conception of theory, even in the helping professions, that so marginalises embodied notions such as hope, affection, humour, love, empathy, compassion or healing, that excludes reconstruction, recovery and matters of the heart as devalued terms within a mind–body binary? Unless we can rectify these troubling omissions, our theory may not be worth practising. Despite this caution I find it hard to resist ending on a triumphal, almost utopian note, but will do my best to remain pragmatic. I have been suggesting that the characteristic postmodern orientation, emphasising pluralism and difference – a willingness to engage with complexity, acknowledge undecideability, suspend prejudgement, work with the creative tension between incommensurable positions and so forth – might have a particularly constructive contribution to make in areas such as gender and 'mental health', where intense personal and political sensitivities arise, and where multiple interests converge. Such an approach offers the possibility of grounding an ethic of non-violence, co-operation, mutuality and care within a strong sense of the complexity of socially configured subject positions, subjectivities and consciousness, and could have significant implications in terms of social, cultural, political and professional practice. It is up to us to improvise on these themes. Unless we are able to bring such principles and intentions to bear, certain kinds of people and experiences, events and phenomena, are likely to remain unrecognised and politically unthinkable.

I have suggested, in particular, that critical postmodern perspectives offer a quite powerful set of insights into the philosophical foundations of both hegemonic masculinity and biomedical psychiatry. By combining postmodern and critical orientations 'we' can hopefully retain a sense of the open-ended play of difference and signification, of the wealth and diversity of human stories, while also conceptualising, and trying to do something about, persistent overarching patterns of social oppression. I have identified two interconnected themes in relation to men's experiences of distress or madness. Firstly there is a pervasive tension between various imperatives towards disclosure and towards self-protection. As the foregoing material demonstrates, this is not a simple single dynamic. Neither are the related sets of tensions between expressiveness and self-containment, emotion and reason, the Dionysian and Apollonian, as straightforward as over-arching critiques of masculinist modernity might seem to suggest. Secondly, I have drawn attention to the heterogeneity of men and masculinities, and in particular to problems posed by men's dual and often contradictory orientations and positionings in relation to discourses of gender-based domination and privilege. Both sets of issues necessitate local understandings and debates that will vary across time and between widely divergent communities of interest, and need to be approached accordingly.

I have also suggested that critical postmodern perspectives pose interesting questions about the dynamics of resistance and personal transformation, in terms of moving towards new forms of democratic pluralist/post-identity politics whose energy no longer derives from allegiance to monolithic collectives or moral binaries, and looks beyond simple reversals of an old order. But perhaps the most distinctive strength of these (and other similar) perspectives is their acknowledgement that we humans are not simple rational creatures, that the adventure of pluralism necessarily involves chaotic disagreement, within and between both individuals and communities. They offer the post-utopian promise that coalition and co-operation will survive our inevitable misunderstandings, mistakes and disagreements. My hope for this book is that it might prove helpful as a resource for those interested in developing new ways of thinking about and working with some fairly difficult and potentially intractable issues. I remain optimistic because of the example of many men who have survived personal crises and emerged with impressive generosity, compassion and political awareness.

Notes

1 Approaching the politics of complexity

1 Questions of language are pivotal to experiences of distress or madness, in diagnosis, in therapy and also in the politics of 'mental health'. Distress and madness have been adopted as alternatives to 'mental illness' in a political process prioritising self-determination and self-definition, comparable to that from which political definitions of 'impairment' and 'disability' have emerged. Such debates are inevitably open-ended and I expect my own use of language to evolve in response to new analyses of new situations (Church, 1995).

2 Church wrote as a former psychologist working with a movement whose members she describes as oppressed by the service system in which she worked. I had previously been in crisis, had not been a mental health professional, but of course am a man. Her account chronicles 'the collapse of the liberal humanist subject' as she experienced physical and emotional breakdown, for the first time, once she opened herself up to 'survivor pain' (Church, 1995).

3 Price and Shildrick also argue that they are directed to construct themselves as women by 'a disciplinary power that shapes being-in-the-world' from a position of privileged disembodiment, based upon assumptions about an idealised standard (healthy white heterosexual, male) body (Price and Shildrick, 1998).

4 Related, of course, to emotional injury, poverty, discrimination and difficulties with the psychiatric system. Although I had access to the social insulation of significant privilege allotted by gender, class, 'race' and sexual orientation, this may seem scant consolation when actually in crisis.

5 The term 'overwhelm' is borrowed from Breggin (1993). One effect of surviving a crisis 'underground' is that there can be very little public acknowledgement that anything at all has happened. This, although no doubt preferable to the experiences of many people who end up in hospital, reinforces an internalised cultural denial of experiences of distress. Helping someone close through their crises can also be intensely stressful, and result in feelings of bereavement.

6 The 'undecideable stranger . . . can no longer be included within philosophical (binary) opposition, resisting and disorganising it, *without ever* constituting a third term, without ever leaving room for a solution in the form of speculative dialectics' (Bauman, 1991 p. 55, citing Derrida, 1974).

7 One of the effects of this divide, which has so defined the institutional architecture of the 'mental health' field, has been to construct survivors' experience as a source of anecdotal colour, useful mainly for enlivening the serious analytic deliberations of 'neutral' experts (Campbell, 2001).

8 For Bly, soft men are sensitive and 'feminine', but lack vitality, ferocity and resolve, so need to discover an inner 'wild man' by severing ties with the mother and undergoing a process of initiation into the male-defined world of the father (1991). Whitehead argues that this account is based on a simplistic and deterministic Jungian model of male–female subjectivity, and assumptions about an inner core of masculinity (2002 pp. 157–8).

9 The idea of paths towards masculinisation comes from Liddle (1993). Sarup (1996) includes a series of autobiographical vignettes in *Identity, Culture and the Postmodern World*.

10 Standard critical works on men and masculinities lacked index references to madness, 'mental health', schizophrenia, depression, psychiatry, suicide, etc., and what little discussion there was tended not to engage with the 'politics of the madhouse'. Similarly, where the 'mental health' literature dealt with men's mental distress there was limited reference to feminist and pro-feminist critiques of masculinity. Miller and Bell's mapping exercise was an exception to this trend (Miller and Bell, 1996). Discussion of the interface between disablism/'mental health' oppression and masculinities also seemed quite limited.

11 The observation that because gender socialisation harms men, 'we' suffer too, tends to be given prominence at the expense of a sense of the costs of hegemonic power to women and to marginalised groups of men. One such article, for example, entitled 'Putting the Men into Mental Health', concluded that 'we do not necessarily see the men's movement as being in conflict with the women's movement, but we do think that Mind should begin to redress the balance' (Rodgers and Mathias, 1996).

12 For example, noting that aggressive behaviour might cause rather than be caused by testosterone (Clare, 2001). Young boys with very little testosterone can be aggressive, and there is evidence that testosterone is not significantly higher in men who are violent and abusive towards women. Females can be aggressive despite significantly lower testosterone levels (Whitehead and Barrett, 2001 p. 16; and see Edley and Wetherell, 1995).

13 Associated claims (about the feminisation of labour etc.) have been rebutted by reference to men's continuing social and material privilege, the persistence of traditional forms of masculinity, and the diversity, fluidity and political nature of masculinities (Whitehead and Barrett, 2001 pp. 16, 21, 8–10).

14 Busfield counters arguments that an exclusive focus on women is justified because of a previous concentration on men's experiences, or because men are positioned and regulated mainly through criminal justice discourse (Ussher, 1991; Chesler, 1972). Barnes and Maple have commented that understandings of the significance of gender for men's mental health were 'undeveloped if not non-existent', and that they would leave this for male colleagues (Barnes and Maple, 1992 p. 3).

15 Discussions of risk and dangerousness that barely mention gender include, on homicide, Taylor and Gunn (1999), and reviewing inquiry reports, Ward and Applin (1998); Parker and McCullogh (1999).

16 For example, an issue of *Sociology of Mental Health and Illness* (2000), devoted to the sociology of mental health, had no contributions from, and very little recognition of, the survivor movement as a source of understanding and theory.

17 On gender and medical professionalisation, see Witz (1992).

18 *National Service Framework* (Department of Health, 2000a). For some critical responses to both the content and the limitations of the 'user involvement' process entailed, see *OpenMind* no. 110, July/August, 2001.

19 A recent survey of psychiatric in-patients reported that many are getting only fifteen minutes' contact with staff per day in ward environments (Hunter, 2000).

20 The use of advance directives, crisis cards, support and advocacy networks or referral systems hopefully means that such men will become more likely to already be known to people running crisis houses. Statutory services may be uncomfortable about such services taking on 'self-referrers', about whom they hold no case notes, but new coercive legislation means that crisis support is more likely to go underground, exacerbating tensions around undecideable male strangers (Faulkner et al., 2000 pp. 51, 55).

21 In Madness and Civilisation Foucault's analysis of the patriarchal authority of the asylum doctor is a striking but secondary theme. Like Foucault, Hillman interpreted Pinel's celebrated removal of asylum inmates' chains as a prelude to further oppression, arguing that 'psychic phenomena still await their liberation from the subtler chains of psychological language' (Hillman, 1972 p. 164). Foucault had written that 'the dialogue of delirium and insult gave way to a monologue in a language that exhausted itself in the silence of others' (Foucault, 1961/1971 p. 261). In talking about the need for liberation from the lap of the mother, however, Hillman was also paving the way for Bly (1991, pp. 15–17).

22 Chesler demanded reparation for women whose abuse had been compounded by hospitalisation. Women, she argued, were being 'punitively labelled, overly tranquillised, sexually seduced while in treatment, hospitalised against their will, given shock therapy, lobotomised, and above all disliked' by mental health professionals (Chesler, 1990 p. 314).

23 Chesler noted that, for men, 'incorporation into the Oedipal father is purchased at great emotional expense', that male 'policing' of other men is 'rooted in an anguish of power', and cited a study in which men diagnosed as schizophrenic were described as giving 'female' responses (McClelland and Watt, 1968). The eagerness of her male colleagues to claim that sexism hurt men, however, seems to have foreclosed discussion of men's experiences of distress (Chesler, 1972 pp. 248, 276–7).

24 Including grief, loss and healing; or female identity and premature separation.

25 Given the recent neo-colonial devastation of modern Iraq, questions about Western appropriations of Sumerian mythology now arise more forcefully.

26 During a subsequent process of patriarchal appropriation Enki appears to have undergone the familiar metamorphosis from son/consort to father god, illustrating the alchemy of cultural construction (Baring and Cashford, 1991).

27 There are some versions, however, in which a goddess searches for her sacrificed son-lover in the underworld, and in a striking reversal of the imagery of Sleeping Beauty, finds him asleep, and eventually wakens him.

28 Hearn redefines domestic violence as 'men's violences to known women', and notes that such violence constitutes a 'kind of legitimated taboo' (Hearn, 1998 p. vii).

29 For instance, Bly distinguishes between grief, as voluntary descent, and depression, in which we resist but are somehow pulled under, and concludes that a lack of initiatory teaching may lead 'some power in the psyche' to arrange a severe katabasis (or 'drop') for us (Bly, 1991 p. 70). Women, however, reportedly experience 'depression' about twice as much as men, a prevalence that would be difficult to explain in terms of resistance to grieving, since feminist accounts have attributed it to being in 'a continual state of mourning' for suppressed power (Nairne and Smith, 1984 p. 178).

30 Though the snake was once revered as a symbol of death and rebirth, or of the phallus as adjunct to a female deity, Kerenyi in his discussion of the mythological motif of incest, interprets its image as 'eminently suited to a male, a son and husband, who forces his way uninterruptedly down through the generations of mothers and daughters – the generations of living beings – and so discloses his continuity, just as zoë does' (Goodison, 1990; Kerenyi, 1976 p. 114).

31 Like the empathetic Enki, he is bisexual, and teaches us about heterosexism. Representations of him as a child symbolise the value of retaining a childlike sense

of 'both/and', as a way of overcoming 'the male habit' of constantly seeing things in terms of winning or losing, right or wrong, true or false (Rowan, 1997 p. 259).

32 Goodison argues that the men paid the price for creating a culture of domination in terms of 'loss of the body, the learning of shame about sexual feelings, and hatred for the woman who arouses those feelings' (Goodison, 1990 p. 164).

33 Whitmont describes helping a woman who heard voices telling her to dismember her child, but goes on to argue that only a prudery comparable to Victorian attitudes towards sex prevents us from acknowledging that violence is 'one of mankind's most profoundly moving experiences' (Whitmont, 1982/1997 p. 17).

2 Why postmodernism? Conceptualising the politics of complexity

1 Lyotard introduced the term 'postmodern condition' to refer to a configuration of technological, economic and social changes characterising contemporary life, and used 'postmodernism' to identify a 'sensibility' or set of responses to this changing condition, notably involving an opposition to totalising theory in any field (Lyotard. 1984). Since both power and resistance assume postmodern forms, no particular political position is implied (Brown, 1995).

2 Some authors often cited as postmodern balk at defining their work in that way. Haraway, for instance, agrees that 'something is going on in the world vastly different from the constitutional arrangements that established the separations of nature and society proper to "modernity"', but resists naming it (Haraway, 1997 pp. 42–3). Brown is reluctant to concede 'the existence of a doctrine or school of thought often more usefully called into question as such', so tends to use 'late modernity' (Brown, 1995 p. 30). Others, such as Foucault, Hall, Bordo and Weedon, prefer post-structuralism, a tradition emphasising the constitutive function of language in social institutions, political processes and the formation of subjectivity, and challenging the belief that phenomena such as society or the human mind can be explained in terms of deep underlying structures.

3 Advocates of critical realism, for example, see the difficulty of Bhaskar's texts as an obstacle (Collier, 1994). bell hooks stresses the importance of abandoning essentialist notions of 'race', but notes the exclusive style of much postmodern writing (cited in Weedon, 1999 p. 171). Best and Kellner suggest that postmodern theory has functioned in the interests of intellectuals needing to position themselves as avant-garde (1991 p. 297). Parker et al. use Foucault extensively but admit that his termi-nology can be 'exceedingly difficult to understand', while Geerz likens his work to an Escher drawing (Parker et al., 1995 p. 131; Dreyfus and Rabinow, 1982 p. xiv).

4 Professor Adrian Raine, in The Science of Crime, Equinox, Channel Four, 7 December 2000. Rose cites an earlier documentary in which Raine claimed that two PET scan images demonstrated an innate difference between a 'normal' brain and that of a murderer (Rose, 1997 p. 290).

5 On a new 'Mental Health Act from Hell', impending at the time of writing, see 'Mad Pride' Website, (www/ctono.freeserve.co.uk/index.htm – accessed 12 December 1999) and Plumb (1999). Similar proposals provoked the first psychiatric survivor demonstration in the UK in 1988.

6 Giddens comments that, although the progenitors of modern thought expected to establish secure foundations for knowledge, the reflexivity of modernity, a constant process of doubt and revision in the light of new information, has actually under-mined the establishment of certainty, even in the natural sciences (Giddens, 1991).

7 We should avoid slipping into an essentialising and utopian view of postmodern ten-dencies as wholly desirable, and remind ourselves that postmodernity is ambivalent,

tense, provisional and contradictory. Re-enchantment may awaken demons and ghosts as well as ancestors and angels. Acceptance of mystery might open up spaces for poetic and metaphorical understandings of experience, but can shade into flight from the effort of analysis and engagement with scientific discourse. Ironic detachment might take the heat out of conflict and help us come to terms with difference, but can lead to indifference towards social oppression (Bauman, 1991).

8 Rabinow argues, however, that the alleged collapse of metanarratives, big stories about smaller ones, has simply not happened in key fields such as technoscience or transnational capitalism (cited by Haraway, 1997 p. 42). The persistence of pre-modern religious grand narratives also needs to be accounted for.

9 Although social class remains an important consideration, much has been suppressed in the universalising notion of class struggle (Spivak, in Harasym, 1990; Nicholson and Seidman, 1995; Hall, 1992; Brah, 1996). There has been debate over whether the postmodern preoccupation with diversity and deconstruction puts the emancipatory gains of modernity at risk by dissolving consensus, eroding commitment to universal provision, and even rendering politics impossible (Harasym, 1990). Critics also identify an unwillingness to move beyond analysis of what is wrong (Nicholson and Seidman, 1995 pp. 8–9).

10 Many theorists integrate elements from critical and poststructuralist or postmodern perspectives, and some use the term 'critical postmodern' (Warren, 1988; Jackson, 1990; Pease 1999, 2000).

11 Bhaskar nonetheless finds substantial areas of agreement with Rorty (1989 pp. 155–7). Although critical realism is favoured by some commentators on the 'mental health' field (Busfield, 1996; Pilgrim and Rogers, 1997), I prefer critical postmodernism, mainly because of its stronger suspicion of knowledge claims about structure, causation, truth and reality.

12 See also Laclau and Mouffe (1985 p. 108), who remind us that Wittgenstein's language games included 'actions', and talk about 'the material character of every discursive structure'.

13 Raymond Williams uses 'structure of feeling' to identify a collective subject which unites the individual and social without reducing either to the terms of the other, and expresses a significant community, or way of seeing, being and acting in the world (Williams, 1965, 1980).

14 Henry Oldenburg, the first secretary of the Royal Society, even exhorted his members to 'root out the woman in us' (Roszak, 2000 p. 56).

15 Like the atom, whose name means 'that which cannot be divided', this 'separative self' is said to be internally solid, admitting of no unconscious or irrational dynamics. The notion of a 'monadic' individual became a core assumption of Enlightenment thought, but by the late nineteenth century the classical Newtonian atom was shown to have been a fiction. The 'indivisible' building block of matter opened out to reveal an exquisite internal architecture enfolding ever smaller and stranger particles. Roszak describes this growing sense of the 'depth, complexity and organic subtlety of nature', and the consequent realisation that we live among 'patterns that interlock to infinity', as 'ethically wrenching' (Roszak, 2000 pp. 51, 55–6, 151, citing Keller, 1986).

16 These include 'mind–body' problems, problems of reference and truth, of other minds, and scepticism about knowledge of the external world. Scheman argues that these problems will remain unsolvable so long as the subject's identity is constituted by such estrangements.

17 The master identifies with the eternal order of the mind, and despises the bodily and manual sphere of compulsion, represented by the slave, the woman and the animal (Plumwood, 1993 p. 97).

18 The distinction is repeated in various accounts of Dionysos cited by Hillman, for whom the presence of the archetypal is what gives madness meaning (1972 p. 273).

3 Genealogy and biography: how we become who we are

1 Artaud has been celebrated as a forerunner of the survivor movement, but also dismissed as 'the residue of psychosis curated by the comfortable' (Curtis et al., 2000 pp. 8, 112).
2 Connell draws on Gramsci to define hegemonic masculinity as 'the masculinity that occupies the hegemonic position in a given pattern of gender relations', and as a 'configuration of gender practice' that currently best legitimises patriarchy. The cultural dynamic by which this leading position is maintained will include strategic concessions in response to challenges (Connell, 1987, 1995 pp. 76–7).
3 Allison notes that two post-mortem examinations failed to identify any syphilitic infection, but says that the course of his illness was consistent with such a cause (Allison, 2001 p. 251, note 13). Hayman discusses the problems in interpreting the evidence, and concludes that Nietzsche's 'delusions of grandeur' and breakdown were unlikely to have been associated with syphilis (Hayman, 1997). Porter finds no convincing proof that growing paralysis was a long-term effect of syphilis but points out that 'Nietzsche himself seems to have given this view currency', and argues for 'a largely psychogenic impetus' for the descent into insanity (1987 p. 137).
4 The title Ecce Homo, 'Behold the Man', are the words of Pilate presenting Christ in a crown of thorns before his crucifixion. Nietzsche catalogues the detail of his bodily ailments, and prepares for immortality through his works (Lionnet, 1989 pp. 80–1). Particularly in England and America, Nietzsche's entire philosophical output was often dismissed retrospectively as the product of an insane mind (Gilman, 1987).
5 Flax argues that epistemology should be reconceived as genealogy, and 'the study of the social and unconscious relations of the production of knowledge', thus introducing the notion of unconscious processes into genealogical enquiry (Flax, 1992 p. 457).
6 Similarly Eribon asserts that although Foucault repeatedly challenged the conventional notion of an author, he did function as one, not just by producing a powerful body of writing but by 'playing the commentary game' (Eribon, 1991 p. ix).
7 Against this we might set the vigour of popular art forms such as carnival, and the transformative, critical and emancipatory potential of art, not least for some survivors.

4 Behold in me the tyrant of Turin! Nietzsche, madness and postmodernism

1 That Nietzsche has become the most widely read philosopher in the Western world (Rosen, 1989), and that his aristocratic philosophy has exerted such an influence on progressive critics, have been sources of amazement and alarm to various commentators (Ansell-Pearson, 1993 pp. 27–8).
2 Allison argues that the association between Nietzsche and National Socialism stems from the activities of his sister, Elizabeth Forster-Nietzsche, who married a leading anti-Semite, adopted an ideology of racial purity, and posthumously edited and published various notes and drafts as The Will to Power. Having previously forged and altered letters, she ignored extensive material in which Nietzsche expressed 'toleration, even praise, of racial and ethnic equality, political internationalism, and cultural diversity' (Allison, 2001 pp. 2–3, 250; Kaufmann, 1950/1974 pp. 42–5).

3 At the age of thirty-four, Nietzsche's health deteriorated to the point where he resigned his professorship and became 'incapacitated for normal social life'. Two years later he wrote 'Five times I invoked death as my only physician. I hoped that yesterday would be my last day – hoped in vain' (Larvin, 1971 pp. 31–2, 40–1, 50; see also Hollingdale, 1965/1999 p. 115).

4 Ronald Laing and David Cooper were two of the leading figures in the anti-psychiatry movement of the 1960s.

5 e.g. Hollingdale (1965/1999); Allison (1977/1985); Sedgwick (1995).

6 The worryingly myopic Nietzsche made acquaintance with a boy from another fraternity for the express purpose of asking him 'in the politest way' for a duel.

> Nietzsche's opponent managed to cut in low *carte* at the bridge of his nose. . . . Within two or three days our hero fully recovered except for a small slanting scar . . . which remained there throughout his life and did not look at all bad on him.
>
> (Deussen, cited in Hayman, 1980 p. 62)

7 In *Zarathustra* we find: 'Men shall be trained for war, and women for the recreation of the warrior; all else is folly' (Nietzsche, 1887/1969 p. 51). At the end of his creative life, he reflects on bitter personal frustration, referring to 'the eternal war between the sexes' and bristling at the notion of love, 'in its methods war, in its foundation the mortal hatred of the sexes' (1888/1979 p. 46).

8 See Schrift on the need for a democratic *agon* (Schrift, 2000). Said applies Nietzsche's 'mobile army of metaphors' in relation to Orientalism (Said, 1978).

9 Reich made a similar case, that the masses *wanted* fascism. Deleuze and Guattari incorporated this with Nietzsche's account of the will, concluding that unless the social field allows for desire to be productive in non-repressive forms, it will produce in whatever forms are available to it (Schrift 1995 p. 269).

10 Feminism here referred to 'the development of female characteristics in a man' (feminisation). Nietzsche set feminismus, denoting 'weakness, cowardice, mendacity, and "rule of feeling"', against self-overcoming (Stringer, 2000 p. 259).

11 In *Zarathustra*, for example, Nietzsche confronts his prophet-like protagonist with the 'temptation' of a 'great cry of distress', that has to be resisted as 'a seduction against allegiance to himself' (Nietzsche, 1887/1969 p. 14).

12 From a letter to his closest long-term friend, Franz Overbeck, written on Christmas Day, 1882. Attempts to find a wife for him had failed, and at the age of thirty-seven he had fallen for, and proposed marriage to, the twenty-one-year-old Lou Salomé. Allison describes this as 'his only real love'. Another friend, Paul Rée, also proposed to her, and was rebuffed. The three discussed forming a Platonic ménage à trois and studying together, but Lou eventually left with Rée. Nietzsche's family was scandalised, and he was ostracised from Wagner's circle (See Allison, 2001 pp. xiii, 113–14, 157, 289 and Warner, 1986.)

13 In this latter sense hardness refers to the independence of mind needed to assert difference, and resist convention. His critique challenged those needing metaphysics as a prop, or for whom the 'impetuous demand for certainty . . . discharges itself . . . in a scientific-positivistic form'. Paradoxically, such demands for conceptual 'firmness' demonstrate a conformist 'instinct of weakness' (Allison, 2001 p. 102).

14 Hollingdale moves from speculation upon the psychosomatic origins of Nietzsche's health problems to suggest that in desiring what harmed him, he became what he himself would describe as 'decadent' and what 'we should . . . speak of as "neurotic"', during the 1870s (Hollingdale, 1965/1999 p. 86).

15 Meta von Salis-Marschlins, poet and women's rights advocate, who obtained a PhD and wrote a book on Nietzsche, noted that he would often tell her about women who had distinguished themselves in their field. (See Gilman, 1987 pp. 159, 199–200.)

16 See also Irigaray (1991); Ansell-Pearson (1993); Gane (1993).

17 Hollingdale includes an extract from the fourteen-year-old Nietzsche's account of his childhood grief (1965/1999 p. 9). In *Ecce Homo*, Nietzsche claimed that his debility started on his thirty-sixth birthday – the age at which his father had died – and wrote 'I am merely my father once more, and as it were, the continuation of his life after an all too early death' (Nietzsche, 1888/1979 p. 14). Lionnet points out that the dates are inaccurate, but constitute a mythic identification with his father, which the autobiography completes by immortalising his work (Lionnet, 1989 pp. 75–6). The legacy of the death may be traceable in Nietzsche's emotionally intense relationship with Wagner, who was born in the same year as his father, and played a 'quasi-paternal' role. This moved through adulation, conflict and finally rejection, and when Wagner died, Nietzsche responded by becoming violently ill, and separating the 'good' from the 'bad' Wagner. He even had unrealisable 'oedipal' feelings for Cosima Wagner (Hollingdale, 1965/1999 p. 213; Kaufmann, 1954 pp. 33–5). His father's death might also have coloured the elusive figure of the 'overman', who embodies unattained human potential, and in whose *absence* the prophetic and oracular Zarathustra must speak. Allison describes Zarathustra as 'a figure of exceptional character, generosity, and independence: full of self-esteem and at once remote and isolated, yet again compassionate, seeking to help with a missionary zeal'. At one point Nietzsche writes 'God died; now we want the overman to live' (Allison, 2001 pp. 117–19).

18 Kaufmann describes him 'condemned' to live in the 'intolerable situation' of a fatherless household, 'alone' with five women (1954 p. 33). The fathers of two friends took an active interest in his education however.

19 The young Nietzsche was intensely homesick at first, but soon conformed to the 'sadistic authoritarianism', winning approval for good behaviour (Hayman, 1980 pp. 28–9). There is limited detail on this, but Jackson's discussion of institutionalised violence in a boys' boarding school in the 1950s shows how such regimes police the norms of hegemonic masculinity (Jackson, 1990).

20 For Tacey the demise of the practice of fathers introducing sons into the traditions of a patriarchal public world marks a fundamental difference between pre- and postmodern times (Tacey, 1997 p. 44).

21 In one recent study nearly all the male respondents described their fathers as 'absent' and 'emotionally distant'. Many influential books on masculinities compound the problem by ignoring fatherhood, or treating it only briefly (Lupton and Barclay, 1997 pp. 144, 3).

22 Clare cites studies claiming that sons of absent fathers have difficulty controlling aggressive and impulsive behaviour, are more likely to fail at school, to have emotional or behavioural difficulties that bring them to psychiatry, or to develop addictions (Clare, 2001 pp. 167, 175).

23 Frosh comments on the irony that proof of paternity then relied on the *word* of the woman (1994 p. 72).

24 Nietzsche outlined the 'double gesture', firstly overturning a binary hierarchy, then interrupting and moving beyond the binary system itself, which Derrida developed with the notion of 'deconstruction'.

25 Gane (1993) cites Warner (1986) on the importance of biographical contingencies in the work of social theorists.

26 See also Seidler, who writes that it took him years to recognise the anger he felt about the early childhood experience of the death of his father, and that blocking this

anger had blocked a process of grieving that was already inhibited by the masculine injunction to 'be strong'. He had, at some level, felt responsible for the death, had felt he had to prove himself to the lost father, and had withdrawn into an inner life of thought (Seidler, 1997 pp. 158–60).

27 Warren argues that Nietzsche 'shows how subjects are possible as historical achievements', and has a detailed discussion of 'will to power' as a nuanced understanding of human agency (Warren, 1988 pp. 126ff.).

28 Allison sees this as Nietzsche's way of establishing a meta-critique of values and beliefs, comparable with Descartes's 'evil demon'. *Human, All Too Human* (1878) is dedicated to these spirits (2001 p. 175).

29 In one of the decisive letters he pushed the notion, and perhaps the experience, of self-dissolution to godlike proportions, declaring: 'the unpleasant thing, which offends my modesty, is that fundamentally I am every name in history'. His old friend Overbeck arrived just in time to prevent the landlord calling the police, and 'they threw themselves into each other's arms and burst into tears. Nietzsche, especially, broke into a convulsive trembling and groaning.' Given a bromide, he calmed down, and playing the piano very softly, 'spoke of himself as the successor to the dead god'. As the calmative wore off he resumed his 'clowning', 'leaping about, dancing, shouting, gesturing obscenely'. Overbeck wrote that 'so far' he was 'quite harmless – in many ways like a child . . . not at all dangerous' (Hayman, 1980 pp. 334–7).

30 A dentist 'experienced in handling the insane' devised the ruse to persuade Nietzsche to travel, and when he wanted to address the crowds at Turin station, 'convinced him that he was too eminent not to travel incognito' (Hayman, 1980 pp. 336–7). Overbeck was so shocked by these developments that he felt 'it would have been a far more genuine act of friendship' to have taken Nietzsche's life than to have handed him over to an asylum (Hollingdale, 1965/1999 p. 239).

31 Heidegger argues that *Ecce Homo* is not an autobiography, and that 'if anything culminates in it, it would be the final moment of the West, in the history of the era of modernity'. Nietzsche is 'the carrier' of the destiny of the West (Derrida, 1995 p. 60).

32 See Gilman (1987 pp. 167, 205–6). Hollingdale argues that all the published works of 1888 (his forty-fourth year) are coherent and well organised (1965/1999 p. 199).

33 Similarly, when, in the clinic at Basel, Nietzsche apologised for the bad weather – 'For you, good people, I shall prepare the loveliest weather tomorrow' – the possibility that this could be humour, self-mockery or bitter irony, rather than literal 'madness', is not entertained. Hollingdale (and others) reports that a conversation with his mother about family matters, was interrupted when he 'suddenly cried: Behold in me the Tyrant of Turin!' Again there is no sense that Nietzsche might have been protesting about having been deemed 'mad' for trying to protect a cart horse, and making too much noise in his lodgings (Hollingdale, 1965/1999 p. 239). Hayman tells us that, on his arrival at the asylum in Jena, Nietzsche 'strode majestically into the room, thanking the attendants for "the magnificent reception"', but overlooks the possibility that this could have been an ironic reference to the promise of a grand reception, used to lure him away from Turin (1980 p. 339).

34 By this time Nietzsche had mentally completely withdrawn from the world, and seemed unaware of her death. A maid then cared for him until he died, after a stroke, on 24 August 1900, seven weeks before his fifty-sixth birthday.

35 For Nietzsche, 'the will to power and life . . . presupposes that one's drives and passions are given free play. The real test of a man's maturity therefore, consists in finding again the seriousness one had as a child at play' (Zeitlin, 1994 p. 40).

36 Nietzsche says little about Apollo as patron of music in order to emphasise the difference with Dionysos (Allison, 2001 p. 24). Neither does he mention that Apollo's arrows could bring disease and death, as when seizing oracle at Delphi (Goodison, 1990 p. 158).

37 Nietzsche felt that tragedy would be reborn when science had been 'pushed to its limits' and 'forced to renounce its claim to universal validity' (Nietzsche, 1871/ 1956 p. 104).

38 In 2001 a memorial was finally established to 306 British soldiers 'judicially murdered' by their own side during the First World War. Most would have been suffering from 'shell shock', or were young men who would now be thought of as having learning impairments. The memorial takes the form of a statue of a blindfolded teenage soldier, surrounded by a semi-circle of stakes bearing the names of the other victims, arranged in the format of a chorus from Greek tragedy (Sengupta, 2001).

39 In his late preface, Nietzsche suggests that the Socratic rational mind is merely a flight into the 'softness' of optimism, 'a clever bulwark against truth', and the product of a waning and weakened culture (Nietzsche, 1871/1956 pp. 4–5, 8–9).

40 In *Ecce Homo* he described *Human, All Too Human* (1878) as 'a monument to rigorous self-discipline' in which he put an end to 'all my infections with "idealism", "beautiful feelings", and other effeminacies', and linked the Dionysian destruction with pronouncements about the need for 'a party of life' to eradicate all that is parasitical and degenerate (Sadler, 1995 p. 139; Safranski, 2002 pp. 268–9).

41 As dragon-slayer Apollo appropriated the oracle of the earth goddess, and took control of prophecy for a new patriarchal order (Baring and Cashford, 1991; Goodison, 1990). He also symbolised a tendency in Greek culture to deny the role of mothers in generation (Gane, 1993, citing Irigaray, 1991).

42 Some men try to compensate for the powerlessness of being labelled 'mad' by exploiting the expectations and prejudices of gender privilege. On his arrival at the clinic a doctor wrote of Nietzsche that he 'claims to be a famous man and asks for women all the time' (Hayman, 1980 p. 337).

5 The scream of life itself? Language and power in the life of Antonin Artaud

1 Foucault's later view was that the notion of a deep meaning behind appearances is an important mythic construction in modern power/knowledge (Dreyfus and Rabinow, 1982 p. 12).

2 'La Parole Soufflée' means 'the word spirited away', or 'stolen'. The term 'exemplar' can refer either to a model – to be emulated or copied – or a typical instance, but both kinds of 'case' might reduce experience in the service of various explanatory discourses.

3 Nietzsche died when he was fifty-six years old, Artaud when he was fifty-one.

4 Some of his intimate relationships became turbulent, however. Anais Nin, who was a friend, reported becoming frightened when he said 'What a divine joy it would be to crucify a being like you, who are so evanescent, so elusive', and 'Between us, there could be a murder' (Barber, 1993 p. 64).

5 In a five-year relationship with Génica Athanasiou, Artaud would alternate between 'violent rage and abjectly apologetic professions of need', echoing his relationship with his mother. In 1925 he writes that he 'needs a woman who belongs exclusively to him and who can always be found at home – a woman who will devote her life to looking after him. She need not be very pretty or intelligent' (Hayman, 1977 pp. 38, 60).

6 e.g. Esslin (1976 p. 116). Artaud claimed to be reintroducing 'an idea of the sacred theatre not despite but thanks to the eviction of God and the destruction of the theatre's theological machinery' (Derrida, 1967/1978 p. 243). Nietzsche foresaw the possible emergence of a 'divine way of thinking' from the intellectual tradition he helped form (Berry and Wernick, 1992 p. 3; Jantzen, 1998 p. 13).

7 Artaud's familiarity with the Gnostics, his interest in acupuncture and non-Western mystical traditions, his experimentation with drugs, and his pioneering ideas on the theatre (the use of 'pile-driving or unbearably piercing' sound, 'brilliant' lighting, etc.) make him a precursor of the counter-culture of the 1960s and beyond (Artaud, 1938/1970).

8 See Artaud (1938/1970 pp. 22, 58, 65, 22).

9 After his own last performance, Artaud, who by then had much to be furious about, wrote:

> I left because I realised that the only
> language I could use on the audience was to
> take bombs out of my pocket and throw them
> in their faces in a gesture of unmistakable aggression.
>
> (Dale, 1997 p. 590)

10 An actress, Paule Thévenin, wrote: 'He gave me exercises to do . . . I learned to scream, to sustain the cry to the point of annihilation, to move from falsetto to a lower pitch, to prolong a syllable till breath was totally spent' (cited in Hayman, 1977 p. 100).

11 Although Artaud insistently opposed the God-like dominion of the author, he demanded absolute directorial control of his 'total theatre'.

> I propose to treat the audience just like those charmed snakes and to bring them back to the subtlest ideas through their anatomies . . . the secret is to irritate those pressure points as if the muscles were flayed . . . the rest is achieved by screams.
>
> (Artaud, 1938/1970 pp. 61–2)

During this period Artaud was undergoing detoxification treatment for opiate addiction. It never seemed to occur to him that other people might have quite different needs. Many people experiencing distress or madness will need to proceed gently, and avoid 'dramatic confrontations of life experiences or deep emotions' (Plumb, 1999 p. 472).

12 Both his playlet The Spurt of Blood, and John Ford's Tis Pity She's a Whore, which he regarded highly, deal with brother–sister incest. The Cenci describes the rape of a daughter by her father, who is then murdered (Artaud, 1938/1970 pp. 19–20: Esslin, 1976 p. 100). Heliogabalus, or the Crowned Anarchist includes incest between the Emperor and his mother (Hayman, 1977 p. 93). Note that Kristeva cites Artaud when writing about the semiotic, and links poetic language to the theme of incest (Kristeva, 1977/1980 pp. 133, 136). The plays also contain much potentially lurid violence. Artaud moved from an early celebration of and curiosity about sexuality to outright renunciation, to the point of elaborating a mythology in which man (sic) had been created by God without sexual or digestive organs, but had degenerated into a sexual and defecating being through the intervention of malign extraterrestrial forces (Esslin, 1976).

13 When he was eight years old the death of an infant sister, Germaine, seems to have been even more troubling. Hayman suggests that he must have wondered whether his

mother, who overwhelmed him alternately with affection and with rage, was a source of life, or death (1980 pp. 37–8).

14 Artaud's father, a prosperous shipping agent, was often away from home (Barber, 1993 p. 14).

15 But emphatically opposed the Surrealists' surrender to unconscious processes. Far from being a theatre of the unconscious, the Theatre of Cruelty was about 'the application of consciousness', about 'exposed lucidity' (Derrida, 1967/1978).

16 Breton also became a father-like figure, their friendship persisting despite his 'often brutal, and patronising insensitivity' towards Artaud. Later he was one of the few people who gave Artaud money and food when he most needed it (Barber, 1993 pp. 22, 86).

17 Near the end of his life, in a 1946 introduction to the *Collected Works*, Artaud even makes characteristically graphic use of the metaphor of hammering. 'If I drive in a violent word like a nail, I want it to suppurate in the sentence like a hundred holed ecchymosis' (Atteberry, 2000 p. 722).

18 Although as early as 1925 Artaud had edited an edition of *La Révolution Surréaliste* in which he published five open letters to public figures, including the Pope ('We are thinking of another war on you Pope, Pope, dog') and the Dalai Lama. This gesture was reminiscent of the 'mad' Nietzsche in content as well as style, in that he displayed 'a yearning for the destruction of the Western world, and the creation of a new, liberated flesh' (Barber, 1993 p. 25).

19 The strange and extreme imagery of the piece, not least an exposition of the notion of a 'Body Without Organs', is, once again, best understood in relation to biographical experience. When offered the services of the best radio producer in Paris, he insisted upon the worst, in order to ensure minimal interference. Barber finds the resulting work 'ferociously funny' (see Barber, 1993 pp. 151–5).

20 The literary editor Rivière used a rhetoric of healing in his correspondence with Artaud, straining to empathise, console and reassure. Atteberry discusses the complicity of the literary community in the social exclusion and medicalisation of Artaud (Atteberry, 2000).

21 Although Foucault is not criticised here, Derrida confronts his mentor's discussion of madness and the work in 'Cogito and the History of Madness' (Derrida, 1967/1978 pp. 170, 31ff.).

22 Pireddu notes that in 'La Parole Soufflée' Derrida alludes to Lacan without explicitly mentioning him. The reference to parricide comes in 'The Theatre of Cruelty', where he notes Artaud's statement 'For even the infinite is dead, / infinite is the name of a dead man / who is not dead', adding 'It is not the living God, but the death-God that we should fear' (Derrida, 1967/1978 p. 246). Lacan's 'Name of the Father' has been likened to the dead 'father of individual prehistory' invoked by Freud in *Totem and Taboo*, whose authority is never so strong as in his absence (Grosz, 1990 p. 68).

23 Lacan was extending Freud's Oedipal theory, which states that the price of eventual accession to power, for a boy, is that he must appease a jealous father by renouncing desire for his mother, along with any affinity with the 'feminine'. As he makes this transition, the structuring power of patriarchy wrenches him away from the 'imaginary', and aligns him with the symbols and codes of power. He must then engage in a continuing struggle to 'have' the 'phallus' (Lacan's term for a defining cultural symbol of patriarchal authority, the 'universal signifier' that stabilises the otherwise ceaseless play of language), and avoid the continuing threat of metaphorical 'castration' (Frosh, 1999 pp. 219–25, 1994 pp. 85, 111–12). The 'normal' subject achieves this by replacing desire for the mother with this paternal signifier, the 'Name' or function of the Law prohibiting that desire. The 'psychotic', however, fails to assimilate the paternal symbolic law, and fills the space left by the foreclosed signifier with a

'cascade of reshapings of the signifier, from which the increasing disaster of the imaginary proceeds'. Rather than being integrated, foreclosed signifiers are said to be projected externally (Pireddu, 1996 p. 51).

24 Feminist critics argue that an in-built phallocentrism and universalism limit the relevance of Lacan's work when attempting to envisage subjectivity in non-patriarchal environments (Urwin, 1984/1998). His appeal to the supposedly universal structure of language masks historically variable relations of domination and, in particular, the social context that gives possession of a penis/phallus such charged significance (Flax, 1990 pp. 90–107). Lacan concludes that women can neither be the subjects of desire nor speak for themselves. Jantzen comments 'the problem is not that women do not/cannot have language, but that men, Lacan foremost amongst them, refuse to listen' (Jantzen, 1998 p. 51–3).

25 Lacan influenced the post-1968 French left, and anti-psychiatry's celebration of the language of madness. From postmodern perspectives, any use of his ideas would entail rescuing them from a strongly scientistic and universalising tendency in his work, e.g. an assumption that language is universally structured.

26 The Oedipal story revolves around castration and penis envy, and 'hinges on the idea of sexual difference', which produces gender-differentiated subjectivities associated with active and passive sexual desire (Hollway, 1996 p. 95). Masson has argued that in relation to women's experience, Freud's mis-interpretation of memories of sexual abuse as 'imaginings', understood in terms of the 'Oedipal complex', has had particularly devastating effects (Masson, 1984/1992, 1992b p. 15). While psychoanalytic accounts of the Oedipal drama were being criticised for overlooking the earlier formative relationship between the child and its mother, most commentators were still ignoring the emotional consequences of fatherhood (Flax, 1990; Lupton and Barclay, 1997). Because Freud posited a narcissistic state, in which the young child constructs a same-sex love object based on the self, and said that homosexual desire would 'normally' be repressed in the process of emerging from the Oedipal struggle, some analysts continued to reduce homosexuality to a pathology of 'narcissism'. This may explain Allendy's conclusion that Artaud was 'a dangerous homosexual drug addict' (Barber, 1993 p. 59). Even if the Oedipus story were unproblematical, evocations of the 'depths' of early biographical experience would be insufficient as an account of men's habitual disavowal of vulnerability.

27 See Chapter 7 below on the Schreber 'case'. Berger likened psychoanalysis to religious conversion, insofar as it provides 'a method of ordering the discrepant fragments of biography in a meaningful scheme'. Whilst actually being inducted into a socially constructed meaning system, the patient comes to believe he [sic] is 'discovering' truths about himself (Berger, 1963 pp. 76–9).

28 Even Masson values many of Freud's theoretical contributions, e.g. 'the reality of the unconscious', and certain psychological devices that protect us from emotional pain (transference, resistance, repression), the importance of trauma and of early childhood experiences, the need to repeat early sorrows, and the significance of dreams, though he rejects their translation into therapeutic devices (Masson, 1984/1992 p. 189, 1992b pp. 15–16).

29 Although The Theatre and Its Double had recently been published, Artaud was described as having 'literary pretensions, which are perhaps justified to the extent to which the delirium may serve as an inspiration'. Barber notes various parallels between the writings of Artaud and Lacan, who had also been active in the Surrealist movement, and also published material that notoriously resisted the reader. Artaud's close friend, Roger Blin, went to see Lacan, who told him 'that Artaud's case did not interest him, that Artaud was "fixed", [and wrongly] that he would live to be eighty, but would never write another line'. Artaud reported being held in solitary confine-

ment there, being silenced and poisoned. He was put in a straitjacket once again for the journey to the next asylum (Ville Evrard), and repeatedly claimed that one of the male nurses kicked him in the testicles during the journey (Barber, 1993 pp. 9, 99–100).

30 By 1938/9 Lacan had written a doctoral thesis on paranoia and developed his concept of the mirror stage, but he did not discuss the importance of the symbolic until the 1950s. In *Ecrits* (1966/1977), Lacan wrote 'Man's being cannot be understood without reference to madness, nor would he be man without carrying madness within as the limit of his freedom.' His work is said to have gone furthest in distancing psychoanalysis as a process of knowledge-seeking from medical notions of cure or adaptation, e.g. by dispensing with admission requirements and hierarchical rules at his Freudian School of Paris (Turkle, 1981 pp. 153, 156–7).

31 Along with 'thought disorder' and 'schizophrenia'. The medical model diverts attention from the context in which disturbed thought and speech occur, resulting in a damaging emphasis on physical treatments (Parker *et al.*, 1995).

32 The term 'psychosis' is highlighted by its introduction at the outset of her account. 'In fact, however, according to the self-contradictory logic of psychosis, the mark of his alphabet of cruelty can only disfigure but not tear off the mask that disguises the authority of tradition' (Pireddu, 1996 pp. 43–4).

33 Foucault's belated reply to 'Cogito et la Histoire de la Folie' provoked a break in relations between Derrida and his former teacher, which lasted for ten years (Eribon, 1991 pp. 120–1). In these essays Derrida doesn't pursue a positive deconstruction of the sane/mad binary beyond Artaud's impassioned and necessary reversal. Boyne develops an analogy between the position of 'the mad' and that of black people under Apartheid, but concludes that 'these situations may not seem strictly comparable, because the mad, by definition (if the definition is right) cannot speak for themselves.' Unlike Derrida, however, he was writing at a time when the psychiatric survivor movement was well established (Boyne, 1990 pp. 58–60; Campbell, 1989; Chamberlin, 1990).

34 He argued that, unlike the European, the Indian knows that much of what is going on inside him [sic] is not himself, but the Other. The Indian is also different from the madman, however, in using peyote to 'reinforce his will power in the work of separation and internal distribution' (Hayman, 1977 p. 113).

35 After being arrested in Dublin for vagrancy, he spent six days in Mountjoy Prison and was deported as an 'undesirable'. During the voyage he is said to have attacked two members of the crew who entered his cabin with a monkey-wrench, either to carry out repairs or to threaten him for making too much noise, and was put in a straitjacket. Artaud commented 'I was accused of hallucinating, according to the usual procedure of all police forces' (Barber, 1993 pp. 95–6). According to the French consulate, the Irish police sent him back to France because he was 'without resources and in an over-stimulated state' (Hayman, 1977 p. 122).

36 At Ville Evrard he had to wear an inmate's uniform, and was continually moved 'without motive or reason' between the maniacs' ward the epileptics' ward, the cripples' ward, and the undesirables' ward. For almost four years no attempt was made to treat him, and he was largely left to himself 'as a patient who calmly complied with orders'. By the spring of 1942 his weight was down to fifty-two kilograms (Barber, 1993 pp. 100–1).

37 Ferdière told him that he planned to restore him to Parisian life. The doctors knew his work, and encouraged him to write, draw and do translations. He was well fed, wore second-hand suits and was allowed to go into the town to meet local artists (Hayman, 1977 pp. 124ff.; Barber, 1993 pp. 105ff.). The warmth of this reception was deceptive, however. Despite talking about restoring to Artaud 'the quality of

human dignity of which he had so long been deprived', Ferdière admitted that 'my wife helped me to play this little game' by inviting him to lunch, and even 'allowing herself to be kissed by this repulsive-looking creature'. While organising this liberal charade, Ferdière was diagnosing Artaud as suffering from 'a chronic and extremely intense delirium characterised by [ideas of] persecution' (Esslin, 1976 pp. 53–4; Hayman, 1977 p. 124; Barber, 1993 p. 106).

38 Ferdière was probably aware that there had been fights with the police in Ireland, though Artaud was only arrested for vagrancy. These, and the struggle on board ship when he was being deported, had taken place almost six years previously (Barber, 1993 pp. 94–5).

39 Ferdière insisted that the shocks were painless, but delegated administration of the treatment to a young assistant. Artaud reported that he had to threaten to strangle Ferdière in order to convince him to abandon the idea of embarking upon another series. Though ECT is now given under general anaesthetic and with a muscle relaxant, its use remains highly contentious, and the consensus among most survivor and advocacy groups is that its use, without consent, should be banned. See for example Frank (1990); Breggin (1993); MIND (2001). And in favour of ECT with well-informed consent, Perkins (1996).

40 During her period of treatment, Plath was given manuscripts to type, and designed a hospital newspaper, but was discouraged from 'unrealistic expectations' about what she could achieve (Wagner-Martin, 1987). Showalter compares Plath's *The Bell Jar* with some accounts in male fiction that portray ECT as taming, and hence feminising, violent men.

41 Though Artaud's 'works' remain wilder and more fragmentary than Plath's. In 'Electroshock, Fragments', which opens with the words 'I died at Rodez under electroshock', he recalls a coma that lasted for ninety minutes, and being told by a young intern that two attendants had been summoned to take his body to the mortuary. He says that he witnessed the scene, in nightmarish detail, 'not from this side of the world but from the other'. As if to underline the importance of this information, he temporarily abandons the relative opacity of poetic language at this point, in favour of vividly direct prose. He then returns to poetic language in order to veil the source of inspiration for the next painfully personal fragment, which suggests incest and mentions 'the notorious father' (Hirschman, 1965 pp. 183–6).

42 These sentiments prefigure Cooper's argument, in the foreword to the English version of *Madness and Civilisation*, that 'we choose to conjure up this disease in order to evade a certain moment of our own existence – the moment of disturbance, of penetrating vision into the depths of ourselves, that we prefer to externalise on to others' (Foucault, 1961/1977 p. viii).

43 At the age of seventeen Artaud had a 'crisis of depression', and was sent away to sanatoria for a five-year period. A prescription for opium initiated a lifelong addiction. He was then transferred to the care of Dr Toulouse, a Parisian psychiatrist researching artistic genius, and lodged with him for six months (Barber, 1993 p. 15). Artaud contributed to, and helped produce, a literary review that Toulouse was editing, and the psychiatrist introduced him to contacts that led to acting work. Some years later he approached Dr Allendy, founder of the French psychoanalytical society, orientalist and beneficiary of a substantial inheritance, to fund the Theatre Alfred Jarry, and then, deeply depressed, booked in for some therapy sessions with him. Artaud may have borrowed his key metaphor of the plague from Allendy, who was writing a book on the black death. He presented his ideas for a Theatre of Cruelty at the Sorbonne as part of a series of lectures organised by the analyst (Hayman, 1977; Barber, 1993). Dr Ferdière, the psychiatrist responsible for Artaud's electroshock treatment at Rodez, was 'a Surrealist poet with anarchist tendencies',

who initially involved him in art and literary criticism, and subsequently claimed to be a pioneer of art psychotherapy (Barber, 1993 pp. 104, 111).

44 *Heliogabalus, or the Crowned Anarchist* was Artaud's first full-scale work, written in 1933 when he was desperate about his poverty-stricken life. It links the theme of premature accession to power, and gross misuse of it, – in a reign characterised by debauchery and cruelty, with contradictory images of sexuality. Heliogabalus was effeminate and homosexual, as well as high priest of a phallic solar religion. Artaud attempted to justify the young emperor's frequent use of castration as a punishment, wrote himself into the story, and emphasised the constant danger of assassination which he compared with his own sense of impending catastrophe (Hayman, 1977 pp. 92–3; Barber, 1993 pp. 60–1).

6 Deconstructing sovereignty: the post-revolutionary toolbox of Michel Foucault

1 According to Macey, Foucault was adjusted to his sexuality from an early age, and was out to his brother and friends, but Eribon cites medical testimony that his often suicidal distress was related to the circumstances in which he was exploring his sexuality. Factors such as anxiety about his appearance, and fear of failure in a highly competitive environment, may have contributed to his distress (Macey, 1993 pp. 27–8; Eribon, 1991 pp. 26–7; Miller, 1993 p. 56).

2 The term 'queer theory' was coined by de Lauretis in 1990 in order to open up a homogenising discourse of homosexual difference to a problematic of multiple sexual differences. Halperin discusses Foucault's influence on the associated politics (1995 pp. 113, 15–16, 31ff., 57–62). These debates are of interest in relation to 'mad pride', and the notion of coming out as disabled or 'mad' (Shakespeare *et al.*, 1996; Faulkner and Sayce, 1997).

3 In France in the 1940s rumours of homosexuality could be sufficient to terminate academic careers, and discriminatory legislation fuelled a fearful atmosphere. The stigma surrounding psychiatric treatment was also considerable. When Louis Althusser, a tutor and then secretary of the arts side at the ENS, was repeatedly admitted to hospital for psychiatric treatment, his absences were passed off as holidays (Macey, 1993 pp. 27–9, 81).

4 Had Foucault lived longer, he might have wanted to relax the habit of reticence imposed by oppression, and reflect publicly upon his early experiences. In an interview conducted from his deathbed, he admitted having used 'somewhat rhetorical methods of avoiding one of the fundamental domains of experience', that of the subject, of the self, of individual conduct (Miller, 1993 p. 31).

5 See the interview appended to Foucault's book on Raymond Roussel (Foucault, 1963/ 1987 pp. 184–5).

6 His new questions are: 'What are the modes of existence of this discourse? Where does it come from; how is it circulated; who controls it? What placements are determined for possible subjects? Who can fulfil these diverse functions of the subject?' (Bouchard, 1977 p. 138).

7 *Madness and Civilisation, Discipline and Punish* and *History of Sexuality* were, albeit often indirectly, influential in their respective 'sectors'. None of the books are narrowly specialist, however, and the works on power and knowledge, and on prisons, contain interesting material relevant to the politics of 'mental health'.

8 Halperin reviews three biographies (1995).

9 Even in 1989 some of Foucault's contemporaries resisted discussion of his homosexuality, but Eribon argued that Foucault's 'entire oeuvre' was 'a revolt against the powers of normalisation' and sought to avoid either suppression or 'exhibitionism'

and voyeurism (Eribon, 1991 p. x). Miller has been criticised for encouraging the latter, and effectively arming hostile critics with excessive revelations. In relation to sexuality, Foucault's late work was informed by his contact with the burgeoning cultures of lesbian and gay communities in the USA (Halperin, 1995). Unfortunately we have no late commentaries from him informed by the nascent psychiatric survivor movement of the time. For accounts of his experiences of distress, biographers have relied on the testimony of contemporaries, including the doctor who described a suicide attempt to Eribon. The ethical questions that arise around how much biographical detail can legitimately be revealed or utilised are complex, but I feel there is a good case for establishing a reasonably informed view of a philosopher whose contribution, based on a variety of personal experience, amounts to a considerable resource on the political uses of experience.

10 Foucault finds ambiguity rather than the simple 'sameness' between the place left empty by the father and the place made radiant by the unfaithful presence of the gods, which seems to guarantee analysts 'easy passage between the work and what lies outside the work'. For Hölderlin, the 'unapproachable' Schiller, who 'observes, declares and protects the Law from his infinite reserve', occupies such a place (Bouchard, 1977 pp. 70, 76, 85).

11 The question is posed as to whether the 'mythical forces [of]) divine violence' which penetrate mortals, are *also* 'Hölderlin's forces as a child' that are 'confiscated out of avarice and withheld by his mother, forces of which he requested the "full and unimpaired use" as a paternal inheritance . . . [to] . . . dispose of as he liked'. Foucault does nothing to distance himself from this speculation that the image of a devouring mother is rooted in a real emasculation of sons by mothers, and by implication, of men by women (Bouchard, 1977 p. 81).

12 After a 'delusional attack' during a period when he feared political persecution, Hölderlin was confined in a hospital at Tubingen, and then, in what Foucault referred to (in an interview) as a small 'Basaglia experiment in the romantic age', Hölderlin spent forty years living in 'the Hölderlin Tower' (Kritzman, 1988 p. 198). A contemporary visitor paints a less happy picture, however, recording that Hölderlin raged whenever he met anyone from the hospital, was regularly taunted when he went out, and would reply by throwing stones and dung (Wallblinger, 1830).

13 At the end of a doctoral thesis on Kant completed in 1961, he turns to Nietzsche, and asks whether the death of God implies 'the murder of man himself' (Macey, 1993 p. 90). *The Birth of the Clinic* closes with further references to Hölderlin and Nietzsche.

14 *Madness and Civilisation* had already been completed, but was published after the death.

15 His style at this time reflects that of the writers (Bataille, Blanchot and De Sade) whose experiments at the limits of language preoccupy him, and contrasts markedly with his first book, *Mental Illness and Personality*, where Sheridan finds prose that is 'dull by a superhuman effort of the will', and refers to a stylistic 'straitjacket' that would soon snap (Sheridan, 1980 p. 6).

16 Dews notes that the gaze appears in *Madness and Civilisation*, in relation to the York Retreat, but the 1967 Tavistock translation uses 'observation' here, and in this passage the gaze is not yet the 'deeply implanted' concept it later becomes (Dews, 1987 pp. 157–8).

17 See Jones and Porter (1994 p. 28).

18 Foucault took up literature, history and philosophy instead of medicine, but Eribon comments on the 'astonishing convergence of the two registers' literature and the history of science, in his work at this point (Eribon, 1991 p. 152). Near the end of *Birth of the Clinic* Foucault argues that the 'irruption of finitude' dominates a relation

to death that simultaneously authorises knowledge derived from the rational scientific discourse of pathological anatomy, while also opening up 'the source of a language that unfolds endlessly in the void left by the absence of the gods' (Foucault, 1963/1973 p. 198).

19 In Foucault's case, the gesture was made when he was still at school, and the change proved permanent. Other explanations don't account for his opting for Michel, the part of his name that his mother had insisted upon adding. Foucault described his father as a bully, and Daniel Defert, his partner of more than twenty years, said that he was 'a violent man' and 'very commanding' (Miller, 1993 pp. 39, 63).

20 Note that in Madness and Civilisation, which contemporaries regarded as autobiographically inspired, Foucault discussed a 'parental complex' that accounted for the 'obscure (but marvellous) powers' of the doctor (Foucault, 1961/1971 pp. 252–3, 276; Eribon, 1991 pp. 27–8).

21 In Birth of the Clinic Foucault describes the epistemic gaze of medicine in admiring and almost affectionately ambivalent detail, sometimes portraying it in a positive light (Foucault, 1963/1973 pp. 65, 107, 84, 121). Twelve years later he concentrates on the menacing and power-saturated subtlety of a totalising political gaze in Discipline and Punish.

22 When Foucault was a student, his father's interventions on his behalf suggest a continuing and sympathetic interest. He seems to have made an informed, if privileged, choice of helper, arranging for, and according to Eribon taking, his son to see an eminent and supportive psychiatrist, and also probably securing his exemption from military service on health grounds. The biographies are silent on his response to his son's sexuality, but had he been more supportive in this respect it seems likely that more would have been said, and unlikely that Foucault would have told friends that he had hated him (Macey, 1993 pp. 15, 28, 81; Eribon, 1991). The anatomists' insights about life, ironically, depend upon death.

23 Foucault used Bentham's plan for the 'Panopticon', a centripetal prison based on these principles, as paradigm and metaphor for modern forms of power that would rely much less on overt displays of force to maintain internal discipline (Foucault, 1975/1977 p. 214). The panoptic principle would enforce rigid segregation of inspected, defined and disciplined populations (Bowring, 1962 pp. 45, 47, 106).

24 Individual description had once been solely about heroisation, a prerogative of power. Disciplinary methods reversed this relation, turning chronicles of ordinary lives that once 'fell below the threshold of description' into documents for use, in a process of objectification and subjection (Foucault, 1975/1977 pp. 190–1). Foucault's conception of an 'axis of individualisation' overlooks the continuing function of heroic biography within hegemonic masculinities, however (Jackson, 1990).

25 Unlike Weber's comparable tale of origins of the state in predatory men's warrior leagues, and correspondingly defensive 'patrimonial' household formations, gender is left unspecified here. Brown finds Weber suggestive for mapping the overt masculinism of external state action, and the internal values of state-ruled societies (Brown, 1995 p. 187).

26 In biographical terms, it was written at the close of a period during which Foucault had expressed his own nostalgia for a violent form of 'popular justice.' (Macey, 1993 pp. 299–300; Foucault, 1980 p. 28).

27 Frosh, however, cites Grosz, arguing that masculinity constructs the illusion of 'a space of pure reflection . . . a mirroring surface that duplicates, re-presents everything but itself.' (Grosz, 1990 p. 173). Foucault argues that the sciences of man instil the habits of introspection, but this will be of a kind that, like Foucault's text, censors any reference to the positioning of individual men in relation to masculinity.

28 Grosz summarises this as

> an internalised image or map of the meaning that the body has for the subject, for others in its social world, and for the symbolic order conceived in its generality. It is an individual and collective fantasy of the body's forms and modes of action.
>
> (Grosz, 1994 pp. 39–40)

29 Unlike in the Panopticon, surveillance here was visible, and performed by a keeper whose authority derived from his not being mad (Foucault 1961/1967 pp. 251–2).

30 Freud 'exploited the structure that enveloped the medical personage; he amplified its thaumaturgical [miracle-working] virtues, preparing for its omnipotence a quasi-divine status.' The analyst, concealed behind and above the patient 'in an absence that is also a total presence', embodied and transformed the powers that had been deployed in the asylum, 'absolute Observation, a pure and circumspect silence a judgement that does not even condescend to language' (Foucault, 1961/1967 pp. 277–8).

31 Robert Hurley's translation for Penguin gives 'loss of parental authority'. There is some support for Foucault's historical assertion about a crisis in parental (paternal) authority at this time, for example in the argument that late Victorian scientific theories of an essential female passivity and the popular artistic and moral theme of woman-as-ministering-angel were a reaction to a 'pervasive sense of manhood in danger.' (Bordo, 1988 pp. 107–8). These changes can be viewed in relation to major economic transformations and the development of public patriarchies (Hearn, 1992 p. 219).

32 Against this, an understanding of power as productive of desire, and of identification with oppression, may help explain women's collusion (Sawicki, 1991 pp. 85–6). Foucault's view that even those who exercise power are 'caught up in a machine' can help explain how men can continue to dominate while appearing neither to wish or intend to (Ramazanoglu and Holland, 1993 p. 247). Where he argues that 'power comes from below', Foucault says that 'major dominations are the hegemonic effects' sustained by local confrontations (Foucault, 1976/1978 p. 94). Rather than a binary structure of 'dominators' and 'dominated', there is 'a multiform production of relations of domination' (Foucault, 1980 p. 142).

33 Aphoristic declarations, such as 'power comes from below', have provoked considerable debate. Inconsistencies between various formulations mean that anyone using them must to some extent improvise. The coercive imagery of power in *Discipline and Punish* contrasts with the more abstract theorisation about a 'liberal' form, immanent in various kinds of relations, in *Will to Knowledge*, where the distinctions between power, force and domination also cause difficulties (Halperin, 1995 pp. 18–22; Foucault, 1976/1978 pp. 92–6).

34 Althusser's notion that individuality is called forth in an ideological process of 'interpellation' transposes easily to the domain of gender, in which men are called up or conscripted, in various ways, into hegemonic positions and identities (Rustin, 1995 pp. 228–9; Connell, 1995). Lacan's internalised 'imaginary ideal self' can be linked with Connell's argument that exemplars, such as film actors or fantasy figures, are important in defining masculinity's 'circle of legitimacy', and that heroism is strongly associated with the reproduction of hegemony (Connell, 1995 pp. 77–9, 234). On Foucault's abandonment of the notion of ideology, not least because it implies privileged access to the truth, see Foucault (1980 p. 118); McNay (1992 pp. 153–4).

35 Although Foucault was aware that Pinel's symbolic act of unchaining some inmates may not have happened, and indicated that he had treated the story as a 'legend of

foundation' within professional discourse, this is not made clear in the shortened English text. Gordon reviews other problems caused by English language readers' unfamiliarity with *Déraison et Folie* (Foucault, 1961/1971 p. 243; Gordon, 1990 p. 16).

36 Ironically it was at this time that he became 'quite possibly the only French philosopher to have had his ribs broken by the CRS riot police' (Macey, 1995 p. 13; Eribon, 1993 p. 260).

37 In a 1967 interview Foucault had defended the use of drugs as a means of entering into 'a state of "nonreason" in which the experience of madness is outside the distinction between the normal and the pathological', and for their dissolution of fixed categories of thought. Miller adds, presumably as a health warning, that Artaud spent most of following decade in asylums (Miller, 1993 p. 248). Whereas Artaud had set out to transgress personal and cultural limits at a time of mounting personal crisis, Foucault, at this stage in his life, was enjoying material success and emotional stability, and was with supportive companions. Protracted incarceration was not, of course, an inevitable or proportionate response to Artaud's condition.

38 The 'repressive hypothesis' refers to the assumption popularised by Reich and various Freudo-Marxists, that there has been a historical movement towards ever-increasing sexual repression linked to the rise of capitalism in the West. Foucault accounts for the popularity of this discourse in terms of 'the speaker's benefit', noting how attractive a proposition it is 'to utter truths and promise bliss' from a position ostensibly untouched by power, when merely to speak seems an act of transgression. Since power is not only negative, a constraint polarised against and separate from some pristine realm of truth, apparently liberating discourses can function to uphold the very power they profess to overturn (Dreyfus and Rabinow, 1982 pp. 129–31).

39 'It seems to me that power *is* "always already there", that one is never outside it, that there are no "margins" for those who break with the system to gambol in' (Foucault, 1980 p. 141).

40 Halperin draws attention to Foucault's often courageous activism during this period, and points out that this is a critique of a liberal form of power that requires us to be 'free', the better to normalise and 'responsibilise' us (Halperin, 1995 pp. 29, 15ff.).

41 Foucault's youthful memories of growing up in occupied France included not knowing whether he would die in the bombing, and witnessing the silence in the street as the Gestapo were taking people away (Macey, 1993 pp. 6–7).

42 While living in Tunis, Foucault became, quite literally for a while, a 'coloniser who resists', taking personal risks supporting radical students who faced far more severe consequences for their actions than their counterparts in Paris (Macey, 1993 pp. 203–6). Butler points out, in the context of the 1991 Gulf War, 'we saw "the Arab" is figured as the abjected Other as well as a site of homosexual fantasy' (Butler, 1995 p. 46). Clearly Foucault could not be seamlessly included among such colonisers.

43 Eribon describes the Ecole Normal Supérieure, an exclusive all-male residential college (women attended a sister institution), as a 'pathogenic environment' that encouraged eccentric behaviour at the personal, intellectual and political levels. To enter the ENS was to enter an intellectual lineage, a highly competitive and pressurised environment in which students were numerically graded from the outset, and the slang term for a philosophy tutor was *caiman* or crocodile (Eribon, 1991 p. 25; Macey, 1993).

44 Such as the globalising and totalitarian theories of psychoanalysis and scientific Marxism (Foucault, 1980 p. 81).

45 Foucault was deterred from going into hospital to seek help with his depression on the advice of his friend, Louis Althusser, who spoke from considerable direct experience. His thinking about madness was coloured by the fate of another friend, Jacques

Martin, a gay man and highly regarded ENS student, who fell into poverty and depression and took his own life after the collapse of his plans for an academic career. For Foucault he became a 'philosophe sans oeuvre', a philosopher who personified his familiar definition of madness as the absence of works (Macey, 1993 pp. 23–6).

46 While Church recalls a survivor colleague pointedly avoiding the term 'discourse', it has since been adopted by some survivor writers (Church, 1995 p. 141; cf. Rose, 2001; Coleman, 1999 p. 18; Wallcraft and Michaelson, 2001).

47 Patients were harnessed to an armchair and wired up with electrodes that monitored their bodily reactions. The young Foucault was thus able to witness two forms of exclusion, that of 'madmen' and 'delinquents'. Because the Sainte-Anne was one of the best hospitals in Paris, and 'not terrible', its effects could be attributed to psychiatry rather than to poor institutional practice (Eribon, 1991 pp. 48–9).

48 Binswanger was, coincidentally, the nephew of the director of the clinic in which Nietzsche had been treated (Eribon, 1991 p. 47). Foucault played an active role in producing a French version of the Colli-Montinari edition of Nietzsche, which aimed to reconstruct the texts according to Nietzsche's own intentions rather than those of his sister (Macey, 1993 pp. 153–4).

49 Reversing Clausewitz's aphorism, Foucault called the notion that 'politics is war continued by other means', 'Nietzsche's hypothesis'. In lectures given in 1976 on his return from California, he reconsiders this, along with the repressive hypothesis, in order to imagine some 'new form of right' beyond subjugating relations (Foucault, 1980 pp. 90–2).

50 'Pervasive and multiform strategies of homophobia . . . saturate the entire field of cultural representation, and like power in Foucault's formulation, are everywhere.' Foucault teaches us to analyse discourse in terms of what it does and how it works rather than simply what it says (Halperin, 1995 pp. 30–1).

7 Like a marble guest: the nervous illness of Daniel Paul Schreber

1 Interestingly, Foucault bemoans the transition from the more heroic earlier 'adventure' accounts of individuality to disciplinary power, so that 'in place of Lancelot we have Schreber'.

2 Up to that point she had been spending several hours a day with him, and taking meals in the asylum.

3 We might add that only some four days after Flechsig welcomed him back to the asylum with a long interview extolling recent advances in psychiatry, Schreber found himself 'pulled out of bed by two attendants in the middle of the night', overpowered and taken, without explanation, to a cell fitted only with an iron bedstead and some bedding. There he made an unsuccessful suicide attempt. He writes 'I was naturally terrified in the extreme by this event' (Schreber, 1903/2000 pp. 50–2).

4 Schatzman points out that intense physical ordeals, bisexuality, cross-dressing, a sense of calling, and access to the language of birds, supernatural language and a spirit world are all features of shamanism (Schatzman, 1973 p. 5). The idea that birds somehow symbolise or embody departed souls is common in folklore, which Schreber tells us is the source of his notion of 'soul murder' (Rowland, 1978; see also Freud, 1911/1979 pp. 168–70). The notion of rays, so prominent in Schreber's cosmology, is important in theosophy, which had an international following in his time, influenced Rudolf Steiner, and are sometimes reminiscent of the 'vibrations' of 1960s drug culture. Arguments that his belief system was not shared and therefore not comparable with spiritualism neglect the conditions of enforced isolation in

which he was thinking and writing. Strategies such as playing the piano, 'picturing' or bellowing in order to cope with troublesome voices have only recently begun to be acknowledged by psychiatry (Romme and Escher, 1993). The idea of 'unmanning' was taken up by Otto Gross, an advocate of the 'inner wealth of bisexuality' in men, who was influential in early counter-cultural circles, and anticipates the experimental effeminacy of some anti-sexist men. Santner argues that Schreber's theories anticipate Foucault in some respects, albeit in a highly intuitive manner (Santner, 1996).

5 At the time of his appointment Flechsig had little experience of psychiatry. Chronic patients were quickly moved on to make room for patients who were near to death and whose brains could be dissected (Santner, 1996 p. 71).

6 Sass talks about an 'inner panopticism', but contrives to retain the language of medicalisation (disease, symptom, schizophreniform, etc.). After reviewing psychoanalytic interpretations of 'cognitive structures', such as Schreber's world of rays, in terms of a regression to infancy, or the instinctual quality of the 'wildman', he interprets them as attempts to escape the self-alienation of modernity, rather than as core facets of madness (Sass, 1987).

7 A tutelage order was intended to protect an individual from the effects of their actions, whether financial or likely to cause them to lose face (Leudar and Thomas, 2000).

8 See Leudar and Thomas (2000) for a discussion of how this and other aspects of his 'madness' were debated and evaluated in the court case.

9 This also leads to a simplistic additive understanding of identity, in which 'race', class and gender are seen as operating separately, so that, for example, differences in the contexts in which black women and white women experience sexism (or indeed disablism or 'mental health' oppression) are neglected (Nicholson, 1999).

10 And of 'psychosis', though most subsequent commentators find a 'schizophrenic' element of 'passivization and boundary confusion' too developed, and therefore invoke a more profound regression (Sass, 1992 p. 245).

11 Freud assumed that hatred of another man was a projection concealing forbidden love. Schatzman questions Freud's hypothesis that Schreber's desire was homosexual, and points out that the father is only considered as an object, not as an agent whose actions almost certainly induced hatred in his sons (Schatzman, 1973 pp. 94–8). Bloch accepts that Schreber did have such fantasies, but argues that Freud overlooked their defensive function in relation to his understandable terror of a threatening father (Bloch, 1989). Lothane attributes this theory to a current of latent homosexuality among the male pioneers of psychoanalysis, and argues that it has no basis in Schreber's life or text (Lothane, 1992).

12 Great emphasis was placed on straightness. One of these devices, a *kopfhalter* or headholder, was designed to pull a child's hair when the head was not held straight. At one point in his madness Schreber complained of a sensation of pain 'like a sudden pulling inside my head . . . [which] may be combined with the tearing off of part of the bony substance of my skull'. The regimen included eye exercises, and Schreber writes 'my eyes and the muscles of the lids which serve to open and close them were an almost uninterrupted target for miracles'. Dr Moritz Schreber felt it crucial to develop character as 'a protective wall against the unhealthy predominance of the emotional side, against that feeble sensitiveness the disease of our age, which must be regarded as the usual reason for the increasing frequency of depression, mental illness, and suicide'. His *Medical Indoor Gymnastics* sold nearly forty editions and was translated into seven languages (Schatzman, 1973 pp. 44–5, 36, 16–17, 142).

13 Locating agency only where repetition is disrupted risks allowing perpetrators of routinised abuse to plead that they are 'only following discourse'. Another difficulty

with Butler's work is that it conveys little sense of lived, material or productive bodies. Sociological accounts of emotion as performative, and implicated in power relations, challenge quasi-mechanical, essentialist and expressive understandings (Burkitt, 1999). Such understandings often overlook the effects of somatic disturbance on our capacity to perform, however. Schreber's madness seems to have been much less comprehensively policed than that of Artaud. Schatzman notes that modern psychiatric treatments would have hindered or prevented his writing (Schatzman, 1973).

14 During this period his refusal of food might be seen as a passive and 'feminine' form of resistance, but his 'whole sense of manly honour' led him to fight with the attendants who were forcing food and medication upon him. For Schreber, femaleness seems to have been about experiencing passivity and sensuality, about 'voluptuousness' (Schreber, 1903/2000 pp. 64, 164). Foucault reminds us that public discourse about sex and sexuality was quite rich and detailed during this period (Foucault, 1976/1978)

15 Schreber's engagement in the discovery and naming of various phenomena, in publishing his own truths, and attempting to contribute to psychiatric progress, mirrored the power/knowledge practices of public masculinity exemplified in the figures of his various doctors.

16 That this took the form of the surgical removal of the ovaries and uterus of women diagnosed with hysteria, would have been unlikely to reassure Schreber, given his intense identification as a potential woman (Santner, 1996 p. 71). Schreber may also have known that some authorities had recommended castration for 'masturbational insanity'.

17 Discussing the possibility of childhood sexual abuse, Schatzman cautiously points to Dr. Moritz Schreber's references to 'penetrating' children with love (Schatzman, 1973 p. 88).

18 Freud felt that since 'paranoiacs' 'only say what they want to say', yet reveal in distorted form those things that 'other neurotics' keep secret, this was precisely a disorder where a case history could take the place of personal acquaintance (Freud, 1911/1979 p. 138).

19 Bloch notes the identification of both fathers with Bismarck. In his retelling of the Oedipus myth Freud omitted the parents' attempt to kill their child (Bloch, 1989).

20 Schreber felt that his skin was softening, his male organ retracting, his stature shrinking, his bosom periodically swelling, that hairs from his beard were being removed, and that scientific examination would confirm the reality of these changes (Schreber, 1903/2000 pp. 90, 142, 248).

21 Ahmed cites Derrida's response to a passage in Nietzsche on 'Women and their Effect at a Distance', in which a great sailing ship glides silently, like a ghost amidst surging breakers, and 'calm enchanting beings' appear, 'whose happiness and retirement he longs for' – women (Ahmed, 1998 pp. 83–4, citing Derrida, 1979). In *Madness and Civilisation* Foucault invokes a 'ship of fools' gliding along 'the calm rivers of the Rhineland', associated with a time when 'madmen led an easy wandering existence' (Foucault, 1961/1971 pp. 7–8). Nietzsche made very different use of Brant's *The Ship of Fools* (Allison, 2001 pp. 128–9, 282 note 56).

22 Deleuze and Guattari specify Schreber alongside Artaud when discussing the Body-Without-Organs, but give no sense of the circumstances under which the two men arrived at the necessity of desiring or experiencing extreme bodily transformation (Deleuze and Guattari, 1972/1977 p. 8). Deleuze's recommendation of Lewis Carroll's Alice, as an exemplar of becoming-woman, is particularly ironical given that Artaud was given this work to translate as part of the psychiatric restoration of his masculine identity (Grosz, 1994 p. 175).

23 *Luder* translates as 'wretch', but for Schreber it carried connotations of scoundrel, whore or dead animal flesh used as bait, and expressed his fears of sexual abuse or being left to rot (Santner, 1996 p. 40).

24 Another reason for the enduring popularity of this story among arbiters of reason may well be its susceptibility to readings that obscure the other major dimensions of social oppression that significantly contribute towards the distress and madness of most psychiatric survivors.

8 Politics and experience: engaging with complex subjectivity

1 Within the user/survivor movement the term 'schizophrenia' has been both rejected and reclaimed. Bracken and Thomas have called on psychiatrists to abandon it (Bracken and Thomas, 1999), and Robin Murray, described as a world authority on schizophrenia, has done so in clinical practice (*All in the Mind*, BBC Radio 4, 1 July 2002). Fernando regards it as a racist construct (Fernando et al., 1998).

2 Alternatively, for Tarnas, a masculinist tradition essential to the evolution of the Western mind has 'painstakingly prepared the way for its own self-transcendence'. Postmodern radical uncertainty characterises an evolutionary crisis in which conditions are analogous to those described in Bateson's double-bind theory of schizophrenia, and the world functions like a 'schizophrenogenic' mother. Since this is a crisis of masculinity, its resolution entails 'modern man' seeking integration with the archetypal feminine ground of his being (Tarnas, 1996 pp. 416–22, 440–5).

3 Transversality was originally intended 'to express the capacity of an institution to remodel the ways of access it offers to the superego so that certain symptoms and inhibitions are removed'. This was to be achieved by ensuring the institution didn't produce 'Oedipalizable objects' in the form of quasi-parental authority figures (Genosko, 2000 pp. 132–3).

4 At the La Borde clinic, doctors, nurses and staff were 'all daddy', and service-users became analysands, whose criticisms of the head doctor's power were interpreted as 'alienation phantasy'. Institutional tasks were rotated, so that even the 'imbecile on the ward' could take a turn in this game of interpretation. Patients' clubs were established in the hope that they would become 'subject' rather than 'subjected' groups, but permitted only limited autonomy, and analysed in a giddily inaccessible and self-referential argot (Genosko, 2000 pp. 117, 133–5).

5 Interestingly, Guattari's critique of the concept of transference as an artefact of analysis, in which there is always also a real situation, the mediating object of institutional life, was shaped by his experience as pupil and analysand in a sycophantic 'cult of the absolute master' around Lacan (Genosko, 2000 p. 117).

6 Others, however, continue to talk about an 'Age of Anxiety' (Dunant and Porter, 1996). Bracken uses Heidegger's understanding of anxiety as 'the mood that reveals the groundlessness of the world' (Bracken, 2002 pp. 136ff.). Increasing suicide rates inter alia strongly suggest that, masculinity and postmodernity notwithstanding, men do remain haunted by 'feeling rooted in personal biography'.

7 The location chosen for *The Scream*, originally called *Despair*, a renowned suicide spot within earshot of Oslo's Asylum, suggests a strand of latent personal meaning, since Munch's sister was to be a patient there and Munch himself was to experience a severe breakdown, becoming a psychiatric patient in Copenhagen in 1908–9 (*The Private Life of a Masterpiece*, BBC2, 8 December 2001).

8 A sense of overwhelming meaningfulness is said to coincide with meaninglessness. Things appear as never before, yet there can also be a feeling of déjà vu. Nietzsche's

term 'Stimmung' has been used by the 'severely schizoid' artist DeChirico, to describe the associated mood (Sass, 1992 pp. 44–5).

9 He talks about the importance of self-reflexivity, of affirming the other, and of co-constituting understandings and actions. Methods such as 'third person listening' may help in relation to conflicts where the modernist tradition of unified egos tends to polarise dialogue into a confrontation between 'my position and your position' (Gergen, 1999).

10 Flax notes that diagnostic categories are constructs that carry certain consequences, but refers to 'borderline people' and 'schizoid people' in terms that sound essentialist. She reports that her patients want her to understand their inner worlds well enough to help them name and differentiate between the various fragments, but says little about the power relations implicit in such work, and sometimes appears to reduce critique to therapy (Flax, 1993, 1990, 1987).

11 For example, women receive twice as much ECT as men, and 'a patient's age and gender are often a determining factor' in its use (Thomas, 1996; Johnstone, 2003). Elderly women, who may have little more than memories left, are the group most likely to receive a treatment which risks erasing memory (ECT Anonymous 1998 pp. 12–13; MIND 1995). Once again, however, the extreme vulnerability of some male recipients should be noted (Frank, 1990). A recent report found 50 per cent of respondents unaware that they could have refused consent (MIND, 2001).

12 Feminist professionals and survivors have applied critiques of the gendered nature of Enlightenment science and rationality to white middle-class male psychology and psychiatry. Such arguments have practical implications, for instance leading some feminists to point out that being in touch with uncomfortable, even uncontrollable emotion, is part of a continuum of ordinary experience.(Hollway, 1989 pp. 110, 124; Foner, 1995 p. 141; Barnes and Maple, 1992 pp. 27–8).

13 Campaigns against oppressive service systems, and calls for alternatives, have generally been made within a context that attends to equal opportunities issues (Plumb, 1993; Lindow, 1994; Read and Wallcraft, 1995).

14 The DSM or *Diagnostic and Statistical Manual* of the American Psychiatric Association (APA) sets out definitions of 'mental disorders' and functions as a global reference work. Feminist campaigns against this victim-blaming diagnostic category were successful. Linkages have been made between the greater incidence and severity of women's experiences of child sexual abuse and, for instance, the finding that women are twice as vulnerable to depression as men (Whiffen and Clark, 1997). Estimates indicate that up to 10 per cent of men have experienced sexual abuse during childhood, compared with 20–30 per cent of women (Department of Health, 2003b). A relatively higher proportion might be expected in psychiatric settings, with one study finding that 41 per cent of a sample of male outpatients reported physical abuse, 13 per cent sexual abuse and 6 per cent both, despite possible under-reporting (Swett et al., 1990 p. 35). In another study, 23 of 100 male psychiatric patients reported sexual activity with an adult before the age of 16 (Metcalfe et al., 1990). It should perhaps also be noted that some radical feminists have written about men as victims of rape (Brownmiller, 1975).

15 See debates about 'False Memory Syndrome' and collusion with the recovered memory movement's psycho-pathologisation of survivors (Brown and Burman, 1997; Showalter, 1997).

16 Feminists have long spoken out against the retraumatisation of rape victims by a system in which further abuse by therapists has not been uncommon (Chesler, 1972; Walker, 1984 p. 197; Sayce, 1995 p. 142).

17 Church, a psychologist-turned-sociologist, writes as an 'outsider' about a movement challenging oppression by a service system in which she had worked, but notes that

very few feminists were then involved (Church, 1995 p. 3). The prominence of women as theorists and leaders within the American psychiatric survivor movement has been compared favourably with the civil rights and anti-war movements, however (Kalinowski and Penny, 1998 p. 128). Another local difference is that the term 'self-advocacy' does not appear to have been in use in Canada.

18 It should be noted that in the Canadian context, there appears to have been a cultural emphasis on valuing emotional expression. Church contrasts a survivor colleague's demands to see her 'pain and passion', with the emotional censorship characteristic of professional discourse (Church, 1995 pp. 25–6, 74, 104). Many individuals, however, want a supportive environment, free of demands for 'dramatic confrontations with life experiences or deep emotions' (Plumb, 1999 p. 472).

19 Chesler writes that a feminist therapist tries to believe what a woman is saying, and knows she will need to be told she is 'not crazy'. Where the woman really is 'crazy', the feminist therapist will want to 'try to avoid hospitalising her against her will, if at all', and will try to provide information and advocacy (Chesler, 1990 pp. 319–20). Some users/survivors reluctantly conclude that compulsory treatment may, in extreme circumstances, be necessary and beneficial.

20 I take this to include violence and oppression against 'Othered' groups of men. Ramazanoglu includes mental health amongst variations in experience where women from different racial, ethnic and national groups and social classes may have more interests in common with men of the same group than with women of different groups (1989 p. 132). Mouffe calls for a political project directed against all forms of subordination, in which homogeneous identities such as 'men' and 'women' would be replaced by a multiplicity of social relations (1992 pp. 372–3).

21 Applied to the violence literature, the feminist standpoint perspective has arguably produced an unrealistically monochrome analysis with limited value in relation to the complexities of social work practice (Featherstone and Trinder, 1997).

22 This term, connoting a multiplicity of influences or causes, comes from Althusser who, as already noted, was a colleague and friend of Foucault and long-term recipient of inpatient psychiatric treatment.

23 There are difficulties with the conventional social model of disability and the associated notion of impairment. Wilson and Beresford argue that ideas based on perceived impairment underpin modernist psychiatry, often with very harmful results, and that adapting a social model against discrimination might reinforce the reification of 'impairment of the mind'. This could still apply where 'psychiatric disability' was applied to iatrogenic injury (Wilson and Beresford, 2002; Sayce, 2000; Plumb, 1994; Bangay, 2000; and on a social disablement model, Perkins, 1995). Although the model formulated by Sayce reminds us that postmodern theory has no monopoly on concern for complex identity and diversity of understandings, any abandonment of 'old battles' over medicalisation would risk isolating survivors for whom challenging 'mental illness' diagnoses is a central concern (Plumb, 1999).

24 Westwood describes psychiatry and racism as two mutually reinforcing regimes of power, but uses medical model discourse (Westwood, 1994). From within the survivor movement, Sassoon and Lindow point out ways in which racism can make speaking out against oppressive psychiatric practice more difficult. Like black disabled people, black psychiatric survivors may need to insist that 'race' is not always prioritised, though racism is likely to be more deeply implicated in distress than in disability (Sassoon and Lindow, 1995).

25 Survivor politics can be located within a broader frame, for instance as a form of 'globalisation from below', and understood in terms of resistance to global developments such as DSM-IV ('the psychiatric equivalent to the World Trade Organisation') that need to be theorised as well as experienced (Carpenter, 2001 p. 71).

26 Brown points out that Nietzsche's value as a diagnostician is circumscribed by his lack of interest in the transformative potential of collective political invention, and that his personal remedy, a process of forgetting, is clearly unhelpful here, given that erased histories and historical invisibility are almost defining characteristics of the politics of subjugated identities (Brown, 1995, p. 74).

27 Attempts to increase compliance with medication can undermine informed choice, and effectively lock people into identification with states of injury, rather than dealing with the causes of their distress or madness (Perkins and Repper, 1999). The effects of stigma mean that those who have recovered rarely become publicly visible as psychiatric survivors (Shaughnessy in Asylum, 2003). After many years of institutional failure to envisage the possibility of recovery, there is a danger of it becoming a buzzword concealing lack of investment in support for those withdrawing from psychiatric drugs, or for independent living (Coleman, 1999; Hart, 2003; Beresford and Hopton, 2003).

28 Church's use of 'unsettling relations' refers to a personally and socially transformative political 'process of self-knowledge' that enables survivors to move 'beyond personal revenge into collective political action' (Church, 1995 pp. 73–4).

29 Bakhtin uses 'authoritative discourse' to refer to pedagogy that brooks no argument, but because of the evident need for excluded groups to reclaim authorship and authority, I would prefer to describe this as 'authoritarian' or 'absolute' discourse (Morson and Emerson, 1990 pp. 218–19).

30 In the context of disability politics, it has been argued that in policing the bounds and deciding 'who counts as the same', politicised groupings 'seem to manifest a nostalgia for the modernist values of separation and exclusion' (Shildrick and Price, 1998 p. 235).

31 Some 'policing' happens even in ostensibly anarchistic subcultures. Radical politics may gain vigour at the expense of breadth of political awareness and sensitivity to others' concerns. An anthology of writings from this strand of 'mad culture', influenced by Artaud and punk, for instance, celebrates transgression but includes some material that would widely be regarded as offensively sexist, while managing to exclude comparable vernacular racism (Curtis et al., 2000). Another potential problem with the 'mad culture' approach (as opposed to the theatrically inspired direct action of Mad Pride, in which props such as white coats, straitjackets and giant syringes have been used to dramatic but coherent effect) is that it risks re-energising rather than undermining prejudice against those deemed mad, since, as already noted, hegemonic sanity needs lurid 'performances' of madness to mask the performative nature of its own 'normality'.

32 The argument that reclaiming 'madness' constitutes a radical advance over using the more inclusive and hence euphemistic term 'distress', and that the latter colludes with oppression by not properly acknowledging and celebrating difference, has been debated within the user/survivor movement (Perkins, 1999). Another position reclaims the term 'distress' to cover any of the wide variety of experiences and conditions labelled as 'mental illness' (Distress Awareness Training Agency (DATA); see Lindow, 1994).

33 For men survivors, a return to conspicuously rational modes of expression through political engagement may also represent 'returning to normal' in terms of gender expectations (of relative power and privilege) as well as in terms of 'mental health' status. Proponents of equality who speak as allies may strongly prefer to maintain a rigid binary distinction (often based on essentialist assumptions that the excluded condition is innate) as protection against the charge that oppressive relations create 'madness', or against contamination by the excluded quality. This tendency was noted in relation to the politics of sexuality, for instance where 'fixity narratives'

dominated mainstream discourse during recent debates around reforming age of consent legislation in the UK (Waites, 2003).

34 Gerschick and Miller theorise disabled men's responses to the demands of hegemonic masculinity, suggesting three strategies, reformulation, reliance and rejection, which are typically combined in the lives and practices of individual men (Gerschick and Miller, 1994).

35 I am uncomfortable with the bracketing of racists, anti-gay bigots or paedophiles alongside their respective male victims within an all-encompassing category that implies that all men are alike. The notion that men can become 'gender-class traitors' encapsulates the value of adopting strategies that allow access to the hidden talk and agendas of powerful men (Hearn, 1992, 1994, 1998). I find this terminology worryingly evocative of phenomena such as the Chinese Cultural Revolution, however. Foucauldian perspectives question the ontological and epistemological assumptions of revolutionary discourse based upon sovereignty, unitary classes and single axes of oppression (Rajchman, 1985 pp. 62–5). Once again we are in the terrain of necessary errors, needing to find a language that describes men's collective political responsibility without 'fixing' rigid and essentialist over-generalisations about 'men' (Connell, 1987).

36 When they say men are damaged, Miller and Bell are referring to the effects of masculinity in 'predisposing men to exploit, dominate, and abuse – not only as boys, as partners and fathers, but as priests, teachers, therapists, lawyers, nurses, psychologists and psychiatrists' (1996 pp. 317–18).

37 At issue, once again, are the implications of situating critical insights (about how men internalise an ideology of domination) within the disciplinary apparatus of psychology. Though there are important issues here, such as the protectiveness of marriage for men, in mental health terms (Barnes and Maple, 1992, p. 12), psychologising sexism may simply divert attention from men's practices.

38 Cartesian discourses of mind–body dualism separate the supposedly disembodied consciousness of universal reason from biological essence imagined at the heart of male power (Seidler, 1994). A divided view of masculinity (as rational yet driven by primordial instinct) is reflected in some accounts of child sexual abuse and domestic violence in which men are portrayed, paradoxically, as both cerebral individuals who know exactly what they are doing (and are conspiratorially intent on rape), yet also as mysteriously susceptible to ill-defined predatory impulses, and 'governed by a kind of ceaseless determinism'. Liddle criticises the implicit suggestion that even relatively enlightened men 'should keep their fingers crossed – who knows, they may at any moment find themselves abusing children sexually', as unconvincing and counter-productive. Such discourses serve to bolster flight from responsibility, and overlook the potential for self-critique to individually or collectively transform gendered selves and bodies (Liddle, 1993, p. 119).

39 Hearn summarises various feminist theorisations of patriarchy and its links with capitalism, and of the development of public patriarchies, in which state policies, public support and professional caretaking increasingly mean that male-headed families are no longer needed to maintain patriarchy. The power of the individual father has been complicated by men's public power, but within this movement he finds the seeds of the destruction of patriarchies, not least in the new reality that all is potentially public (Hearn, 1994 pp. 19–20, 52–64, citing Brown, 1981; O'Brien, 1981; Walby, 1990). Within the political economy of reproduction, men can be seen to variously participate in, manage, organise or avoid processes including birth, childcare, adult nurturance, sexuality, violence and death (Hearn, 1994 pp. 81–3).

40 Witz writes that 'medical professionalisation is perhaps one of the best examples of a male professional project', and traces the historical construction of professional closure here (Witz, 1992 pp. 73–4).

41 After 1973, the category 'ego-dystonic homosexuality' was retained for individuals unhappy about their identity. Findings indicating that lesbian and gay youth are between two and six times as likely to attempt suicide as their heterosexual counterparts suggest that continuing prejudice will have made this a fairly likely occurrence (Golding, 1997 p. 3). Kutchins and Kirk stress that empirical data played a negligible role in the twenty-year debate about the inclusion of homosexuality within the DSM, and that participants on both sides were aware that the deletion of homosexuality as a mental disorder would usher in a new era of pluralism (1997/1999 p. 56). Declassification by the WHO happened as recently as 1992 (Pilgrim and Rogers, 1993/1999).

42 If we take oppression to refer to the systematic subjugation, deliberately or unintentionally, and by various means, of disadvantaged individuals and groups, then most individuals in late or postmodern Western societies have identities that are not just hyphenated but contradictory in this sense (e.g. black or working-class men, white women, middle-class gay or disabled men, etc.). Connell's analysis of an overarching gender order makes it clear, however, that hegemonic men have historically instigated, maintained and policed the exclusions of colonial, female and homosexual 'others' with particular vigour, and often violence (Connell, 1995).

43 Service responses to instances where men report a history of physical and, in a small minority of cases, sexual abuse by women need to be carefully addressed and contextualised. They render simplistic understandings of gender relations inadequate, and suggest the need for good supervision and support for those working with the consequences (cf. Featherstone, 1997).

44 Although Hollway adapts Lacan's concept of misrecognition to describe patterns of desire established during infancy, the term can usefully be defined in a much broader manner.

45 For instance, despite Laing's important critique of medicalisation, he retains medicalising discourse (sometimes enclosing it in distancing quotation marks), and case-study presentation (albeit from an anti-psychiatric angle). There is considerable irony in describing someone's state of mind in terms of Kierkegaard's 'shutupness', while excluding them from the process of analysing their own predicament. Laing's discussion focuses on the sense of disembodiment and splitting between a remote 'real self' and a 'false-self system' comprising a number of 'partially elaborated fragments of what might constitute a personality' (Laing, 1959/1965 pp. 73–4).

46 He tends to focus on the individual level, and doesn't say much, for instance, about racism and 'schizophrenia'. Although the 'borderline' diagnosis is one that has been applied predominantly to women (Kutchins and Kirk, 1997/1999), his examples of 'borderliners' are all dissenting men.

9 Masculinities and risk: negotiating the politics of complexity

1 The provisions introduced in a 1999 consultation document produced by the New Labour government, entitled *Managing People with Severe Dangerous Personality Disorder*, are seen as designed to circumvent the European Convention of Human Rights which prohibits preventive detention, except of people judged to be of unsound mind (Mullen, 1999).

2 Almost half of all respondents to a survey conducted by MIND had experienced verbal or physical abuse because of being identified as having mental health problems, and discrimination is commonplace (Sayce, 2000; Read and Baker, 1996).

3 Because this mostly occurs within intimate relationships and can occur in public places, and in order to distinguish it from violence carried out by women and/or directed against men or children, Hearn refers to 'men's violence against known women' rather than 'domestic violence' (Hearn, 1996).

4 The highly problematic term 'dangerousness' misleadingly suggests a permanent trait capable of objective measurement, and disguises processes of socio-political judgement imbued with prevailing mythology and misconception, particularly in relation to black people (Fernando et al., 1998). Clinicians and social workers, who are more often accused of under-reporting violence, have concerns about the 'normalisation' and reintegration of patients who may be refused services or accommodation if labelled violent. They are also less likely than nurses to experience violence directly.

5 Commenting on the tendency to invoke madness and resort to psychiatry in the face of horrific acts, Beresford suggests that it is the relationship between psychiatry and violence that demands attention, rather than that between service-users and violence (Beresford and Hopton, 2001).

6 These characteristically involve an obligation to discover and disclose 'the truth' in the context of constituting and transforming the self. Foucault uses the term 'governmentality' to describe the encounter between technologies of domination and those of the self (Rabinow, 1994/2000 pp. 177–8, 225).

7 Foucault's point is that such questions would have seemed completely out of place in such a tribunal 150 years earlier. A book of 1835, 'I, Pierre Rivière, Having Slaughtered my Mother, my Sister, and my Brother . . .' (Foucault, 1973/1975), deals with a case at that point in time. Despite his reputation as an imbecile, the young peasant accused of three murders produced a remarkably articulate memoir that was ignored by the court. Foucault prioritised an imperative to let this repressed voice speak across the centuries, rather than discussing the complex operations of gender here, even though a medical memorandum that secured a commutation of the death penalty identified Rivière as 'prey to the singular monomania namely aversion to women and female animals' (Foucault, 1973/1975 pp. ix–xiv, 167).

8 But not with constructions of black masculinity apparently, since although ethnic minority recipients are heavily over-represented in British Special Hospitals, comparatively few are detained under the legal category of psychopathy (Stowell-Smith and McKeown, 1999).

9 NBC journalists described a 'hell hole' housing 2,000 'mentally ill' men among 18,500 inmates (6,000 of whom are on medication) (NBC4 – Report, 3 May 2003, www.nbc4tv -Team4Reports – Trapped Inside.htm). The American Civil Liberties Union say that 'supermax' prisons are now being used as a dumping ground for people with serious mental health problems, many of whom report difficulties getting appropriate medication and are in solitary confinement for twenty-three hours a day (Campbell, 2003).

10 Rose discusses the tripartite division into zones of low, medium and high risk that has become standard within British psychiatric policy, the techniques of control applied within each, and the new archipelago of 'islands of confinement' (expanded medium secure units run by the NHS and private sector, locked acute wards and the detention of people diagnosed as suffering from a 'psychopathic disorder' in prisons). Diagnosis might be said to have become postmodern insofar as it is about location on a continuum rather than binary states, and with a continuous process of risk management rather than with the identification of 'something fixed stable, inherent, and hence predictable to all futures'. It also takes place across a complex institutional

topography within the community, so that the asylum walls no longer mark a simple and fixed distinction between those within and outside the system (Rose, 1998 pp. 182–4, 179).

11 In England, formal admissions under the 1983 Mental Health Act rose from 16,000 to 27,000 between 1988/9 and 1998/9, an increase of 69 per cent in ten years. The number of men admitted under part 2 of the Act almost doubled, compared with a 47 per cent increase in the number of women (Department of Health, 2000b). During the early 1990s there were a number of high-profile homicide cases and inquiry reports. In the USA, a ruling in the *Barefoot v. Estelle* court case insisted that however unreliable clinicians' predictions were, they were still admissible. This was at a time when 300,000 people were subjects of involuntary civil commitment on grounds of dangerousness (Rose, 1998 p. 187).

12 Environments equipped with 'locks, alarms and barriers at every point' induce fear that can lead to aggression (Langan and Lindow, 2000). Lindow notes that in user-controlled services, out-of-control behaviour tends to be much less evident. Although critics claim that such projects cater for less severely impaired people, those with minimal difficulties are highly unlikely to use them (Lindow, 1999). Projects set up for African-Caribbean and African clients, with substantial numbers of black staff and a democratic ethos, report an absence of violence (Francis and McKenzie in evidence to Blofeld *et al.*, 2004). Rotov attributes about 40 per cent of violent incidents on wards to insensitive rule enforcement. He cites evidence that higher staffing levels can be counter-productive, including instances from Israel and the USA where 'patient functioning' improved when staff went on strike and were almost totally absent. Positive results were reported from moving patients identified as 'most difficult' between hospitals, and giving them a welcoming ceremony where no references to previous troubles was permitted. Rotov warns of an increasingly 'tough' culture in American hospitals in which 'broken and demoralised patients' are counted among therapeutic successes. One man reported as 'chronically violent' was found to have begun flailing about only when staff ordered him to get up off the floor (Rotov, 1994 pp. 262–3). A study that consulted service-users about violence on wards highlighted cramped environments with little opportunity to discuss problems or get help when feeling distressed, and staff aggression. Preventive strategies suggested include provision of punch bags or pillows, a gym, somewhere to run and shout without being treated like an escapee, quiet space, more TV's and separate rooms, relaxation and debriefing after incidents. The authors note that a greater awareness of these perceptions would enable staff to anticipate and understand conflict better. They find general implementation of detailed risk assessment impracticable due to staffing constraints (Bhui *et al.*, 2001).

13 Many kinds of behaviour that are 'dangerous to self or others' are disregarded as evidence of 'mental illness' (Sayce, 1995; Foner, 1995 p. 139). Simpson points out that Peter Sutcliffe, who killed thirteen women in the 1980s, would not have been picked up by the proposed Mental Health Act, 'since he held down a job, paid a mortgage and did all the respectable things that in our culture signify "sanity"'. During this period suggestions for a late night curfew on men were greeted with indignation, but would arguably have been no more oppressive than introduction of Community Treatment Orders (Simpson, 1999).

14 Methodological difficulties are discussed by Mulvey (1994); Crichton (1995); Taylor and Monahan (1996); Rogers and Pilgrim (2003). Hopton, who elsewhere advocates preventive detention, somewhat confusingly proposes a rigorously mathematical and research-based profiling approach, but warns that such profiles should still be regarded as 'best guesses' (Hopton, 1998 pp. 252–4; Beresford and Hopton, 2001). Individuals who arrive identified as violent sometimes respond positively once they feel confident

that their interests are being taken seriously. Being subject to formal assessment by a wary professional at an inevitably tense moment may induce further distrust and exacerbate the problem.

15 People who are violent during psychotic episodes may never be violent otherwise, and usually don't want to harm others. They may well feel very upset by their violence, and this should be acknowledged (Campbell and Lindow, 1997).

16 Walker and Seifert cite three studies that found women to be more violent in ward contexts, and three in which neither sex was significantly more violent. Their own study was of violence in a six-bed psychiatric intensive care unit in inner London, established in 1990 when an open ward policy was abandoned because of increasing levels of violence, and catering mainly for detained patients judged to pose an immediate danger to themselves or others. The study only considered physical assaults, and found that an incident happened every five days. Despite finding neither sex significantly more violent, all three instances of violence causing major injuries involved men, and 50 per cent of all assaults were committed by four men, all of whom abused drugs, had criminal records, and were single and unemployed. Most attacks took place when medication was being administered (Walker and Seifert, 1994).

17 Studies published in the 1990s began to conclude that psychiatric patients were rather more prone to violence than average, but methodological difficulties contribute to a lack of consensus over their findings (Monahan, 1993 p. 299; Guite, 1994 p. 246; Mulvey, 1994 p. 663; Langan, 1999). Coid, in a paper calling for greater compulsory powers, reported that five out of six international epidemiological studies show that people suffering from 'major mental illnesses' are more 'dangerous' than the general public. He neglected to mention, however, that the exception was a study from Switzerland, where community facilities were in place, and there was little homelessness (Coid, 1996 p. 985; Modestin and Amman, 1995 p. 673). This 'Swiss effect' repeats an earlier contrast between Bleuler's relative optimism about 'schizophrenia' (he worked in Switzerland, believed in active community rehabilitation, and talked about 'the natural healing of psychoses'), and the balefully self-fulfilling pessimism of Kraeplin that prevailed elsewhere in a context of poor practice and intolerant communities with higher unemployment (Warner, 1985/1994 p. 15). Being young, male, of low socio-economic status, and involved in substance abuse, are regarded as much stronger risk factors for violence than being a psychiatric patient (Hiday, 1995).

18 Men are more likely to be handcuffed when suspected of being mentally disordered in a public place, are more likely to experience forced admission and seclusion, and are over-represented in secure facilities (Pilgrim, 1997 p. 60). Women, however, are proportionately more likely to be diverted from the criminal justice system into special hospitals and to be detained there longer for more minor offences (Warner, 1996 pp. 99–100).

19 This American study concluded that mothers were 'at high risk of being the targets of repeated violence', not least because they do most of the 'caring' for people the researchers construct as their 'adult children' (rather than sons and daughters), and because of a comparative absence of fathers from these households. They report that 31.8 per cent of their sample had experienced childhood sexual abuse, but found that these people were less likely to have threatened or attacked others as adults (Estroff et al., 1994 pp. 674, 677).

20 The importance of alcohol and drug abuse, as well as personality disorder, in this population has been highlighted. Appleby (Department of Health, 2001) finds 90 per cent of homicides committed by men, while 83 per cent of Morrall's sample of 'mad murders' were committed by men (Morrall, 2000). Media discourse surrounding these

discussions relies on categories and statistics dependent upon institutional and conceptual contingency. Coverage of the Boyd report, for example, portrayed patients being 'freed to kill', when half of those who did kill had been seen in the preceding month, and fewer than one in four were being seen less frequently than professionally recommended. Crepaz-Keay argues that greater levels of support rather than compulsory medication, which can have highly damaging effects, is likely to reduce risk (Crepaz-Keay, 1996; Sayce, 1995). Adverse effects of antipsychotic medication in men can include erectile dysfunction and galactorrhoea (milk secretion through the nipples) (Krabbendam and van Os, 2002).

21 At various points before and after a previous armed assault, on a young woman with whom he had a brief and mutually unsatisfying sexual encounter, as a student, Robinson had stated that an air pistol would make him look more macho, and that women can only respect someone who dominates them. He identified the woman as a source of evil, and felt that maiming her would enable his suicide (Blom-Cooper et al., 1995).

22 According to doctors, Andrew Robinson had had an earlier encounter with a young woman who rejected him and broke confidence about an intense preoccupation he had with the shape of his nose, and this resulted in him being taunted by other students. So convinced was he that his nose made him unattractive to women that he arranged for plastic surgery on several occasions. (Note that Freud referred a woman patient for nasal surgery for irregular or painful menstruation assumed to be related to masturbation, on the basis of his 'nasal reflex neurosis' hypothesis. See Masson, 1984/1992 p. 59.) Robinson had talked at length about his sexual difficulties during a first admission, and consulted sex therapists and a psychologist. It would seem pertinent, therefore, to ask how sexual distress is approached within patriarchal psychiatric environments, and why services had been unable to engage with his distress during a period when he was actively seeking help. He may have managed to conceal his rage at this time, of course, but since on discharge he rehearsed an attack on his prospective victim, it seems unlikely that he was in any meaningful sense 'well'. The implications of reliance on neuroleptics, which can exacerbate sexual difficulties, may also be relevant, particularly during the later stages of this story (Blom-Cooper et al., 1995).

23 Nor does it express concern about his discharge into the care of landladies, commenting only that had they been informed, 'it is always possible that Andrew might not have been viewed as a suitable tenant'. Given that he had by that time almost killed, had harassed and intimidated female staff, and subsequently developed sadistic homicidal fantasies about women, this seems a remarkable understatement, especially in view of the report's comments on professionals becoming 'seduced' and minimising both serious incidents and habitual violence in their accounts (Blom-Cooper et al., 1995 p. 186). The inquiry report has also been criticised as both misleading and damaging for advocating community treatment orders (involving indefinite reliance on potentially harmful medication, and use of the 1983 Act to detain former patients who have stopped taking medication, even if 'asymptomatic'), on the basis of a murder committed by a patient who was both on medication and in hospital (Harrison and Kessler, 1995).

24 Griffin, for example, refers to people in secure units as 'the underclass of the underclass' (Griffin and Sayce, 2003 p. 19). Pete Shaughnessy, who became involved in advocacy within the English Special Hospitals, partly because of the murder of his sister by a boyfriend who was judged to have been in a state of paranoid psychosis, felt that inmates in Rampton are not 'different from us' (Olden, in Asylum, 2003 pp. 13–14).

25 There have been histories of gross abuse, many individuals are detained long after the decision that they no longer pose a threat, and black and ethnic minority patients are over-represented (see, for example, Sayce, 1995). Warner reports that in an environment where sexual assaults continue, women patients have been made to socialise with sex offenders as part of 'treatment' presumably designed to inculcate feminine heterosexuality (Warner, 1996 p. 107).

26 Sayce reviews the pure libertarian position adopted by some American survivor activists who see an insistence upon 'mad' offenders taking responsibility for their crimes as a price worth paying for an end to coercive treatment. A more multifaceted approach might call for 'problem-solving' policing, taking account of the effects of victimisation and poverty, less punitive criminal justice systems, and a range of measures such as advance directives, advocacy and survivor-informed crisis support within state provision of safe spaces for people experiencing extreme distress (Sayce, 2000).

27 Boys outnumber girls in diagnoses of childhood behavioural syndromes by about four to one. Mariani cites the notorious 'monkey remarks' made by a former director of the National Institute for Mental Health, but notes that white middle-class boys appear to be disproportionately targeted by biobehavioural research since they are more likely to be referred to clinics rather than being channelled into the criminal justice system. 'If white boys are out of control', she writes, 'how can they be expected to *maintain* control as white men?' (Mariani, 1995 pp. 137–40, 153; see also Rose, 1997 p. 290; Breggin and Breggin, 1994; Breggin, 1995/1996).

28 Hare's popularising manual *Without Conscience*, in which the classically 'paranoid' motif of a pair of eyes in photographic negative is repeated throughout, is based upon a fear-anxiety paradigm derived from work in which experimental subjects are given aversive or painful stimulation (electric shocks) to test their capacity for 'anticipatory fear' (Hare, 1993). The psychopathy checklist has been recommended as 'a measuring tool that was not made of out rubber' (*The Science of Crime*, Equinox, Channel 4, 7 December 2000).

29 Just as ECT was first used experimentally on a man arrested in a Rome railway station, such men may also become the first experimental subjects of radical developments in social control technology such as the installation of microchip brain implants.

30 After these losses in 1984 and 1985 he began to show signs of odd behaviour, and was hospitalised in Jamaica. Because his mother had died when he was away, he had been unable to attend the funeral. He was twenty-two years old at this time (Ritchie, 1994).

31 Such services would be staffed by people who could engage with users and see the world from their perspective. This would not depend upon ethnic matching (Ritchie, 1994 p. 65).

32 David 'Rocky' Bennett died while being held face down on the floor for some twenty-five minutes in a medium secure unit in Norwich. He had told his sister that it was not unusual for him to be racially abused and physically attacked by other patients, and the events leading to his death were the culmination of a long history of discrimination and angry, sometimes violent, retaliation. During an altercation with another patient he had been racially abused, and he felt aggrieved that he, rather than the other man, had been removed to another ward and seriously assaulted a female nurse (Blofeld et al., 2004). More than a decade earlier, a report into the deaths of Orville Blackwood and two other black patients in Broadmoor hospital had identified institutional racism (Prins, 1999 pp. 84–7; Fernando et al., 1998 pp. 190–4).

33 Though according to Shah, older men remain the demographic group at highest proportional risk (Shah and De, 1998).

34 In 1992 Pritchard drew attention to a rapid rise in young male suicide, and noted that the trend was more marked in the UK than in the rest of Europe (Pritchard, 1992). People categorised as social class five are approximately four times more likely to take their own lives as those in social class one (Department of Health, 2002). Smith and Leon state that suicides among 15–24-year-olds rose by 75 per cent in the 1980s (Smith and Leon, 2001). Katz et al. cite a 60 per cent rise in suicide rates for this group between the periods 1976–81 and 1986–1991 (Katz et al., 1999). Swanwick and Clare found that the suicide rate for young men in Ireland had doubled since 1977 while that for women had levelled off (Swanwick and Clare, 1997). In a four-year study of notified suicides by people defined as having a mental illness in England and Wales 75 per cent (or a ratio of 3 : 1) overall, and 82 per cent of all 25–34-year-olds, were men (Department of Health, 2001). Stack concludes that the major trend internationally has been a shift from converging male and female suicide rates (between 1919 and 1972) to a widening gender gap since the 1970s (Stack, 2000).

35 The authors conclude that despite some evidence of reluctance to classify female deaths as suicide any understatement is insufficient to vitiate the overall pattern of higher male mortality rates from suicide, and that the gender gap is real, at least where the male–female ratio of deaths is high (Canetto and Sakinofsky, 1998, pp. 8, 4).

36 A study of 174 young suicides in the UK (85 per cent male) found that less than half the overall sample had ever had any contact with mental health services (Hawton et al., 1999).

37 One factor has been that drugs commonly used in overdoses have become less toxic. It is also noted that a decline in marriage, increases in divorce, and increasing income inequality have been consistently associated with young male suicide but have had little effect on suicides by young women (Schapira et al., 2001).

38 For Durkheim, anomie referred to the loss of societal norms regulating individual goals and aspirations in relation to the means available to fulfil them. For young men, Pritchard suggested that the effects of having an unemployed father at home might be significant (Pritchard, 1992).

39 This linkage occurs in the story of Andrew Robinson (Blom-Cooper et al., 1995).

40 A medical study concluded that, despite privations, family bereavements, and terrifying bombing raids, wartime experience (during the Second World War) had been beneficial for the mental health of women, if only as a cure for 'hypochondria' (Hemphill, 1941, cited in Bracken, 2002 pp. 67–8). Some of these women will have benefited from the absence of violent men, and in war, of course, men's suicidal acts are readily mistaken for, or transmuted into, Durkheimian altruism.

41 The suicidal intent of psychiatric patients tends to be treated as irrational, regardless of people's reasons for feeling devalued and desperate (Pilgrim and Rogers, 1993/1999 p. 184). Some psychiatric drugs have been found to induce suicide (Healy, 2001).

42 For Heidegger, ontological enquiry concerns itself with the question of being, the 'holding together' of things that gives our life-world meaning (Bracken, 2002 pp. 12–3).

43 They were found to be four times as likely to have experienced violence (70 per cent of this group had experienced violence from an adult), three times as likely to have been threatened with violence by an adult, and six times as likely to have been beaten. Bullying was a common problem, and they were ten times as likely to be using drugs to relieve stress (Katz et al., 1999).

44 The political map of research relationships in this study is characteristically complex. Given concerns about power/knowledge practices that focus upon detailed interpretation of service-users' utterances, use of discourse analytic methods in research

with recipients must be regarded as problematic. Against this, however, the position of female researchers needs to be considered vis-à-vis a male participant admitted to the unit because of physical aggression towards his mother.

10 Reconstructing men's lives: power/knowledge, personal recovery and social transformation

1 For example, the Vancouver Emotional Emergency Centre focused on intensive emotional support and help with life changes (Chamberlin, 1977/1988). Breggin advocates a democratised psychotherapy. People experiencing their first 'schizophrenic break' were successfully helped at Soteria House with relatively little use of potentially damaging medication by staff who mostly had no formal qualifications and were chosen primarily for their egalitarian values (Breggin, 1993 pp. 475–7). Access to counselling has long been included among the political demands of the user/survivor movement.

2 He made this point in the context of Mannoni's claim that the Malagasy were susceptible to an inferiority complex from childhood, and that this was merely activated by the colonial experience in exceptional individuals who aspired beyond their station, and appears to have been dismissive of such explanations of psychosis (Fanon, 1952/1986, citing Mannoni, 1964).

3 His response, 'I felt knife blades open within me. I resolved to defend myself', is interesting in relation to the Clunis case (Fanon, 1952/1986 p. 118). Although he was conventional in making extensive use of ECT, which had not yet been widely contested, Fanon developed a strong interest in psychoanalysis, literature and culture. He also worked in the context of the Algerian War, where his patients included both torturers and their victims, and he declared colonial psychiatry impossible. 'The social structure existing in Algeria was hostile to any attempt to put the individual back where he belonged.' (Macey, 2000 pp. 144–53, 210–11).

4 Some gay men report having been assertively heterosexist before they were able to come out, and repression has driven some men to seduce or rape, and then assault or even kill a gay man (Hopkins, 1996 pp. 101–2).

5 Reasonable responses to oppression thus become labelled as 'phobias' as lesbians and gay men given this apparently supportive diagnosis are encouraged to examine how they may have adopted a victim attitude and perpetuated their own social isolation (Kitzinger, 1997).

6 That phobia has currency beyond and apart from clinical usage, that these terms are not strongly associated with the sharp end of the psychiatric system, and that agoraphobia is linked with gender oppression, may have a bearing on these discussions. Usage of the term might also mask variation in the phenomenon, such as the role of sexual abuse in the formation of some of this fear and prejudice.

7 Atmore is replying to a commentary by Scott attributing feminists' difficulty in responding to the False Memory Syndrome as a discourse of disbelief, to a postmodern tendency to deride certainty. Scott's conclusion that there are important political (as opposed to epistemological) questions about the interests served by the production and distribution of that discourse is consistent with critical and social postmodern perspectives, however, as are judgements about the appropriateness, consistency and reliability of memory (understood as perspectival and context specific) (Scott, 1997). Showalter notes some controversial cases among the literature on male 'survivors', and regards PTSD as a euphemism for and part of the cultural denial of 'male hysteria' (Showalter, 1997 pp. 153, 64).

8 The cost of importing experiences of intense emotional injury into the clinical domain includes the adoption of a set of positivist and individualising assumptions

me meaning as individual and internal rather than cultural and historical. ɪg the empirical research, Bracken concludes that 'it would appear that the nent of PTSD after significant trauma such as combat or rape is the excep- ner than the rule'. The aftermath of trauma can take diverse forms and under- sta.ɪ... ɪg can be constrained and distorted by rigidly cognitive Western clinical constructs (Bracken, 2002 p. 77).

9 Tautological because the constellation includes viewing violence as manly and danger as exciting, as well as callous sexuality towards women, toughness and self-control (Zaitchik and Mosher, 1993).

10 Jukes still sees battering and abuse as indicative of sexism rather than individual pathology, however (Jukes, 1996). Frosh manages to challenge the liberal position that 'we are all basically reasonable, and . . . abusive acts are the products of disturbed and criminal personalities', without implying that all men succumb to the potential for abuse inherent in masculine socialisation (Frosh, 1994 pp. 1–4). Jukes's view of a 'gendered psychosis' due to the trauma of separation appears diametrically opposed to Lacan's equally totalising assertion that psychosis results from a failure to separate from (and in the process denigrate) the mother, in order to enter the paternal realm of the symbolic (Frosh, 1994 p. 111).

11 Petersen comments that in magazines such as the British *Achilles Heel* or the Australian *XY* 'discussions about personal identity and experiences of personal "crisis" tend to be given priority over discussions about relations of power' (Petersen, 1998 p. 93).

12 In this analysis, abuse is driven by an 'abhorrence of the feminine within', so that women become symbolic representatives of 'unacceptable' aspects of men, and socially sanctioned recipients of violence that results from psychic splitting. Because the intensity of denied emotion and desire becomes threatening to such men, they often choose the least threatening and most controllable objects – children, rather than adult women (Frosh, 1994 pp. 113–14).

13 More interventionist approaches may re-enact the traditional masculine response of coming in, disrupting the unity between mother and child, saying 'no', and taking control (Frosh, 1992). Frosh notes that the openness of 'reverie' can be too emotion-ally intrusive for some men.

14 Frosh argues that advocacy is not always sufficient since psychological distress involves a non-transparent (presumably distorting) relationship to 'reality', and that because of the opportunity it offers to work on transference, apparently authoritarian therapy can be more subversive than overtly egalitarian forms. The analyst's task is to 'aid the process of reality testing' (Frosh, 1999 pp. 250, 276). On abuse in therapy, see for example Jehu (1994); Hetherington (2000).

15 Introducing an account of unconscious processes and a sense of the continuity of self-hood into the way in which subjects are positioned in discourses addresses limitations imposed by a rationalistic view of agency and the voluntaristic model of change within liberation politics (Henriques *et al.*, 1984/1998).

16 This 'holding' stance entails a state of 'openness to all the projections of the patient', a process of containment that absorbs fragmenting pain and destructiveness, and a willingness to be changed by the other's experience (Frosh, 1992 pp. 157–9).

17 But note that, like Nicholson, Rose cites Freud approvingly in contrast with subse-quent developments in therapeutics that seek to establish a regime of self-mastery in which grief, frustration, disappointment and death are to be managed as challenges to the powers of the self (Rose, 1998 p. 159).

18 Some such work adopts a medicalising approach, however. Real, for example, identi-fies 'covert depression', argues that many men use arrogance to 'medicate' themselves against it, and advocates the use of drugs such as Prozac to provide a 'stable platform from which to undertake the hard work of psychotherapy' (Real, 1997 p. 288).

19 The narrative method seeks to reverse the effects of techniques of power that incite people to constitute their lives through professionally ordained 'truths' by encouraging clients to discard problem-saturated descriptions of their lives and develop more rewarding personal stories (White and Epston, 1990).

20 'This selection has been made with the aim of demonstrating the applicability of literate means to a wide range of presenting problems' (White and Epston, 1990 p. 216).

21 For example, encouraging polysemy, poetic language and multiple perspectives might complicate matters for some people, and in several examples where narrative therapy appears to have helped people deal with problematic voice-hearing, this does not seem to be what has happened (White and Epston, 1990 p. 83).

22 These kinds of activity could be supported under the aegis of self-advocacy, community work/arts/action, action research, consciousness-raising or life-history work. Though often presented as inherently progressive, the direct involvement of therapists in creating contexts in which marginalised voices can be heard raises questions about the therapeutisation of politics. People from working-class and ethnic minority communities, who have long been assumed not to be suitable candidates for counselling (not being articulate enough, and not having interesting enough inner lives?), could find themselves being propelled towards untimely political activism. For an account of feminist 'social action psychotherapy', influenced by both Winnicott and Freire, that blurs boundaries between therapy and political action, see Holland (1992).

23 Despite calls for professional reflexivity, therapists may mark out the language of deconstruction as a professional preserve, reconfiguring the conventional therapist's power to differentiate between normal and abnormal into a deconstructive therapist's privileged insight into the distinction between normalising power and resistance (Parker, 1999; Kaye, 1999).

24 Swan stresses the importance of coming to see self-criticism and a sense of worthlessness as reflections of (and discomfort about) the tools of power, rather than as evidence of unhealed or unresolved damage created by abuse, as evidence of a subconscious need to harm oneself or as a marker of personal weakness. Therapy can be a toxic environment, but can also create 'space for the local, day-to-day problematisation and contestation of the oppressive effects of power' (Swan, 1999 pp. 110, 113).

25 Law mentions working alongside women co-therapists, referring to a 'reflecting team' of women therapists, and using videotapes of the work, with consent of participants, in training (Law, 1999). Issues arise here about sources of political power-knowledge, and about the risk of prescriptive 'correctness' in deconstructive practice (Kaye, 1999).

26 Law makes this argument having considered the difficulties involved in giving space to Don's story, not least that for some women and men it would not be possible, or even desirable, to hear about his pain.

27 For Foucault this typically involved a deciphering of experience in terms of signs and symptoms that would be validated according to scientific discourses of truth within the hermeneutic procedures of the confessional (Foucault, 1976/1978).

28 This entails recognising that his career and professional practices had not been the result of self-determined personal expression and innovation, but 'the semi-products of a social and historical construction', and that his formerly 'thrusting, striving "I", was in effect 'the willing prisoner of a destructive childhood'. He then moves to another paradoxical position, involving 'a much more charged, active grappling, along with other men' to move towards a gentler world in which the fluid and contradictory nature of subjectivity is acknowledged (Jackson, 1990 pp. 257–9).

Grant (1993), he argues that some interpretations of standpoint theory
men's experience within particular historical and discursive contexts and
; notion of a single female perspective. We see the world from the standpoint
ubject positions we take up within discourse (Pease, 2000 p. 140, 1999
p. ₁~

30 In the project Pease describes, men reframed childhood experiences, and looked at
relationships with fathers and mothers, homophobia and the objectification of
women. Speaking from a dominant position, men talked about what it meant to
repress experiences of intimacy with other men, and about the part they had played
in the reproduction of hierarchical heterosexuality (Pease, 2000 p. 149).

31 Developing a systematic critique of social conditions may be a useful way of affirming
non-conventional life stories, involving living alone, non-parenthood, poverty and
unemployment, for example, that hegemonic values about masculinity characterise
in terms of failure.

32 Such as sexually abused men often not feeling safe working with male professionals
(Myers, 1989), the need to address cultural differences, the sensitivity of language
and labelling, the impact of medication in a context of biomedical dominance, the
immediacy of practical problems, and the inappropriateness of attempting to elicit
personal stories from some men who are likely to find such processes unbearably
invasive for a variety of reasons.

33 Introductions to Re-evaluation Counselling (RC) written by psychiatric survivors
can be found in Read (2001) and Foner (1995). These writers neglect to mention
other co-counselling organisations, however. When evaluating co-counselling from
an advocacy perspective, I talked to people who had moved both ways between RC
and Co-Counselling International (CCI) because of their contrasting strengths and
weaknesses. Any basic training entails opting into a set of ideas, such as particular
versions of identity politics and a 'hydraulic' model of emotions and human distress.
Questions need to be asked about informed consent, accountability, ideological
content and methods taught, not least since critics of RC highlight suppression of
criticism, and somewhat cult-like organisational features (Tourish and Irving,
1995). CCI veers towards an entrepreneurial/personal growth model of leadership.
RC devotes specific attention to psychiatric survivor issues, and people involved in
it have been highly influential in the psychiatric survivor movement, but for a critical
history written by a founder of the breakaway CCI, see Heron (1980).

34 The ability or desire to open up and examine memory, about what will often be a
history of harrowing experience, may well depend upon the privileges of enjoying
relative emotional and material stability, being free from the adverse effects of
medication and from routine demands to provide summaries of intimate biographical
experience to caring professionals or officialdom. Recent accounts reflecting the
diversity of sources of support include a user-led research project by a group of British
Muslims on the effects of attendance at mosque during times of distress (Bobat,
2001), a disabled Vietnam veteran who has devoted himself to environmental
restoration work (Lyman, 2004), and a young man who believed aliens were monitoring his activities and thoughts, and who found emotional support and practical
strategies from an on-line support group for alien abductees (Knight, 2004).

35 Some critical writings about masculinity seem to imply that men actually liking other
men amounts to a lapse in proper scepticism. Given that groups of men tend to be
predisposed by masculinity towards competitiveness, mutual suspicion and fear of
intimacy, such a view would clearly be unhelpful in 'mental health' settings.

Bibliography

Ahmed, S. (1998) *Differences that Matter, Feminist Theory and Postmodernism*, Cambridge, Cambridge University Press.

Alcoff, L. and Gray, L. (1993) 'Survivor Discourse: Transgression or Recuperation?', Signs, Winter, pp. 260–90.

Alcoff, L. and Potter, E. eds (1993) *Feminist Epistemologies*, New York, Routledge.

Allen, J. and Laird, J. (1991) 'Men and Story, Constructing New Narratives in Therapy', pp. 75–100 in *Feminist Approaches for Men in Family Therapy*, New York, Harrington Park Press.

Allison, D. ed. (1977/1985) *The New Nietzsche: Contemporary Styles of Interpretation*, Cambridge, Mass., MIT Press.

Allison, D. (2000) 'Musical Psychodramatics, Ecstasis in Nietzsche', pp. 66–78 in Schrift, A. ed. *Why Nietzsche Still?*, Berkeley, University of California Press.

Allison, D. (2001) *Reading the New Nietzsche*, Lanham, Md, Rowman and Littlefield.

Ansell-Pearson, K. (1993) 'Nietzsche, Woman and Political Theory', pp. 27–48 in Patton, P. ed. *Nietzsche, Feminism and Political Theory*, London, Routledge.

Archer, J. and Lloyd, B. (2002) *Sex and Gender*, 2nd edition, Cambridge, Cambridge University Press.

Armstrong, D. (1997) 'Foucault and the Sociology of Health and Illness, A Prismatic Reading', pp. 15–30 in Petersen, A. and Bunton, R. eds *Foucault, Health and Medicine*, London, Routledge.

Armstrong, L. (1996) *Rocking the Cradle of Sexual Politics*, London, Women's Press.

Artaud, A. (1938/1970) *The Theatre and Its Double*, London, Calder and Boyars.

Artaud, A. (1976) *Collected Works*, ed. Paul Thévenin, Vol. 8, Diverse texts, letters and journalism, *Revolutionary Messages*, Paris, Gallimard.

Ascheim, S. (1992) *The Nietzsche Legacy in Germany, 1890–1990*, Berkeley, University of California Press.

Atmore, C. (1997) 'Commentary: Conflicts over Recovered Memories – Every Layer of the Onion', Feminism and Psychology, Vol. 7, No. 1, pp. 57–62.

Atteberry, J. (2000) 'Reading Forgiveness and Forgiving Reading: Antonin Artaud's Correspondance avec Jacques Rivière', Modern Language Notes, Vol. 115, Sept., pp. 717–40.

Baldwin, J. (1964) *Notes of a Native Son*, London, Corgi.

Bangay, F. (2000) 'An Uphill Struggle, But It's Been Worth It', pp. 101–4, in Curtis, T., Dellar, R., Leslie, E. and Watson, B. eds *Mad Pride: a Celebration of Mad Culture*, London, Spare Change Books.

Barber, S. (1993) *Antonin Artaud, Blows and Bombs*, London, Faber and Faber.

Baring, A. and Cashford, J. (1991) *The Myth of the Goddess: Evolution of an Image*, London, Viking Press.

Barker, P., Campbell, P. and Davidson, B. eds (1999) *From the Ashes of Experience: Reflections on Madness, Survival, and Growth*, London, Whurr Publishers.

Barnes, M. and Bowl, R. (2001) *Taking over the Asylum: Empowerment and Mental Health*, Basingstoke, Palgrave.

Barnes, M. and Maple, N. (1992) *Women and Mental Health, Challenging the Stereotypes*, Birmingham, Venture Press.

Baron-Cohen, S. (2003) *The Essential Difference*, London, Penguin.

Bartky, S. (1988) 'Foucault, Femininity, and the Modernisation of Patriarchal Power', pp. 61–86 in Diamond, I. and Quimby, L. eds *Feminism and Foucault, Reflections on Resistance*, Boston, Mass., Northeastern University Press.

Bauman, Z. (1991) *Modernity and Ambivalence*, Cambridge, Polity Press.

Bauman, Z. (1992) *Intimations of Postmodernity*, London, Routledge.

Bauman, Z. (1993) *Postmodern Ethics*, Oxford, Blackwell.

Bauman, Z. (1997) *Postmodernity and its Discontents*, London, Polity Press.

Bauman, Z. (2000) 'Social Issues of Law and Order', British Journal of Criminology, Vol. 40, pp. 205–21.

Beilharz, P. (2001) *The Bauman Reader*, Oxford, Blackwell.

Benjamin, J. (1995) 'Sameness and Difference, Toward an 'Over-Inclusive' Theory of Gender Development', pp. 106–22 in Elliot, A. and Frosh, S. eds *Psychoanalysis in Contexts*, London, Routledge.

Benvenuto, B. and Kennedy, R. (1986) *The Works of Jacques Lacan, An Introduction*, London, Free Association Books.

Beresford, P. (2000) 'What Have Madness and Psychiatric System Survivors Got to Do with Disability and Disability Studies?', Disability and Society, Vol. 15, No. 1, pp. 167–72.

Beresford, P. and Croft, S. (1998) 'Postmodernity and the Future of Welfare: Whose Critiques, Whose Social Policy?', pp. 103–17 in Carter, J. ed. *Postmodernity and the Fragmentation of Welfare*, London, Routledge.

Beresford, P. and Croft, S. (2001) 'Mental Health Policy: A Suitable Case for Treatment?', pp. 10–22 in Newnes, C., Holmes, G. and Dunn, C. eds *This is Madness Too: Critical Perspectives on Mental Health Services*, Ross-on-Wye, PCCS Books.

Beresford, P and Hopton, J. (2001) 'Who's in Danger Anyway?', OpenMind, 108, March/April, pp. 20–1.

Beresford, P. and Hopton, J. (2003) 'Recovery or Independent Living?', OpenMind, 124, Nov./Dec., pp. 16–17.

Berger, P. (1963) *Invitation to Sociology, A Humanistic Perspective*, Harmondsworth, Penguin.

Berger, M., Wallis, B. and Watson, S. (1995) *Constructing Masculinity*, London, Routledge.

Berry, P. and Wernick, A. eds (1992) *Shadow of Spirit, Postmodernism and Religion*, London, Routledge.

Bersani, L. (1995) 'The Gay Daddy', in *Homos*, Cambridge, Mass., Harvard University Press.

Best, S. and Kellner, D. (1991) *Postmodern Theory, Critical Interrogations*, Basingstoke, Macmillan Press.

Bhabha, H. (1994) *The Location of Culture*, London, Routledge.

Bhabha, H. (1995) *Are You a Man or a Mouse?*, pp. 57–65 in Berger, M., Wallis, B. and Watson, S. eds *Constructing Masculinity*, New York, Routledge.

Bhaskar, R. (1989) *Reclaiming Reality: a Critical Introduction to Contemporary Philosophy*, London, Verso.

Bhui, K et al. (2001) 'Implementing Clinical Practice Guidelines on the Management of Imminent Violence on Two Acute Psychiatric In-Patient Units', Journal of Mental Health, Vol. 10, No. 5 pp. 559–69.

Bhui, K. ed. (2002) *Racism and Mental Health, Prejudice and Suffering*, London, Jessica Kingsley.

Bion, W. (1962) *Learning from Experience*, London, Maresfield.

Bloch, D. (1989) 'Freud's Retraction of his Seduction Theory and the Schreber Case', Psycho-analytic Review, Vol. 76, No. 2, Summer, pp. 185–201.

Blofeld, J., Sallah, D., Sashidharan, S., Stone, R. and Struthers, J. (2004) *Independent Inquiry into the Death of David Bennett*, Cambridge, Norfolk, Suffolk, and Cambridgeshire Strategic Health Authority, Fulbourn.

Blom-Cooper, L., Hally, H. and Murphy, E. (1995) *The Falling Shadow: One Patient's Mental Health Care 1978–1993*, London, Duckworth.

Bly, R. (1991) *Iron John, A Book About Men*, Shaftesbury, Element.

Bobat, H. (2001) 'A User-Led Research Project into Mosque, Exploring the Benefits that Muslim Men with Severe Mental Health Problems Find from Attending Mosque', London, Mental Health Foundation.

Bock, G. and James, S. eds (1992) *Beyond Equality and Difference: Citizenship, Feminist Politics, Female Subjectivity*, London, Routledge.

Bordo, S. (1988) 'Anorexia Nervosa: Psychopathology as the Crystallisation of Culture', pp. 87–117 in Diamond, I. and Quinby, L. eds *Feminism and Foucault, Reflections on Resistance*, Boston, Mass., Northeastern University Press

Bordo, S. (1990) 'The Body and the Reproduction of Femininity: a Feminist Appropriation of Foucault', in Jagger, A. and Bordo, S. eds *Gender/Body/Knowledge: Feminist Reconstructions of Being and Knowing*, New Brunswick, Rutgers University Press.

Bordo, S. (1990b) 'Feminism, Postmodernism, and Gender-Scepticism', pp. 133–56 in Nicholson, L. ed. *Feminism/Postmodernism*, New York, Routledge.

Bordo, S. (1999) 'Feminism, Foucault, and the Politics of the Body', pp. 246–57 in Price, J. and Shildrick, M. *Feminist Theory and the Body, A Reader*, Edinburgh, Edinburgh University Press.

Bouchard, D. (1977) *Michel Foucault. Language, Counter-Memory, Practice*, Ithaca, NY, Cornell University Press.

Bowring, J. ed. (1843/1962) *The Works of Jeremy Bentham*, New York, Russell and Russell.

Boyd, W. D. (1994) *A Preliminary Report on Homicide*, London, Steering Committee of the Confidential Inquiry into Homicides and Suicides by Mentally Ill People.

Boyne, R. (1990) *Foucault and Derrida: the Other Side of Reason*, London, Routledge.

Bracken, P. (1993) 'Post-Empiricism and Psychiatry: Meaning and Methodology in Cross-Cultural Research', Social Science and Medicine, Vol. 36, No. 3, pp. 265–72.

Bracken, P. (1995) 'Beyond Liberation: Michel Foucault and the Notion of Critical Psychiatry', Philosophy, Psychiatry, and Psychology, Vol. 2, pp. 1–13.

Bracken, P. (2002) *Trauma, Culture, Meaning and Philosophy*, London, Whurr.

Bracken, P. and Thomas, P. (1999) *Cognitive Therapy, Cartesianism and the Moral Order*, European Journal of Counselling and Health, Vol. 2, No. 3, Dec., pp. 325–44.

Bracken, P. and Thomas, P. (1999b) 'Let's Scrap Schizophrenia', OpenMind, Sept./Oct., p. 17.

Bracken, P. and Thomas, P. (2001) 'Postpsychiatry: a New Direction for Mental Health', British Medical Journal, Vol. 322, 24 March, pp. 724–7.

Bracken, P. and Thomas, P. (forthcoming) Postpsychiatry, Oxford, Oxford University Press.

Brackx, A. and Grimshaw, C. (1989) Mental Health Care in Crisis, London, Pluto.

Brah, A. (1996) Cartographies of Diaspora, London, Routledge.

Breggin, P. (1993) Toxic Psychiatry, Drugs and Electroconvulsive Therapy: the Truth and Better Alternatives, London, Fontana.

Breggin, P. (1995/1996) 'Campaigns Against Racist Federal Programs by the Center for the Study of Psychiatry and Psychology', Journal of African American Men, Vol. 1, No. 3, Winter, pp. 3–22.

Breggin, P. and Breggin, G. (1994) The War Against Children: How the Drugs, Programmes, and Theories of the Psychiatric Establishment Are Threatening America's Children with a 'Cure' for Violence, New York, St Martin's Press.

Brod, H. (1998) 'To Be a Man, or Not to Be a Man, That is the Feminist Question', pp. 197–212 in Digby, T. ed. Men Doing Feminism, New York, Routledge.

Broverman, I., Broverman, D., Clarkson, F., Rosenkranz, P. and Vogel, S. (1970) 'Sex Role Stereotypes and Clinical Judgements of Mental Health', Journal of Consulting and Clinical Psychology, Vol. 2, pp. 1–13.

Brown, C. (1981) 'Mothers, Fathers, and Children: from Private to Public Patriarchy', pp. 239–67 in Sergent, L. ed. Women and Revolution: the Unhappy Marriage of Marxism and Feminism, London, Pluto.

Brown, L. and Burman, E. eds (1997) 'Feminist Responses to the "False Memory" Debate', Feminism and Psychology, Vol. 7, No. 1, pp. 7–16.

Brown, W. (1995) States of Injury, Power and Freedom in Late Modernity, Princeton, NJ, Princeton University Press.

Brown, W. (2000) 'Nietzsche for Politics', pp. 205–23 in Schrift, A. ed. Why Nietzsche Still? Reflections on Drama, Culture, and Politics, Berkeley, University of California Press.

Brownmiller, S. (1975) Against Our Will: Men, Women, and Rape, New York, Simon and Schuster.

Bruggen, P. (1997) Who Cares? True Stories of the NHS Reforms, London, Jon Carpenter.

Burkitt, I. (1999) Bodies of Thought, Embodiment, Identity, and Modernity, London, Sage.

Burman, E. et al. eds (1996) Psychology, Discourse, Practice. From Regulation to Resistance, London, Taylor and Francis.

Burman, E. and Parker, I. (1993) Discourse Analytic Research; Repertoires and Readings of Texts in Action, London, Routledge.

Bury, M. (1998) 'Postmodernity and Health', in Modernity, Medicine, and Health: Medical Sociology Towards 2000, London, Routledge.

Busfield, J. (1996) Men, Women, and Madness, Basingstoke, Macmillan.

Busfield, J. (2001) Rethinking the Sociology of Mental Health, Oxford, Blackwell.

Butler, J. (1990) Gender Trouble, Feminism and the Subversion of Identity, London, Routledge.

Butler, J. (1990b) 'Gender Trouble, Feminist Theory and Psychoanalytic Discourse', pp. 324–40 in Nicholson, L. ed. Feminism/Postmodernism, New York, Routledge.

Butler, J. (1993) Bodies that Matter: On the Discursive Limits of 'Sex', London, Routledge.

Butler, J. (1995) 'Contingent Foundations: Feminism and the Question of Postmodernism', in Benhabib, S. ed. Feminist Contentions: a Philosophical Exchange, London, Routledge.
Butler, J. and Scott, J. (1992) Feminists Theorise the Political, New York, Routledge.
Callinicos, A. (1989) Against Postmodernism, a Marxist Critique, Cambridge, Polity Press.
Campbell, D. (2003) '300,000 Mentally Ill in U.S. Prisons', Guardian, 3 March.
Campbell, P. (1989) 'The Self-Advocacy Movement in the U.K.', pp. 206–13 in Brackx, A. and Grimshaw, C. eds Mental Health Care in Crisis, London, Pluto.
Campbell, P. (1990) 'Psychiatry and Personal Autonomy', Critical Public Health, No. 4, pp. 11–15.
Campbell, P. (1992) 'A Survivor's View of Community Psychiatry', Journal of Mental Health, Vol. 1, pp. 117–22.
Campbell, P. (1995) 'The Last Communication', Openmind, 74, April/May, pp. 18–19.
Campbell, P. (2001) 'Surviving Social Inclusion', pp. 93–102 in Newnes, C., Holmes, G. and Dunn, C., This Is Madness Too: Critical Perspectives on Mental Health Services, Ross-on-Wye, PCCS Books.
Campbell, P. and Lindow, V. (1997) Changing Practice, Mental Health Nursing and User Empowerment, London, Royal College of Nursing and Mind.
Canetto, S. (1992–3) 'She Died for Love and He Died for Glory: Gender Myths of Suicidal Behaviour', Omega, Vol. 26, No. 1, pp. 1–17.
Canetto, S. and Sakinofsky, I. (1998) 'The Gender Paradox in Suicide', Suicide and Life Threatening Behaviour, Vol. 28, No. 1, pp. 1–23.
Carpenter, M. (2001) 'Mental Health Policy under Welfare Capitalism since 1945', pp. 58–75 in Busfield, J. ed. Rethinking the Sociology of Mental Health, Oxford, Blackwell.
Carter, J. ed. (1998) Postmodernity and the Fragmentation of Welfare, London, Routledge.
Chadwick, P. (1997) Schizophrenia: the Positive Perspective, In Search of Dignity for Schizophrenic People, London, Routledge.
Chadwick, P. (2000) 'Bullying and Psychosis', OpenMind, 103, May/June, p. 24.
Chadwick, P. (2002) 'How to Become Better After Psychosis Than You Were Before', OpenMind, 115, May/June, pp. 12–13.
Chamberlin, J. (1977/1988) On Our Own, London, Mind.
Chamberlin, J. (1990) 'The Ex-Patients' Movement: Where We've Been and Where We're Going', The Journal of Mind and Behaviour, Summer and Autumn, pp. 323–36.
Chamberlin, J. (1994) 'A Psychiatric Survivor Speaks Out', Feminism and Psychology, Vol. 4, No. 2, pp. 284–7.
Chambon, A., Irving, A. and Epstein, L. eds (1999) Reading Foucault for Social Work, New York, Columbia University Press.
Champ, S. (1999) 'A Most Precious Thread', pp. 113–26 in Barker, P., Campbell, P. and Davidson, B. eds From the Ashes of Experience: Reflections on Madness, Survival, and Growth, London, Whurr Publications.
Chesler, P. (1972) Women and Madness, New York, Doubleday.
Chesler, P. (1990) 'Twenty Years Since Women and Madness', in Cohen, D. ed. Challenging the Therapeutic State, Critical Perspectives on Psychiatry and the Mental Health System, Journal of Mind and Behaviour, Vol. 11, Nos 3 and 4, April, pp. 965–6.
Church, K (1995) Forbidden Narratives, Critical Autobiography as Social Science, Luxembourg, Gordon and Breach.
Clare, A. (2001) On Men, Masculinity in Crisis, London, Chatto and Windus.

Clifford, J. (1986) 'On Ethnographic Allegory', pp. 98–121 in Clifford, J. and Marcus, G. eds Writing Culture, The Poetics and Politics of Ethnography, Berkeley, University of California Press.

Clifford, J. and Marcus, G. eds (1986) Writing Culture, the Poetics and Politics of Ethnography, Berkeley, University of California Press.

Cohen, D. ed. (1990) Challenging the Therapeutic State, Critical Perspectives on Psychiatry and the Mental Health System, Journal of Mind and Behaviour, Vol. 11, Nos 3 and 4, Summer and Autumn.

Coid, J. (1996) 'Dangerous Patients with Mental Illness, Increased Risks Warrant New Policies, Adequate Resources, and Appropriate Legislation', British Medical Journal, Vol. 312, April, pp. 965–6.

Coleman, R. (1998) Politics of the Madhouse, Runcorn, Handsell.

Coleman, R. (1999) Recovery, An Alien Concept, Gloucester, Handsell.

Collier, A. (1994) Critical Realism: an Introduction to Roy Bhaskar's Philosophy, London, Verso.

Collinson, D. and Hearn, J. (1994/2001) 'Naming Men as Men: Implications for Work, Organisation and Management', pp. 144–69 in Whitehead, S. and Barrett, F. eds The Masculinities Reader, Cambridge, Polity.

Connell, R. (1987) Gender and Power, Cambridge, Polity Press.

Connell, R. (1994) 'Psychoanalysis and Masculinity', pp. 11–38 in Brod, H. and Kaufmann, M. eds Theorising Masculinities, Thousand Oaks, Calif., Sage.

Connell, R. (1995) Masculinities, Cambridge, Polity Press.

Conway, D. (1993) Das Weib an Sich, The Slave Revolt in Epistemology, in Patton, P. ed. Nietzsche, Feminism and Political Theory, London, Routledge.

Conway, D. (1994) 'Genealogy and Critical Method', in Schacht, R. ed. Genealogy, Morality, Essays on Nietzsche's 'On the Genealogy of Morals', Berkeley, University of California Press, pp. 318–33.

Conway, D. (1995) 'Returning to Nature: Nietzsche's Gotterdammerung', pp. 31–52 in Sedgwick, P. ed. Nietzsche, A Critical Reader, Oxford, Blackwell.

Corker, M. and Shakespeare, T. (2002) Disability/Postmodernity: Embodying Disability Theory, London, Continuum.

Couzens-Hoy, D. ed. (1986) Foucault, a Critical Reader, Oxford, Blackwell.

Coyle, A. and Morgan-Sykes, C. (1998) 'Troubled Men and Threatening Women: the Construction of "Crisis" in Male Mental Health', Feminism and Psychology, Vol. 8, No. 3, pp. 263–84.

Crepaz-Keay, D. (1996) 'Who Do You Represent?', in Read, J. and Reynolds, J. eds Speaking Our Minds, An Anthology, Basingstoke, Macmillan and Open University Press.

Crepaz-Keay, D. (1996b) 'A Sense of Perspective: the Media and the Boyd Enquiry', pp. 37–44 in Philo, G. ed. Media and Mental Distress, London, Longman.

Crepaz-Keay, D. (2004) GSOH Required, Sarah Dunn Profiles David Crepaz-Keay, Chief Executive of Mental Health Media, OpenMind, 125, Jan./Feb., p. 24.

Crichton, J. ed. (1995) Psychiatric Patient Violence, Risk and Response, London, Duckworth.

Curtis, T., Dellar, R., Leslie, E. and Watson, B. (2000) Mad Pride, A Celebration of Mad Culture, London, Spare Change Books.

Dale, C. (1997) 'Cruel: Antonin Artaud and Gilles Deleuze', Canadian Review of Comparative Literature, Vol. 24 (15.3), pp. 589–608.

Daly, M. (1984) Pure Lust, Elemental Feminist Philosophy, London, Women's Press.

Darton, K., Gorman, J. and Sayce, L. (1994) *Eve Fights Back*, London, MIND.

Deleuze, G. (1962/1983) *Nietzsche and Philosophy*, trans. Hugh Tomlinson, London, Athlone Press.

Deleuze, G. (1977/1985) 'Nomad Thought', pp. 143–9 in Allison, D. ed. *The New Nietzsche, Contemporary Styles of Interpretation*, Cambridge, Mass., MIT Press.

Deleuze, G. (1990) *Pourparlers*, Paris, Editions de Minuit.

Deleuze, G. and Guattari, F. (1972/1977) *Anti-Oedipus, Capitalism and Schizophrenia*, New York, Viking Press.

Denzin, N. (1989) *Interpretive Biography*, Newbury Park, Calif., Sage.

Denzin, N. (1994) 'Evaluating Qualitative Research in the Post-Structuralist Moment: the Lessons James Joyce Teaches Us', International Qualitative Studies in Education, Vol. 7, pp. 64–88.

Denzin, N. (1999) 'Two-Stepping in the 90's', Qualitative Enquiry, Vol. 5, No. 4, pp. 586–72.

Department of Health (DoH) (2000a) *National Service Framework for Mental Health*, London, Department of Health Publications.

Department of Health (2000b) *National Survey of NHS Patients*, London, Department of Health Publications.

Department of Health (2001) *Safety First, Five Year Report of the National Confidential Inquiry into Suicide and Homicide by People with Mental Illness*, London, Department of Health Publications.

Department of Health (2002) *National Suicide Prevention Strategy for England*, London, Department of Health Publications.

Department of Health (2003a) *Inside Outside, Improving Mental Health Services for Black and Minority Ethnic Communities in England*, N.I.M.H, Leeds, Department of Health Publications.

Department of Health (2003b) *Mainstreaming Gender and Women's Mental Health, Implementation Guidance*, N.I.M.H, Leeds, Department of Health Publications.

Derrida, J. (1967/1978) *Writing and Difference*, Chicago, University of Chicago Press.

Derrida, J. (1974) *Of Grammatology*, trans. G. Spivak, Baltimore, Md., Johns Hopkins University Press.

Derrida, J. (1979) *Spurs: Nietzsche's Styles*, Chicago, University of Chicago Press.

Derrida, J. (1983) 'The Principle of Reason: the University in the Eyes of its Pupils', Diacritics, Vol. XIX, pp. 3–20.

Derrida, J. (1995) *Interpreting Signatures (Nietzsche/Heidegger): Two Questions*, pp. 53–68 in Sedgwick, P. ed. *Nietzsche, a Critical Reader*, Oxford, Blackwell.

Dews, P. (1987) *The Logics of Disintegration, Post-structuralist Thought and the Claims of Critical Theory*, London, Verso.

Diamond, I. and Quimby, L. eds (1988) *Feminism and Foucault, Reflections on Resistance*, Boston, Mass., Northeastern University Press.

Digby, T. (1998) *Men Doing Feminism*, New York, Routledge.

Dobash, R. E. and Dobash, R. P. (1992) *Women, Violence and Social Change*, London, Routledge.

Donaldson, M. (1993) 'What is Hegemonic Masculinity?', pp. 643–57 in Connell, R. ed. Theory and Society, Vol. 22, No. 5, October.

Double, D. (2001) 'Integrating Critical Psychiatry into Psychiatric Training' , pp. 23–34 in Newnes, C., Holmes, G. and Dunn, C. eds, This is Madness Too: Critical Perspectives on Mental Health Services, Ross-on-Wye, PCCS Books.

Dreyfus, H. and Hall, H. (1992) Heidegger: a Critical Reader, Oxford, Blackwell.

Dreyfus, H. and Rabinow, P. (1982) Michel Foucault, Beyond Structuralism and Hermeneutics, New York, Harvester Wheatsheaf.

Dunant, S. and Porter, R. eds (1996) The Age of Anxiety, London, Virago.

Durkheim, E. (1897/1952) Suicide, a Study in Sociology, London, Routledge and Kegan Paul.

E.C.T. Anonymous (1998) Newsletter, Spring/Summer.

Edley, N. and Wetherell, M. (1995) Men in Perspective; Practice, Power and Identity, Hemel Hempstead, Harvester Wheatsheaf.

Elliot, A. and Frosh, S. (1995) Psychoanalysis in Contexts, Paths Towards Theory and Modern Culture, London, Routledge.

Elliot, A. and Turner, B. eds (2001) Profiles in Contemporary Social Theory, London, Sage.

Erben, M. (2004) 'Learning About Suicide: Who Would Bear the Whips and Scorns of Time?', Auto/Biography, Vol. 12, No. 1, pp. 63–76.

Eribon, D. (1993) Michel Foucault, trans. Betsy Wing, Cambridge, Mass., Harvard University Press.

Esslin, M. (1976) Artaud, Glasgow, Fontana.

Estroff, S., Zimmer, C., Lachicotte, W. S. and Benoit, J. (1994) 'The Influence of Social Networks and Social Support on Violence by Persons with Serious Mental Illness', Hospital and Community Psychiatry, July, Vol. 45, No. 7, pp. 669–79.

Fanon, F. (1952/1986) Black Skin, White Masks, London, Pluto Press.

Faulkner, A. (1997) Knowing Our Own Minds: a Survey of How People in Emotional Distress Take Control of Their Own Lives, London, Mental Health Foundation.

Faulkner, A. (1999) Strategies for Living: a Report of User-led Research into People's Strategies for Living with Mental Distress, London, Mental Health Foundation.

Faulkner, A. and Sayce, L. (1997) 'Disclosure', OpenMind, 85, May/June, pp. 8–9.

Faulkner, A., Petit-Zeman, S., Sherlock, J. and Wallcraft, J. (2002) Being There in Crisis: a Report of the Learning from Eight Mental Health Crisis Services, London, Mental Health Foundation.

Fawcett, B. and Featherstone, B. (1994) 'Power and Difference: Perspectives for Practice', pp. 41–52 in Toft, C. ed. Women, the System, and Mental Health, Bradford, Department of Applied Social Studies, University of Bradford.

Fawcett, B. and Featherstone, B. (1998) 'Quality Assurance and Evaluation in Social Work in a Postmodern Era', pp. 67–84 in Carter, J. ed. Postmodernity and the Fragmentation of Welfare, London, Routledge.

Fawcett, B., Featherstone, B., Hearn, J. and Toft, C. eds (1996) Violence and Gender Relations, Theories and Interventions, London, Sage.

Fawcett, B., Featherstone, B., Fook, J. and Rossiter, A. eds (2000) Practice and Research in Social Work: Postmodern Feminist Perspectives, London, Routledge.

Featherstone, B. (1997) 'Familiar Subjects? Domestic Violence and Child Welfare', Child and Family Social Work, Vol. 2, pp. 147–59.

Featherstone, B. (1997b) 'I Wouldn't Do Your Job! Women, Social Work, and Child Abuse', pp. 166–92 in Hollway, W. and Featherstone, B. eds Mothering and Ambivalence, London, Routledge.

Featherstone, B. and Trinder, I. (1997) *Familiar Subjects? Domestic Violence and Child Welfare*, Child and Family Social Work, Vol. 2, pp. 147–59.

Feeley, M. and Simon, J. (1992) 'The New Penology: Notes on the Emerging Strategy of Corrections and its Implications', Criminology, Vol. 30, No. 4, pp. 449–74.

Fernando, S. (1991) *Mental Health, Race, and Culture*, London, Macmillan.

Fernando, S. ed. (1995) *Mental Health in a Multi-Ethnic Society: a Multi-disciplinary Handbook*, London, Routledge.

Fernando, S. (2004) 'Power and Misconceptions', OpenMind, 125, Jan./Feb., p. 25.

Fernando, S., Ndegwa, D. and Wilson, M. (1998) *Forensic Psychiatry, Race, and Culture*, London, Routledge.

Feyerabend, P. (1975) *Against Method*, London, Verso.

Flax, J. (1987) 'Remembering the Selves, Is the Repressed Gendered?', Michigan Quarterly Review, Vol. 26, pp. 92–110.

Flax, J. (1990) *Thinking Fragments, Psychoanalysis, Feminism, and Postmodernism in the Contemporary West*, Berkeley, University of California Press.

Flax, J. (1990b) 'Postmodernism and Gender Relations in Feminist Theory', pp. 39–62 in Nicholson, L. ed. *Feminism/Postmodernism*, New York, Routledge.

Flax, J. (1992) 'The End of Innocence', pp. 445–63 in Butler, J. and Scott, J. eds *Feminists Theorise the Political*, New York, Routledge.

Flax, J. (1992b) 'Beyond Equality: Gender, Justice and Difference', pp. 193–210 in Bock, G. and James, S. eds *Beyond Equality and Difference: Citizenship, Feminist Politics, Female Subjectivity*, London, Routledge.

Flax, J. (1993) 'Multiples, On the Contemporary Politics of Subjectivity', Human Studies, Vol. 16, parts 1–2, pp. 33–49.

Foner, J. (1995) 'A Double Whammy, Sexism, Mentalism, and What We Can Do About It', pp. 133–47 in Grobe, J. ed. *Beyond Bedlam, Contemporary Women Psychiatric Survivors Speak Out*, Chicago, Ill., Third Side Press.

Foote, C. and Frank, A. (1999) *Foucault and Therapy, the Disciplining of Grief*, pp. 157–87 in Chambon, A., Irving, A. and Epstein, L. eds *Reading Foucault for Social Work*, New York, Columbia University Press.

Forrester, J. (1990) *The Seductions of Psychoanalysis: Freud, Lacan and Derrida*, Cambridge, Cambridge University Press.

Foucault, M. (1961/1971) *Madness and Civilisation, a History of Insanity in the Age of Reason*, London, Penguin.

Foucault, M. (1963/1973) *The Birth of the Clinic*, London, Tavistock and Routledge.

Foucault, M. (1963/1987) *Death and the Labyrinth, the World of Raymond Roussel*, London, Athlone Press.

Foucault, M. (1967) *Nietzsche, Freud, Marx*, in Nietzsche, Paris: Cahiers de Royaumont.

Foucault, M. (1971/1984) 'Nietzsche, Genealogy, History', pp. 76–100 in Rabinow, P. ed. *The Foucault Reader*, London, Penguin.

Foucault, M. (1972) *The Archaeology of Knowledge*, London, Tavistock.

Foucault, M. (1973) *The Order of Things: an Archaeology of the Human Sciences*, New York, Vintage, Random House.

Foucault, M. ed. (1973 / 1975) *I Pierre Rivière, Having Slaughtered my Mother, my Sister and my Brother . . . , A Case of Parricide in the 19th Century*, Harmondsworth, Penguin.

Foucault, M. (1975/1977) *Discipline and Punish; the Birth of the Prison*, trans. Alan Sheridan, Harmondsworth, Penguin.

Foucault, M. (1976/1978) *The Will to Knowledge, The History of Sexuality I*, London, Penguin.

Foucault, M. (1980) *Power/Knowledge, Selected Interviews and Other Writings, 1972–1977*, ed. Colin Gordon, New York, Harvester Wheatsheaf.

Foucault, M. (1983) 'On the Genealogy of Ethics: an Overview of Work in Progress', in Rabinow, P. ed. (1984) *The Foucault Reader*, London, Penguin.

Foucault, Michel (1984) 'What Is Enlightenment?', in Rabinow, P. ed., *The Foucault Reader*, London, Penguin.

Fox, D. and Prilleltensky, I. (1997) *Critical Psychology, An Introduction*, London, Sage.

Francis, E. (2004) 'Too Little Too Late', *Society Guardian*, 11 February, p. 9.

Frank, L. (1990) 'Electroshock: Death, Brain Damage, Memory Loss, and Brainwashing', The Journal of Mind and Behaviour, Summer and Autumn, Vol. 11, Nos 3 and 4, pp. 489–513.

Fraser, N. and Nicholson, L. (1994) 'Social Criticism without Philosophy: an Encounter between Feminism and Postmodernism, pp. 242–61 in Seidman, S. ed. *The Postmodern Turn, New Perspectives on Social Theory*, Cambridge, Cambridge University Press.

Freud, S. (1911/1979) *Sigmund Freud, Case Histories II*, London, Penguin.

Freud, S. (1939/1985) *Moses and Monotheism*, in *The Origins of Religion*, Harmondsworth, Penguin.

Freud, S. (1963) *The Standard Edition of the Complete Psychological Works of Sigmund Freud*, London, Hogarth Press and Institute of Psychoanalysis.

Frosh, S. (1991) *Identity Crisis: Modernity, Psychoanalysis and the Self*, London, Macmillan Education.

Frosh, S. (1992) 'Masculine Ideology and Psychological Therapy', pp. 153–70 in Ussher, J. M. and Nicholson, P. eds *Gender Issues in Clinical Psychology*, London, Routledge.

Frosh, S. (1994) *Sexual Difference: Masculinity and Psychoanalysis*, London, Routledge.

Frosh, S. (1995) 'Unpacking Masculinity, From Rationality to Fragmentation', pp. 218–31 in Burck, C. and Speed, B. eds *Gender, Power, and Relationships*, London, Routledge.

Frosh, S. (1997) 'Screaming Under the Bridge, Masculinity, Rationality and Psychotherapy,' in Ussher, J. ed. *Body Talk*, London, Routledge.

Frosh, S. (1997b) 'Father's Ambivalence (Too)', pp. 37–53 in Hollway, W. and Featherstone, B. eds *Mothering and Ambivalence*, London, Routledge.

Frosh, S. (1999) *The Politics of Psychoanalysis, An Introduction to Freudian and Post-Freudian Theory*, 2nd edition, Basingstoke, Macmillan.

Gane, M. (1993) *Harmless Lovers? Gender, Theory, and Personal Relationships*, London, Routledge.

Genosko, G. (2000) 'The Life and Work of Félix Guattari: From Transversality to Ecosophy', in Guattari, F. ed. *The Three Ecologies*, London, Athlone Press.

Gergen, K. (1991) *The Saturated Self*, New York, Basic Books.

Gergen, K. (1999) *An Invitation to Social Constructionism*, London, Sage.

Gershchick, T. and Miller, A. (1994) *Gender Identities at the Crossroads of Masculinity and Physical Disability*, Masculinities, Vol. 2, No. 1, Spring, pp. 34–55.

Gersons, B. P. R. and Carlier, I. V. E. (1992) 'Post-Traumatic Stress Disorder, the History of a Recent Concept', British Journal of Psychiatry, Vol. 161, pp. 742–8.

Giddens, A. (1978) *Durkheim*, London, Fontana.

Giddens, A. (1990) *The Consequences of Modernity*, Cambridge, Polity Press.

Giddens, A. (1991) *Modernity and Self-Identity; Self and Society in the Late Modern Age*, Cambridge, Polity Press.

Gilman, S. ed. (1987) *Conversations with Nietzsche, a Life in the Words of his Contemporaries*, trans. David Parent, New York, Oxford University Press.

GLAD (2003) *Black and Ethnic Minority Mental Health User Groups and User Involvement, Conference Report*, London, Greater London Action on Disability.

Golding, J. (1997) *WithOut Prejudice: Mind Lesbian, Gay and Bisexual Mental Health Awareness Research*, London, MIND.

Goodison, L. (1990) *Heaven and Earth. Sexuality, Spirituality, and Social Change*, London, The Women's Press.

Gordon, C. (1990) 'Histoire de la Folie: An Unknown Book by Michel Foucault', History of the Human Sciences, Vol. 3, No. 1, pp. 3–26.

Grant, J. (1993) *Fundamental Feminism: Contesting the Core Concepts of Feminist Theory*, New York, Routledge.

Greally, H. (1971) *Bird's Nest Soup*, Dublin, Attic Press.

Gregory, D. (1994) *Geographical Imaginations*, Oxford, Blackwell.

Grier, W. and Cobbs, P. (1968) *Black Rage*, New York, Basic Books.

Griffin, A. P. and Sayce, L. (2003) 'Making Rights Real', OpenMind, 124, pp. 18–19.

Grimshaw, J. (1993) 'Practices of Freedom', pp. 50–72 in Ramazanoglu, C. ed. *Up Against Foucault*, London, Routledge.

Grobe, J. ed. (1995) *Beyond Bedlam: Contemporary Women Psychiatric Survivors Speak Out*, Chicago, Ill., Third Side Press.

Grossberg, L. (1996) 'On Postmodernism and Articulation, An Interview with Stuart Hall', pp. 131–50 in Morley, D. and Kuan-Hsing C. eds *Stuart Hall, Critical Dialogues in Cultural Studies*, London, Routledge.

Grosz, E. (1990) *Jacques Lacan, A Feminist Introduction*, London, Routledge.

Grosz, E. (1993) 'Bodies and Knowledges: Feminism and the Crisis of Reason', pp. 187–215 in Alcoff, L. and Potter, E. eds *Feminist Epistemologies*, New York, Routledge.

Grosz, E. (1994) *Volatile Bodies, Towards a Corporeal Feminism*, Bloomington, Indiana University Press.

Guirand, F. and Pierre, A. (1953) 'Roman Mythology', in *New Larousse Encyclopaedia of Mythology*, London, Hamlyn.

Guite, H. (1994) 'Violence and Psychiatric Patients, A View from the Community', Criminal Behaviour and Mental Health, 4, pp. 245–52.

Gutterman, D. (2001) 'Postmodernism and the Interrogation of Masculinity', pp. 56–71 in Whitehead, S. and Barrett, F. eds *The Masculinities Reader*, Cambridge, Polity.

Haar, M. (1977/1985) 'Nietzsche and Metaphysical Language', in Allison, D. ed. *The New Nietzsche, Contemporary Styles of Interpretation*, Cambridge Mass., MIT Press.

Haar, M. (1992) 'Attunement and Thinking', pp. 155–72 in Dreyfus, H. and Hall, H. eds *Heidegger, a Critical Reader*, Oxford, Blackwell.

Haar, M. (1992b) 'The Play of Nietzsche in Derrida', pp. 52–71 in Wood, D. ed. *Derrida, a Critical Reader*, Oxford, Blackwell.

Habermas, J. (1987) *The Philosophical Discourse of Modernity*, Cambridge, Polity Press.

Habermas, J. (1994) 'The Tasks of A Critical Theory', pp. 142–9 in *The Polity Reader in Social Theory*, Cambridge, Polity Press.

Hall, S. (1990) 'Cultural Identity and Diaspora', pp. 222–37 in Rutherford, J. ed. *Identity: Community, Culture, Difference*, London, Lawrence and Wishart.

Hall, S. (1991) 'Old and New Identities, Old and New Ethnicities', pp. 41–68 in King, A. ed. Culture, Globalisation and the World System, Basingstoke, Macmillan.

Hall, S. (1992) 'The New Ethnicities', in Donald, J. and Rattansi, A. eds 'Race', Culture and Difference, London, Sage.

Hall, S., Held, D. and McGrew, T. (1992) Modernity and Its Futures, Cambridge, Polity and Open University Press.

Hallberg, M. (1989/1992) 'Feminist Epistemology: An Impossible Project?', pp. 372–7 in Hall, S., Held, D. and McGrew, T. eds Modernity and Its Futures, Understanding Modern Societies, An Introduction, Cambridge, Polity and Open University Press.

Halperin, D. (1995) Saint Foucault, Towards a Gay Hagiography, New York, Oxford University Press.

Hanmer, J. (1996) 'Women and Violence, Commonalities and Diversities', pp. 7–21 in Fawcett, B. and Featherstone, B. eds Violence and Gender Relations, Theories and Interventions, London, Sage.

Harasym, S. ed. (1990) Spivak, Gayatri Chakrovorty, The Postcolonial Critic, Interviews. Strategies, Dialogues, New York, Routledge.

Haraway, D. (1991) Simians, Cyborgs, and Women. The Re-invention of Nature, London, Free Association Books.

Haraway, D. (1997) Modest_Witness@Second_Millenium. Female Man© Meets OncoMouse™, Feminism and Technoscience, New York, Routledge.

Hare, R. (1993) Without Conscience, The Disturbing World of the Psychopaths Among Us, New York, Pocket Books.

Harris, V. (1994) Review of the Report of the Inquiry into the Care and Treatment of Christopher Clunis, A Lack of Perspective, London, Race Equality Unit.

Harrison, K. and Kessler, E. (1995) 'What Went Wrong in Torbay?', OpenMind, 73, February/March, pp. 6–7.

Hart, L. (2003) 'Recovery, Let's Get Real', OpenMind, 124, p. 15.

Hartstock, N. (1990) 'Foucault on Power. A Theory for Women?', in Nicholson, L. ed. Feminism/Postmodernism, Routledge, New York.

Harvey, D. (1989) The Condition of Postmodernity, An Enquiry in the Origins of Cultural Change, Oxford, Blackwell.

Harvey, D. (1990) 'Between Space and Time, Reflections on the Geographical Imagination', Annals of the Association of American Geographers, 80, pp. 418–34.

Hawton, K., Houston, K. and Shepperd, R. (1999) 'Suicide in Young People', British Journal of Psychiatry, Vol. 175, pp. 271–6.

Hayman, R. (1977) Artaud and After, Oxford, Oxford University Press.

Hayman, R. (1980) Nietzsche, A Critical Life, London, Weidenfeld and Nicolson.

Hayman, R. (1997) Nietzsche, London, Phoenix.

Haywood, C. and Mac an Ghaill, M. (2003) Men and Masculinities, Buckingham, Open University Press.

Healy, D. (2001) 'The SSRI Suicides', pp. 58–69 in Newnes, C., Holmes, G. and Dunn. C. eds This Is Madness Too, Ross-on-Wye, PCCS Books.

Hearn, J. (1987) The Gender of Oppression, Men, Masculinity, and the Critique of Marxism, Brighton, Wheatsheaf.

Hearn, J. (1992) Men in the Public Eye, the Construction and Deconstruction of Public Patriarchies, London, Routledge.

Hearn, J. (1994) 'Research in Men and Masculinities: Some Sociological Issues and Possibilities', Australia and New Zealand Journal of Sociology, Vol. 30, No. 1, April, pp. 47–70.

Hearn, J. (1996) 'The Problem of Men's Violence', pp. 99–114, in Fawcett, B., Featherstone, B., Hearn, J. and Toft, C. eds Violence and Gender Relations, Theories and Interventions, London, Sage.

Hearn, J. (1996b) 'Is Masculinity Dead? A Critique of the Concept of Masculinity/Masculinities', in Mac an Ghaill, M. ed. Understanding Masculinities, Social Relations, and Cultural Arenas, Buckingham, Open University Press.

Hearn, J. (1998) The Violences of Men, London, Sage.

Hearn, J. (1998b) 'Theorising Men and Men's Theorising: Varieties of Discursive Practices in Men's Theorising of Men', Theory and Society, 27, pp. 781–816.

Heidegger, M. (1961) Nietzsche, Pfullingen, Gunther Neske.

Hemphill, R.E. (1941) 'The Influence of the War on Mental Disease; a Psychiatric Study', Journal of Medical Science, 87, pp. 170–82.

Hendin, H. (1999) Suicide in America, New York, W. W. Norton.

Henriques, J., Hollway, W., Urwin, C., Venn, C. and Walkerdine, V. eds (1984/1998) Changing the Subject: Psychology, Social Regulation and Subjectivity, London, Routledge.

Herman, J. (1992) Trauma and Recovery; the Aftermath of Violence – from Domestic Violence to Political Terror, New York, Basic Books.

Heron, J. (1980) 'History and Development of Co-Counselling', Self and Society, Vol. VIII, No. 4, April/May, pp. 99–106.

Hetherington, A. (2000) 'A Psychodynamic Profile of Therapists who Sexually Exploit their Clients', British Journal of Psychotherapy, Vol. 16, No. 3, pp. 274–86.

Hiday, V. A. (1995) 'The Social Context of Mental Illness and Violence', Journal of Health and Social Behaviour, 36, pp. 122–37.

Hill, D. (1983) The Politics of Schizophrenia, Psychiatric Oppression in the U.S., Lanham, Md., University Press of America.

Hillman, J. (1972) The Myth of Analysis, New York, Harper and Row.

Hillman, J. (1979) The Dream and The Underworld, New York, Harper and Row.

Hirschman, J. ed. (1965) Artaud Anthology, San Francisco, City Lights Books.

Hodin, J. (1972) Edvard Munch, London, Thames and Hudson.

Holland, S. (1992) 'From Social Abuse to Social Action, A Neighbourhood Psychotherapy and Social Action Project for Women', pp. 68–77 in Ussher, J. and Nicholson, P. eds Gender Issues in Clinical Psychology, London, Routledge.

Hollingdale, R. (1965/1999) Nietzsche, The Man and His Philosophy, Cambridge, Cambridge University Press, revised edition.

Hollway, W. (1984/1998) 'Gender Difference and the Production of Subjectivity', pp. 227–63 in Henriques, J., Hollway, W., Urwin, C., Venn, C. and Walkerdine, V. eds Changing the Subject, London, Routledge.

Hollway, W. (1989) Subjectivity and Method in Psychology; Gender, Meaning and Science, London, Sage.

Hollway, W. (1996) 'Recognition and Heterosexual Desire', pp. 91–108 in Richardson, D. ed. Theorising Heterosexuality, Buckingham, Open University Press.

Hollway, W. and Featherstone, B. (1997) Mothering and Ambivalence, London, Routledge.

hooks, bell (1989) Talking Back, Thinking Feminism, Thinking Black, London, Sheba.

hooks, bell (1995) Killing Rage, Ending Racism, London, Penguin.

Hopkins, P. (1996) 'Gender Treachery: Homophobia, Masculinity, and Threatened Identities', pp. 95–115 in May, L., Strikwerda, R. and Hopkins, P. eds Rethinking Masculinity: Philosophical Explorations in Light of Feminism, second edition, Lanham, Md., Rowman and Littlefield.

Hopton, J. (1998) 'Risk Assessment Using Psychological Profiling Techniques: an Evaluation of Possibilities', British Journal of Social Work, Vol. 28, pp. 247–61.

Howells, C. (1999) Derrida, Deconstruction from Phenomenology to Ethics, Cambridge, Polity Press.

Huka, G. (1996) 'The Sanctuary Project', pp. 207–16 in Tomlinson, D. and Carrier, J. eds Asylum in the City, London, Routledge.

Hunter, M. (2000) 'Services Need User Input', Community Care, November, 16–22, p. 12.

Ingelby, D. (1981) Critical Psychiatry, The Politics of Mental Health, Harmondsworth, Penguin.

Irigaray, L. (1987/1993) Sexes and Genealogies, trans. G. C. Gill, New York, Columbia University Press.

Irigaray, L. (1991) Marine Lover of Friedrich Nietzsche, trans. G. C. Gill, New York, Columbia University Press.

Jackson, D. (1990) Unmasking Masculinity, London, Unwin Hyman.

Jameson, F. (1991) Postmodernism, or the Cultural Logic of Late Capitalism, London, Verso.

Jantzen, G. (1998) Becoming Divine, Towards a Feminist Philosophy of Religion, Manchester, Manchester University Press.

Jehu, D. (1994) Patients as Victims, Sexual Abuse in Psychotherapy and Counselling, Chichester, John Wiley.

Johnstone, L. (2003) 'A Shocking Treatment?', The Psychologist, Vol. 16, No. 5, pp. 236–9.

Jorm, A. F. ed. (1995) Men and Mental Health, a Reference Document, Canberra, National Health and Medical Research Council.

Jones, C. and Porter, R. eds (1994) Reassessing Foucault; Power, Medicine and the Body, London, Routledge.

Jukes, A. (1993) Why Men Hate Women, London, Free Association Books.

Jukes, A. (1996) 'Working With Men who are Violent to Women', pp. 254–9 in Palmer, S., Dainow, S. and Milner, P. eds Counselling, The BAC Counselling Reader, London, Sage.

Kalinowski, C. and Penny, D. (1998) 'Empowerment in Women's Mental Health Services', in Lubotsky, L., Blanch, A. and Jennings, A. eds, Women's Mental Health Services, A Public Health Perspective, Thousand Oaks, Calif., Sage.

Kant, I. (1992) 'What is Enlightenment?', in Eliot, S. and Whitelock, K. eds The Enlightenment, Texts, II, Milton Keynes, Open University Press.

Karner, T. (1995) 'Medicalising Masculinity: Post Traumatic Stress Disorder in Vietnam Veterans', Masculinities, Vol. 3, No. 4, Winter, pp. 23–65.

Katz, A., Buchanan, A. and McCoy, A. (1999) Young Men Speak Out, London, Samaritans.

Kaufman, M. (1994) 'Men, Feminism, and Men's Contradictory Experiences of Power', pp. 142–63 in Brod, H. and Kaufman, M. eds Theorising Masculinities, Thousand Oaks, Calif., Sage.

Kaufmann, W. (1950/1974) Nietzsche; Philosopher, Psychologist, Antichrist, fourth edition, Princeton, NJ, Princeton University Press.

Kaufmann, W. (1954) The Portable Nietzsche, New York, Viking.

Kaye, J. (1999) 'Towards a Non-Regulative Praxis', pp. 19–38 in Parker, I. ed. Deconstructing Psychotherapy, London, Sage.

Keller, C. (1986) *From a Broken Web: Separation, Sexism, and the Self*, Boston, Mass., Beacon Press.

Kerenyi, C. (1976) *Dionysos, Archetypal Image of Indestructible Life*, trans. Ralph Mannheim, Bollingen Series LXV 2, Princeton, NJ, Princeton University Press.

Kimmel, M. (1987) 'The Contemporary "Crisis" of Masculinity in Historical Perspective', pp. 121–53 in Brod, H. ed. *The Making of Masculinities, the New Men's Studies*, Boston, Mass., Allen and Unwin.

Kimmel, M. (1994) 'Masculinity as Homophobia: Fear, Shame, and Silence in the Construction of Gender Identity', pp. 119–41 in Brod, H. and Kaufmann, M. eds *Theorising Masculinity*, Thousand Oaks, Calif., Sage.

Kimmel, M. (1996) *Manhood in America: a Cultural History*, New York, The Free Press.

Kimmel, M. (1998) *Who's Afraid of Men Doing Feminism?*, pp. 56–68 in Digby, T. ed. *Men Doing Feminism*, New York, Routledge.

Kittler, F. (1990) *Discourse Networks. 1800/1900*, trans. Michael Metteer and Chris Cullens, Stanford, Calif., Stanford University Press.

Kitzinger, C. (1997) 'Lesbian and Gay Psychology: a Critical Analysis', pp. 202–16 in Fox, D. and Prilleltensky, I. *Critical Psychology, an Introduction*, London, Sage.

Knight, T. (2004) 'You'd Better Believe It!', OpenMind, 128, July/August, pp. 12–13.

Koonz, C. (1988) *Mothers in the Fatherland*, London, Methuen.

Krabbendam, L. and van Os, J. (2002) 'Men with Schizophrenia: a Double Disadvantage', Men's Health Journal, Vol. 1, No. 4, pp. 114–17.

Kreiger, D. (1979) *The Therapeutic Touch, How to Use Your Hands to Help or Heal*, Englewood Cliffs, NJ, Prentice Hall.

Kristeva, J. (1977/1980) *Desire in Language, a Semiotic Approach to Literature and Art*, Oxford, Blackwell.

Kritzman, L. ed. (1988) *Michel Foucault; Politics, Philosophy, Culture: Intensities and Other Writings 1977–1984*, New York, Routledge.

Kuhn, T. (1962/1970) *The Structure of Scientific Revolutions*, 2nd edition, Chicago, Ill., University of Chicago Press.

Kumar, K. (1995) *From Post-Industrial to Postmodern Society, New Theories of the Contemporary World*, Oxford, Blackwell.

Kutchins, H. and Kirk, S. (1997/1999) *Making Us Crazy, DSM – The Psychiatric Bible and the Creation of Mental Disorders*, London, Constable.

Lacan, J. (1966/1977) *Ecrits*, London, Routledge.

Laclau, E. and Mouffe, C. (1985) *Hegemony and Socialist Strategy; Towards a Radical Democratic Politics*, London, Verso.

Laing, R. (1959/1965) *The Divided Self, An Existential Study in Sanity and Madness*, Harmondsworth, Penguin.

Laing, R. (1967) *The Politics of Experience and the Bird of Paradise*, Harmondsworth, Penguin.

Land, N. (1992) 'Shamanism Nietzsche', pp. 158–70 in Sedgwick, R. ed. *Nietzsche, a Critical Reader*, Oxford, Blackwell.

Landry, D. and MacLean, G. (1996) *The Spivak Reader*, New York, Routledge.

Langan, J. (1999) 'Assessing Risk in Mental Health', pp. 153–78 in Parsloe, P. ed. *Risk Assessment in Social Care and Social Work*, London, Jessica Kingsley.

Langan, J. and Lindow, V. (2000) 'Risk and Listening', OpenMind 101, Jan./Feb., pp. 14–15.

Laquer, T. (1996) *The Facts of Fatherhood*, pp. 173–92 in May, L., Strickwerda, R. and Hopkins, P. eds *Rethinking Masculinity, Philosophical Explorations in the Light of Feminism*, Lanham, Md., Rowman and Littlefield.

Larvin, J. (1971) *Nietzsche, a Biographical Introduction*, London, Studio Vista.

Law, I. (1999) 'A Discursive Approach to Therapy with Men', pp. 115–31 in Parker, I. ed. *Deconstructing Psychotherapy*, London, Sage.

Lawson, M. (1988) 'Eric', Asylum, Vol. 3, No. 1.

Lawson, M. (1991) 'A Recipient's View', pp. 62–83 in Ramon, S. ed. *Beyond Community Care, Normalisation and Integration Work* London, MIND.

Lembcke, J. (1999) 'The "Right Stuff" Gone Wrong: Vietnam Veterans and the Social Construction of Post-Traumatic Stress Disorder', Critical Sociology, Vol. 24, Nos 1 and 2, pp. 27–64.

Lennon, P. (2001) 'Call to Arms', Guardian, 13 January.

Leudar, I. and Thomas, P. (2000) *Voices of Reason, Voices of Insanity, Studies of Verbal Hallucinations*, London, Routledge.

Levy, O. (1921/1985) *Friedrich Nietzsche, Selected Letters*, trans. A. N. Ludovici, London, Soho Book Company.

Liddle, A. Mark (1993) 'Gender, Desire and Child Sexual Abuse: Accounting for the Male Majority', Theory, Culture, and Society, Vol. 10, pp. 103–26.

Lindow, V. (1993) 'A Vision for the Future', pp. 182–91 in Beresford, P. and Harding, T. eds *A Challenge to Change, Practical Experiences of Building User-led Services*, London, NISW.

Lindow, V. (1994) *Self-Help Alternatives to Mental Health Services*, London, MIND.

Lindow, V. (1999) 'Survivor Controlled Alternatives to Psychiatric Services', pp. 211–26 in Newnes, C., Holmes, G. and Dunn, C. eds *This is Madness, A Critical Look at Psychiatry and the Future of Mental Health Services*, Ross-on-Wye, PCCS Books.

Lionnet, F. (1989) *Autobiographical Voices; Race, Gender, Self-Portraiture*, Ithaca, NY, Cornell University Press.

Littlewood, R. and Lipsedge, M. (1982/1997) *Aliens and Alienists, Ethnic Minorities and Psychiatry*, 3rd edition, London, Routledge.

Lloyd, G. (1984) *The Man of Reason*, London, Methuen.

Lothane, Z. (1992) *In Defence of Schreber: Soul Murder and Psychiatry*, Hillsdale, NJ, Analytic Press.

Lupton, D. and Barclay, L. (1997) *Constructing Fatherhood, Discourses and Experiences*, London, Sage.

Lyman, F. (2004) 'Spiritual Restoration', Resurgence, No. 225, July/August, p. 45.

Lyon, D. (1999) *Postmodernity*, 2nd edition, Buckingham, Open University Press.

Lyotard, J. (1984) *The Postmodern Condition, A Report on Knowledge*, trans. G. Bennington and B. Massumi, Minneapolis, University of Minnesota Press.

Lyotard, J. (1991) *The Inhuman*, trans. G. Bennington and R. Bowlby, Cambridge, Polity Press.

Lyotard, J. (1993) *Jean-François Lyotard: Political Writings*, ed. Readings, B., London, UCL Press.

MacCannell, D. and MacCannell, J. (1993) 'Violence, Power and Pleasure, A Revisionist Reading of Foucault from the Victim Perspective', pp. 203–38 in Ramazanoglu, C. ed. *Up Against Foucault*, London, Routledge.

McClelland, D. and Watt, N. (1968) 'Sex Role Alienation in Schizophrenia', Journal of Abnormal Psychology, Vol. 73, No. 3.

Macey, D. (1988) Lacan in Contexts, London, Verso.

Macey, D. (1993) The Lives of Michel Foucault, London, Hutchinson.

Macey, D. (1995) 'Michel Foucault: J'Accuse', New Formations, No. 25, Summer, pp. 5–13.

Macey, D. (2000) Frantz Fanon, a Life, London, Granta.

MacIntyre, A. (1994) 'Genealogies and Subversions', pp. 284–305 in Schacht, R. ed. Nietzsche, Genealogy, Morality: Essays on Nietzsche's 'On the Genealogy of Morals', Berkeley, University of California Press.

McMahon, A. (1993) 'Male Readings of Feminist Theory: the Psychologisation of Sexual Politics in the Masculinity Literature', pp. 675–95 in Connell, R. W. ed. Theory and Society, Vol. 22/5, October.

McNamara, J. (1996) 'Out of Order, Madness is a Feminist and a Disability Issue', pp. 194–205 in Morris, J. ed. Encounters with Strangers, London, Women's Press.

McNay, L. (1992) Foucault and Feminism, Power, Gender, and the Self, Cambridge, Polity Press.

McQueen, C. and Henwood, K. (2002) 'Young Men in "Crisis": Attending to the Language of Teenage Boys' Distress', Social Science and Medicine, 55, pp. 1493–1509.

Majors, R. (2001) 'Cool Pose, Black Masculinity and Sports', pp. 209–17, in Whitehead, S. and Barrett, F. eds The Masculinities Reader, Cambridge, Polity Press.

Mama, A. (1995) Beyond the Masks, Race, Gender, and Subjectivity, London, Routledge.

Mann, K. (1998) '"One Step Beyond", Critical Social Policy in "Postmodern" Britain', pp. 85–102 in Carter, J. ed. Postmodernity and the Fragmentation of Welfare, London, Routledge.

Mannoni, O. (1964) Prospero and Caliban: the Psychology of Colonisation, New York, Praeger.

Mariani, P. (1995) 'Law-and-Order Science', pp. 135–56 in Berger, M., Wallis, B. and Watson, S. eds Constructing Masculinity, New York, Routledge.

Marriott, D. (2000) On Black Men, Edinburgh, Edinburgh University Press.

Martin, L., Gutnam, H. and Hutton, P. eds (1988) Technologies of the Self: a Seminar with Michel Foucault, Amherst, University of Massachusetts Press.

Masson, J. (1984/1992) The Assault on Truth: Freud and Child Sexual Abuse, London, Fontana.

Masson, J. (1990) Against Therapy, London, Fontana.

Masson, J. (1992) Final Analysis: the Making and Unmaking of a Psychoanalyst, London, Fontana.

Masson, J. (1992b) 'The Tyranny of Psychotherapy', pp. 7–40 in Dryden, W. and Feltham, C. eds Psychotherapy and its Discontents, Buckingham, Open University Press.

May, R. (2000) 'Psychosis and Recovery', OpenMind, 106, Nov./Dec., pp. 24–5.

May, R. (2003) 'Pete Shaughnessy, Tribute Issue – Introduction', Asylum, Vol. 13, No. 4, pp. 4–5.

May, L., Strikwerda, R. and Hopkins, P. eds (1996) Rethinking Masculinity: Philosophical Explorations in the Light of Feminism, Lanham, Md., Rowman and Littlefield.

Medawar, C. (1992) Power and Dependence, Social Audit on the Safety of Medicines, London, Social Audit Ltd.

Memmi, A. (1967) The Colonizer and the Colonized, Boston, Mass., Beacon Press.

Mercer, K. and Julien, I. (1988) 'Race, Sexual Politics, and Black Masculinity: a Dossier', pp. 97–164 in Chapman, R. and Rutherford, J. eds Male Order, Unwrapping Masculinity, London, Lawrence and Wishart.

Messner, M. (1997) The Politics of Masculinities, Men in Movements, Thousand Oaks, Calif., Sage.

Metcalfe, M., Oppenheimer, R., Dignon, A. and Palmer, R. (1990) 'Childhood Sexual Experiences Reported by Male Psychiatric Patients', Psychological Medicine, 20, November, pp. 925–9.

Meth, R. and Pasick, R. eds (1990) Men in Therapy, the Challenge of Change, New York, The Guilford Press.

Mental Health Foundation (2001) Something Inside So Strong, London, Mental Health Foundation.

Miller, J. (1993) The Passion of Michel Foucault, New York, Simon and Schuster.

Miller, J. and Bell, C. (1996) 'Mapping Men's Mental Health', Journal of Community and Applied Social Psychology, Vol. 6, pp. 317–27.

Millet, K. (1990) The Loony Bin Trip, New York, Simon and Schuster.

Millet, K. (1992) NAPS News (Journal of the National Association of Psychiatric Survivors – North America), Winter.

MIND (1995) Making Sense of Treatment and Drugs – ECT, London, MIND.

MIND (2001) Shock Treatment, a Survey of People's Experiences of Electro-Convulsive Therapy (ECT), London, MIND.

MIND (2003) 'Mental Health and Social Wellbeing of Gay Men, Lesbians, and Bisexuals in England and Wales, London, MIND.

Mindell, A. (1988) City Shadows, Psychological Interventions in Psychiatry, New York, Routledge.

Mitchell, J. (1974/2000) Psychoanalysis and Feminism: a Radical Reassessment of Freudian Psychoanalysis, London, Penguin.

Modestin, J. and Amman, R. (1995) 'Mental Disorders and Criminal Behaviour', British Journal of Psychiatry, 166, pp. 667–75.

Moller-Leimkuhler, A. (2003) 'The Gender Gap in Suicide and Premature Death: Why Are Men so Vulnerable?', European Archives of Psychiatry and Clinical Neuroscience, Vol. 253, No. 1, pp. 1–8.

Monahan, J. (1993) 'Mental Disorder and Violence, Another Look', pp. 287–302 in Hodgkins, S. ed. Mental Disorder and Crime, Newbury Park, Calif., Sage.

Morgan, D. (1987) It Will Make a Man of You: Notes on National Service, Masculinity, and Autobiography, Manchester, Department of Sociology, University of Manchester.

Morgan, S. (2000) 'Risk-Making or Risk-Taking?', OpenMind, 101, Jan./Feb., pp. 16–17.

Morrall, P. (2000) Madness and Murder, London, Whurr Publishers.

Morrall, P. (2002) 'Madness, Murder and Media, A Realistic Critique of the Psychiatric Disciplines in Post-Liberal Society', Critical Psychiatry Network Conference, Beyond Drugs and Custody: Renewing Mental Health Practice, Birmingham, 26 April.

Morris, J. ed. (1996) Encounters with Strangers, London, Women's Press.

Morson, G. S. and Emerson, C. (1990) Mikhail Bakhtin, Creation of a Prosaics, Stanford, Calif., Stanford University Press.

Mouffe, C. (1992) 'Feminism, Citizenship and Radical Democratic Politics', pp. 369–84 in Butler, J. and Scott, J. eds Feminists Theorise the Political, New York, Routledge.

Mouffe, C. (1996) *Deconstruction, Pragmatism, and the Politics of Democracy*, London, Routledge.

Muldoon, M. (1995) 'Foucault, Madness and Language', *International Studies in Philosophy*, Vol. 27, Part 4, pp. 51–86.

Mullen, P. (1999) 'Dangerous People with Severe Personality Disorder, British Proposals for Managing them are Glaringly Wrong – and Unethical', *British Medical Journal*, Vol. 319, pp. 1146–7.

Mulvey, E. (1994) 'Assessing the Evidence of a Link Between Mental Illness and Violence', *Hospital and Community Psychiatry*, Vol. 45, No. 7, pp. 663–8.

Myers, M. (1989) 'Men Sexually Assaulted as Adults and Sexually Abused as Boys', *Archives of Sexual Behaviour*, Vol. 18, No 3, pp. 203–15.

Nairne, K. and Smith, G. (1984) *Dealing With Depression*, London, Women's Press.

Newnes, C., Holmes, G. and Dunn, C. (1999) *This Is Madness: a Critical Look at Psychiatry and the Future of Mental Health Services*, Ross-on-Wye, PCCS Books.

Ngai-Ling S. (2000) 'From Politics of Identity to Politics of Complexity', pp. 131–44 in Ahmed, S., Kilby, J., Lury, C., McNeil, M. and Skeggs, B. eds *Transformations: Thinking through Feminism*, London, Routledge.

Nicholson, L. ed. (1990) *Feminism/Postmodernism*, New York, Routledge.

Nicholson, L. (1999) *The Play of Reason, From the Modern to the Postmodern*, Buckingham, Open University Press.

Nicholson, L. and Fraser, N. (1999) 'Social Criticism without Philosophy: an Encounter between Feminism and Postmodernism', pp. 99–115 in Nicholson, N. ed. *The Play of Reason, From the Modern to the Postmodern*, Buckingham, Open University Press.

Nicholson, L. and Seidman, S. (1995) *Social Postmodernism, Beyond Identity Politics*, Cambridge, Cambridge University Press.

Niederland, W. (1984) *The Schreber Case: Psychoanalytic Profile of a Paranoid Personality*, Hillsdale, NJ, Analytic Press.

Nietzsche, F. (1871/1956) *The Birth of Tragedy*, trans. Francis Golffing, New York, Anchor.

Nietzsche, F. (1882/1974) *The Gay Science*, New York, Vintage Books.

Nietzsche, F. (1886/1970) *Beyond Good and Evil*, London, Penguin.

Nietzsche, F. (1887/1956) *The Genealogy of Morals, An Attack*, trans. Francis Golffing, New York, Anchor.

Nietzsche, F. (1887/1969) *Thus Spoke Zarathustra, A Book for Everyone and No One*, Harmondsworth, Penguin.

Nietzsche, F. (1888/1979) *Ecce Homo, How One Becomes What One Is*, trans. R. J. Hollingdale, London, Penguin.

Nietzsche, F. (1968) *The Will to Power*, trans. Walter Kaufmann and R. J. Hollingdale, New York, Vintage Books.

Norris, C. (1987) *Derrida*, London, Fontana.

O'Brien, M. (1981) *The Politics of Reproduction*, London, Routledge and Kegan Paul.

O'Hagan, M. (1996) *Two Accounts of Mental Distress*, pp. 44–50 in Read, J. and Reynolds, J. eds *Speaking Our Minds, An Anthology*, Basingstoke, Macmillan and Open University.

Olden, M. (2003) *An Interview with Pete Shaughnessy*, Asylum, Vol. 13, No. 7, pp. 13–14.

Oliver, M. (1996) *Understanding Disability: From Theory to Practice*, Basingstoke, Macmillan.

OpenMind (1994) *Personal Experiences of Mental Distress, 1983–1994*, London, MIND.

Oppel, F. (1993) 'Speaking of Immemorial Waters, Irigaray with Nietzsche', pp. 88–109 in Patton, P. ed. *Nietzsche, Feminism and Political Theory*, London, Routledge.

Otto, W. F. (1933) *Dionysos: Myths und Kilts*, trans. R. B. Palmer, Frankfurt.

Parker, C. and McCullogh, A. (1999) *Key Issues from Homicide Enquiries*, London, MIND.

Parker, I. (1995) 'Michel Foucault, Psychologist', The Psychologist, pp. 503–5.

Parker, I. (1997) *Psychoanalytic Culture, Psychoanalytic Discourse in Western Society*, London, Sage.

Parker, I. ed. (1999) *Deconstructing Psychotherapy*, London, Sage.

Parker, I., Georgaca, E., Harper, D., McClaughlin, T. and Stowell-Smith, M. (1995) *Deconstructing Psychopathology*, London, Sage.

Parton, N. (2000) 'Some Thoughts on the Relationship between Theory and Practice in and for Social Work', British Journal of Social Work, Vol. 30, pp. 449–63.

Pasley, M. ed. (1978) *Nietzsche, Imagery and Thought*, London, Methuen.

Patton, P. (1993) *Nietzsche, Feminism and Political Theory*, London, Routledge.

Payne, S. and Lart, R. (2004) 'Researching Suicidal Behaviour', Radical Statistics, http://www.radstats.org.uk/no070/index.htm. April 2004.

Pease, B. (1999) 'Deconstructing Masculinity – Reconstructing Men', pp. 97–112 in Pease, B. and Fook, J. eds *Transforming Social Work Practice: Postmodern Critical Perspectives*, London, Routledge.

Pease, B. (2000) *Recreating Men, Postmodern Masculinity Politics*, London, Sage.

Pease, B. (2000b) 'Researching Pro-feminist Men's Narratives, Participatory Methodologies in a Postmodern Frame', pp. 136–58 in Fawcett, B., Featherstone, B., Fook, J. and Rossiter, A. eds *Practice and Research in Social Work, Postmodern Feminist Perspectives*, London, Routledge.

Pease, B. (2002) '(Re)Constructing Men's Interests', Men and Masculinities, Vol. 5, No. 2, October, pp. 165–77.

Pease, B. and Fook, J. eds (1999) *Transforming Social Work Practice: Postmodern Critical Perspectives*, London, Routledge.

Pembroke, L. ed. (1994/1996) *Self-Harm, Perspective from Personal Experience*, London, Survivors Speak Out.

Perera, S. (1981) *Descent to the Goddess, a Way of Initiation for Women*, Toronto, Inner City Books.

Perkins, R. (1995) 'Whose Community Is It Anyway? Doubly Disadvantaged Groups in Rehabilitation and Community Care', Clinical Psychology Forum, Vol. 82, August, pp. 33–8.

Perkins, R. (1996) 'Choosing ECT', pp. 66–70 in Read, J. and Reynolds, J. *Speaking Our Minds, An Anthology*, Basingstoke, Macmillan and Open University.

Perkins, R. (1999) 'Madness, Distress, and the Language of Inclusion', OpenMind, 98, July/August, p. 6.

Perkins, R. and Moodley, P. (1993) 'The Arrogance of Insight?', Psychiatric Bulletin, 17, pp. 233–4.

Perkins, R. and Repper, J. (1999) 'Compliance or Informed Choice', Journal of Mental Health, Vol. 8, No. 2, pp. 117–29.

Petersen, A. (1998) *Unmasking the Masculine, 'Men' and 'Identity' in a Sceptical Age*, London, Sage.

Petersen, A. and Bunton, R. eds (1997) *Foucault, Health and Medicine*, London, Routledge.

Philo, G. ed. (1996) *Media and Mental Distress*, The Glasgow Media Group, London, Longman.

Pilgrim, D. (1997) *Psychotherapy and Society*, London, Sage.

Pilgrim, D. and Rogers, A. (1993/1999) *A Sociology of Mental Health and Illness*, 2nd edition, Buckingham, Open University Press.

Pilgrim, D. and Rogers, A. (1997) 'Mental Health, Critical Realism and Lay Knowledge', pp. 32–49 in Ussher, J. ed. *Body Talk: the Material and Discursive Regulation of Sexuality, Madness, and Reproduction'*, London, Routledge.

Pilgrim, D. and Rogers, A. (2003) *Mental Health and Inequality*, Basingstoke, Palgrave Macmillan.

Pireddu, N. (1996) 'The Mark and the Mask: Psychosis in Artaud's Alphabet of Cruelty', Arachne, Vol. 3, Part 1, pp. 43–65.

Plath, S. (1963) *The Bell Jar*, London, Heinemann.

Plumb, A (1993) 'The Challenge of Self-Advocacy', Feminism and Psychology, Vol. 3, No. 2, pp. 169–87.

Plumb, A. (1994) *Distress or Disability?*, Manchester, GMCDP Publications.

Plumb, A. (1999) 'New Mental Health Legislation. A Lifesaver? Changing Paradigm and Practice', Social Work Education, Vol. 18, No. 4, pp. 459–78.

Plummer, K. (1995) *Telling Sexual Stories; Power, Change, and Social Worlds*, London, Routledge.

Plumwood, V. (1993) *Feminism and the Mastery of Nature*, London, Routledge.

Polt, R. (1999) *Heidegger, An Introduction*, Ithaca, NY, Cornell University Press.

Porter, R. (1987) *A Social History of Madness, Stories of the Insane*, London, Weidenfeld and Nicolson.

Pozatek, E. (1994) 'The Problem of Certainty: Clinical Social Work in the Postmodern Era', Social Work, Vol. 39, No. 4, July, pp. 396–403.

Price, J. and Shildrick, M. (1998) 'Uncertain Thoughts on the Dis/Abled Body', pp. 224–49 in *Vital Signs, Feminist Reconfigurations of the Bio/logical Body*, Edinburgh, Edinburgh University Press.

Price, J. and Shildrick, M. (1999) *Feminist Theory and the Body, a Reader*, Edinburgh, Edinburgh University Press.

Prins, H. (1999) *Will They Do it Again? Risk Assessment and Management in Criminal Justice and Psychiatry*, London, Routledge.

Prior, P. (1999) *Gender and Mental Health*, London, Macmillan.

Pritchard, C. (1992) 'Is There a Link Between Suicide in Young Men and Unemployment? A Comparison of the U.K. with Other European Community Countries', British Journal of Psychiatry, Vol. 160, pp. 750–6.

Rabinow, P. ed. (1984/1991) *The Foucault Reader*, London, Penguin.

Rabinow, P. ed. (1994/2000) *Michel Foucault, Ethics. Essential Works of Foucault 1954–1984, Volume 1*, London, Penguin.

Rajchman, J. (1985) *Michel Foucault, the Freedom of Philosophy*, New York, Columbia University Press.

Rajchman, J. (1995) 'Foucault Ten Years After', New Formations, No. 25, Summer, pp. 14–20.

Ramazanoglu, C. (1989) *Feminism and the Contradiction of Oppression*, London, Routledge.

Ramazanoglu, C. ed. (1993) *Up Against Foucault, Explorations of Some Tensions Between Foucault and Feminism*, London, Routledge.

Ramazanoglu, C. and Holland, J. (1993) 'Women's Sexuality and Men's Appropriation of Desire', pp. 239–64 in Ramazanoglu, C. ed. Up Against Foucault, London, Routledge.

Rattansi, A. (1995) 'Just Framing: Ethnicities and Racisms in a "Postmodern" Framework', pp. 250–86 in Nicholson, L. and Seidman, S. eds Social Postmodernism – Beyond Identity Politics, Cambridge, Cambridge University Press.

Read, J. (1992/1994) 'Real Men Do Cry', in Personal Experiences of Mental Distress, 1983–1994, London, MIND.

Read, J. ed. (2001) Something Inside So Strong, London, Mental Health Foundation.

Read, J. and Baker, S. (1996) Not Just Sticks and Stones. A Survey of the Stigma, Taboos, and Discrimination, Experienced by People with Mental Health Problems, London, MIND.

Read, J. and Reynolds, J. (1996) Speaking Our Minds: an Anthology, Basingstoke, Open University and Macmillan.

Read, J. and Wallcraft, J. (1995) Guidelines on Equal Opportunities and Mental Health, London, Mind and Unison.

Real, T. (1997) I Don't Want to Talk About It: Overcoming the Secret Legacy of Male Depression, Dublin, New Leaf.

Repper, J. and Perkins, R. (1995) 'The Deserving and the Undeserving: Selectivity and Progress in a Community Care Service', Journal of Mental Health, Vol. 4, pp. 483–98.

Ritchie, J. (1994) The Report of the Inquiry into the Care and Treatment of Christopher Clunis, London, HMSO.

Rodgers, P. and Mathias, J (1996) 'Putting the Men into Mental Health', OpenMind, 79, February/March, p. 22.

Rogers, A. and Pilgrim, D. (1991) '"Pulling Down Churches": Accounting for the British Mental Health Users' Movement', Sociology of Health and Illness, Vol. 13, No. 2, pp. 129–48.

Rogers, A. and Pilgrim, D. (2003) Mental Health and Inequality, Basingstoke, Palgrave Macmillan.

Romme, M. and Escher, S. (1993) Accepting Voices, London, Mind.

Rorty, R. (1996) 'Remarks on Deconstruction and Pragmatism', pp. 13–18 in Mouffe, C. ed. Deconstruction, Pragmatism, and the Politics of Democracy, London, Routledge.

Rose, D. (2001) 'Terms of Engagement', OpenMind, 108, March/April pp. 16–17.

Rose, N. (1996) Inventing Ourselves: Psychology, Power, and Personhood, Cambridge, Cambridge University Press.

Rose, N. (1989/1999) Governing the Soul; the Shaping of the Private Self, London, Free Association Books.

Rose, N. (1998) 'Governing Risky Individuals', Psychiatry, Psychology, and Law, Vol. 5, No. 2, pp. 177–95.

Rose, N. (1999) Powers of Freedom, Reframing Political Thought, Cambridge, Cambridge University Press.

Rose, N. (2000) 'Government and Control', British Journal of Criminology, Vol. 40, pp. 321–39.

Rose, S. (1997) Lifelines; Biology, Freedom, Determinism, London, Penguin.

Rosen S. (1989) The Ancients and the Moderns: Re-Thinking Modernity, New Haven, Yale University Press.

Roszak, T. (2000) The Gendered Atom: Reflections of the Sexual Psychology of Science, Totnes, Green Books.

Rotov, M. (1994) 'Ward Environment and Violence', Criminal Behaviour and Mental Health, 4, pp. 259–66.

Rowan, J. (1987) The Horned God; Feminism and Men as Wounding and Healing, London, Routledge.

Rowan, J. (1997) Healing the Male Psyche: Therapy as Initiation, London, Routledge.

Rowland, B. (1978) Birds with Human Souls, a Guide to Bird Symbolism, Knoxville, University of Tennessee.

Roy, A. (2002) The Algebra of Infinite Justice, London, Flamingo.

Rustin, M. (1995) 'Lacan, Klein, and Politics, The Positive and Negative in Psychoanalytic Thought', pp. 223–45 in Elliot, A. and Frosh, S. eds Psychoanalysis in Contexts, London, Routledge.

Sadler, T. (1995) Nietzsche, Truth and Redemption, Critique of the Postmodern Nietzsche, New Jersey, Athlone Press.

Safranski, R. (2002) Nietzsche, a Philosophical Biography, London, Granta.

Said, E. (1978) Orientalism, Harmondsworth, Penguin.

Sainsbury Centre (2002) Breaking the Circles of Fear: a Review of the Relationship between Mental Health Services and African and Caribbean Communities, London, Sainsbury Centre.

Sallis, J. (1991) Crossings, Nietzsche and the Space of Tragedy, Chicago, Ill., University of Chicago Press.

Salomé, L. (1988) Nietzsche, Redding Ridge, Black Swan.

Samaritans (1999) Young Men Speak Out, London, Samaritans.

Santner, E. (1996) My Own Private Germany, Daniel Paul Schreber's Secret History of Modernity, Princeton, NJ, Princeton University Press.

Sardar, Z. (1998) Postmodernism and the Other, the New Imperialism of Western Culture, London, Pluto.

Sargant, W. (1958) 'Discussion on Sedation and Stimulation in Man', Proceedings of the Royal Society of Medicine, Vol. 51, No. 353, pp. 13–18.

Sarup, M. (1996) Identity, Culture and the Postmodern World, Edinburgh, Edinburgh University Press.

Sashidharan, S. and Francis, E. (1999) 'Racism in Psychiatry Necessitates Reappraisal of General Procedures and Eurocentric Theories', British Medical Journal, Vol. 24, 319 (7204), p. 254.

Sass, L. (1987) 'Schreber's Panopticism: Psychosis and the Modern Soul', Social Research, Vol. 54, No. 1, Spring, pp. 101–47.

Sass, L. (1992) Madness and Modernism, Insanity in the Light of Modern Art, Literature, and Thought, New York, Basic Books.

Sassoon, M. and Lindow, V. (1995) 'Consulting and Empowering Black Mental Health System Users', in Fernando, S. ed. Mental Health in a Multi-Ethnic Society: a Multi-disciplinary Handbook, London, Routledge.

Sattel, J. (1976/1989) 'The Inexpressive Male, Tragedy or Sexual Politics', pp. 374–82 in Kimmel, M. and Messner, M., Men's Lives, New York, Macmillan.

Sawick, J. (1991) Disciplining Foucault, New York, Routledge.

Sayce, L. (1995) 'Response to Violence, a Framework for Fair Treatment', in Crichton, J. ed. Psychiatric Patient Violence: Risk and Response, London, Duckworth.

Sayce, L. (2000) From Psychiatric Patient to Citizen, Overcoming Discrimination and Social Exclusion, Basingstoke, Macmillan.

Schapira, K., Linsley, K., Linsley, J., Kelly, T. and Kay, D. (2001) 'Relationship of Suicide Rates to Social Factors and Availability of Lethal Methods: Comparison of Suicide Rates in Newcastle upon Tyne 1961–1965 and 1985–1994', British Journal of Psychiatry, 178. May, pp. 458–64.

Schatzman, M. (1973) Soul Murder, Persecution in the Family, London, Allen Lane.

Scheman, N. (1996) 'Though This be Method, Yet There is Madness in it: Paranoia and Liberal Epistemology', pp. 203–19 in Keller, E. F. and Longino, H. eds Feminism and Science, Oxford, Oxford University Press.

Schneider, M. (2001) 'The Sword and the Bridge; the Anatomical and the Political in Conceptions of Sexual Difference', Radical Philosophy, 106, March/April, pp. 7–14.

Schreber, D. (1903/2000) Memoirs of My Nervous Illness, introduction by Rosemary Dinnage, trans. Ida MacAlpine and Richard Hunter, New York, New York Review of Books.

Schrift, A. (1995) Nietzsche's French Legacy: a Genealogy of Poststructuralism, London. Routledge.

Schrift, A. (2000) Why Nietzsche Still? Reflections on Drama, Culture, and Politics, Berkeley, University of California Press.

Scott, J. (1992) 'Experience', pp. 22–40 in Butler, J. and Scott, J., Feminists Theorise the Political, New York, Routledge.

Scott, S. (1997) 'Feminists and False Memories: A Case of Postmodern Amnesia', Feminism and Psychology, Vol. 7, No. 1, pp. 33–8.

Scourfield, J. (2004) 'Suicidal Masculinities', Paper for the British Sociological Association Conference, York.

Sedgwick, P. ed. (1995) Nietzsche, a Critical Reader, Oxford, Blackwell.

Sedgwick, P. (2001) Descartes to Derrida, an Introduction to European Philosophy, Oxford, Blackwell.

Segal, L. (1990/1997) Slow Motion, Changing Masculinities, Changing Men, London. Virago.

Segal, L. (1993) 'Changing Men: Masculinities in Context', Theory and Society, Vol. 22, pp. 625–41.

Seidler, V. (1994) Unreasonable Men, Masculinity and Social Theory, London, Routledge.

Seidler, V. (1997) Man Enough, Embodying Masculinities, London, Sage.

Seidler, V. (1998) 'Masculinity, Violence, and Emotional Life', pp. 193–210 in Bendelow, G. and Williams, S. eds Emotions in Social Life: Critical Themes and Contemporary Issues, London, Routledge.

Seidler, V. (2001) 'Jean-François Lyotard', pp. 128–39 in Elliot, A. and Turner, B., Profiles in Contemporary Social Theory, London, Sage.

Seidman, S. ed. (1994) The Postmodern Turn; New Perspectives on Social Theory, Cambridge, Cambridge University Press.

Seidman, S. (1994/2004) Contested Knowledge, Social Theory Today, Oxford, Blackwell.

Seidman, S. and Alexander, J. (2001) The New Social Theory Reader, London, Routledge.

Sengupta, K. (2001) ' "Tragic" Statue for the Great War's Executed Soldiers', The Independent, 22 June.

Shah, A. and De, T. (1998) 'Suicide and the Elderly', International Journal of Psychiatry and Clinical Practice, Vol. 2, pp. 3–17.

Shakespeare, T. (1999) 'When Is a Man not a Man? When He's Disabled', pp. 47–58 in Wild, J. ed. Working with Men for Change, London, UCL Press.

Shakespeare, T., Gillespie-Sells, K. and Davies, D. eds (1996) 'The Sexual Politics of Disability: Untold Stories, London, Cassell.

Shaw, C. and Proctor, G. (2004) 'Women at the Margins, a Feminist Critique of Borderline Personality Disorder', Asylum, Vol. 14, No. 3, pp. 8–9.

Sheridan, A. (1980) Michel Foucault, the Will to Truth, London, Tavistock.

Shildrick, M. (1997) Leaky Bodies and Boundaries, Feminism, Postmodernism and (Bio)ethics, London, Routledge.

Shildrick, M. and Price, J. eds (1998) Vital Signs: Feminist Reconfigurations of the Bio/logical Body, Edinburgh, Edinburgh University Press.

Shotter, J. and Gergen, K. eds (1989) Texts of Identity, London, Sage.

Showalter, E. (1987) The Female Malady, London, Virago.

Showalter, E. (1997) Hystories, Hysterical Epidemics and Modern Culture, London, Picador.

Simpson, T. (1996) 'Beyond Rage', pp. 215–16 in Read, J. and Reynolds, J. eds Speaking Our Minds, Basingstoke, Open University and Macmillan.

Simpson, T (1999) 'Risk – The Need for Perspective', Crisis Point, Vol. 1, No. 9, March.

Smith, G., Bartlett, A. and King, M. (2004) 'Treatments of Homosexuality in Britain Since the 1950's: An Oral History: The Experience of Patients', British Medical Journal, Vol. 328, pp. 427–9.

Smith, K. and Leon, L. (2001) Developing Community Based Crisis Services for 16–25 Year Olds Experiencing a Mental Health Crisis, London, Mental Health Foundation.

Spellman, E. (1999) 'Woman as Body: Ancient and Contemporary Views', pp. 32–41 in Price, J. and Shildrick, M. eds Feminist Theory and the Body, Edinburgh, Edinburgh University Press.

Spender, D. (1980) Man Made Language, London, Routledge and Kegan Paul.

Spregnether, M. (1995) 'Mourning Freud', pp. 142–65 in Elliot, A. and Frosh, S. eds, Psychoanalysis in Contexts, London, Routledge.

Stack, G. (2000) 'Suicide, A Fifteen Year Review of the Sociological Literature, Part One', Suicide and Life Threatening Behaviour, Vol. 30, pp. 145–62.

Stanley, L. (1992) The Auto/biographical I, Manchester, Manchester University Press.

Staples, R. (1982) Black Masculinity: the Black Man's Role in American Society, San Francisco, Calif., The Black Scholar Press.

Starhawk (1979) The Spiral Dance: a Rebirth of the Ancient Religion of the Great Goddess, San Francisco, Harper and Row.

Stern, J. P. (1979) A Study of Nietzsche, Cambridge, Cambridge University Press.

Stowell-Smith, M. and McKeown, M. (1999) 'Race, Psychopathy, and the Self: A Discourse Analytic Study', British Journal of Medical Psychology, Vol. 72, pp. 459–70.

Strickland, C. (1993) 'So You're Thinking of Setting up a Crisis Service?', OpenMind, 63, June/July, p. 15.

Stringer, R. (2000) '"A Nietzschean Breed": Feminism, Victimology, Ressentiment', pp. 247–73 in Schrift, A. ed. Why Nietzsche Still? Reflections on Drama, Culture, and Politics, Berkeley, University of California Press.

Swan, V. (1999) 'Narrative, Foucault and Feminism: Implications for Therapeutic Practice', pp. 103–14 in Parker, I. ed. Deconstructing Psychotherapy, London, Sage.

Swanson, J., Holzer III, C., Ganju, V. and Jono, R. (1990) 'Mental Disorder, Substance Abuse and Community Violence: Evidence from the Epidemiological Catchment Area Surveys', Hospital and Community Psychiatry, 41, pp. 761–70.

Swanwick, G. and Clare, A. (1997) 'Suicide in Ireland, 1945–1992: Social Correlates', Irish Medical Journal, Vol. 90, No. 3, pp. 106–8.

Swartz, S. (1996) 'Shrinking, a Postmodern Perspective on Psychiatric Case Histories', South African Journal of Psychology, Vol. 26, No. 3, pp. 150–6.

Swett, C., Surrey, J. and Cohen, C. (1990) 'Sexual and Physical Abuse Histories and Psychiatric Symptoms among Male Psychiatric Outpatients', American Journal of Psychiatry, Vol. 147, No. 5, May, pp. 632–6.

Tacey, D. (1997) Remaking Men: Jung, Spirituality and Social Change, London, Routledge.

Tarnas, R. (1996) The Passion of the Western Mind, Understanding the Ideas that Have Shaped our World View, London, Pimlico.

Tatchell, P. (2000) 'Aversion Therapy Is Like a Visit to the Dentist', Asylum, Vol. 12, No. 3, pp. 21–3.

Taylor, B. (1993/1996) 'Reflections on Therapy', pp. 158–62 in Read, J. and Reynolds, J. eds Speaking Our Minds, An Anthology, Basingstoke, Macmillan and Open University Press.

Taylor, C. (1986) 'Foucault on Freedom and Truth', pp. 69–102 in Couzens-Hoy, D. ed. Foucault, a Critical Reader, Oxford, Blackwell.

Taylor, P. and Gunn, J. (1999) 'Homicides by People with Mental Illness: Myth and Reality', British Journal of Psychiatry, 174, pp. 9–14.

Taylor, P. and Monahan, J. (1996) 'Commentary: Dangerous Patients or Dangerous Diseases?', British Medical Journal, Vol. 312, pp. 967–9.

Taylor-Gooby, P. (1994) 'Postmodernism and Social Policy, a Great Leap Backwards?', Journal of Social Policy, Vol. 232, No. 3, pp. 385–405.

Theweleit, K. (1989) Male Fantasies, Volume 2: Male Bodies, Psychoanalysing the White Terror, Cambridge, Polity Press.

Thomas, P. (1996) 'Electroshock Therapy, More Shock than Value?', What the Doctors Don't Tell You, November, Vol. 7, No. 8.

Timimi, S. (2005) Naughty Boys: Anti-social Behaviour, A.D.H.D. and the Role of Culture, Basingstoke, Palgrave Macmillan.

Tourish, D. and Irving, P. (1995) 'Group Influences and the Psychology of Cultism within Re-Evaluation Counselling, A Critique', Counselling Psychology Quarterly, Vol. 8, No. 1, pp. 15–30.

Trivedi, P. (2002) 'Racism, Social Exclusion and Mental Health, A Black User's Perspective', pp. 71–82 in Bhui, K., Racism and Mental Health, Prejudice and Suffering, London, Jessica Kingsley.

Tudor, K. (1999) 'Men in Therapy: Opportunity and Change', pp. 73–97 in Wild, J. ed. Working with Men for Change, London, UCL Press.

Turkle, S. (1981) 'French Anti-Psychiatry', pp. 150–83 in Ingelby, D. ed. Critical Psychiatry, The Politics of Mental Health, Harmondsworth, Penguin.

Urwin, C. (1984/1998) 'Power Relations and the Emergence of Language', pp. 264–322 in Henriques, J., Hollway, W., Urwin, C., Venn, C. and Walkerdine, V. eds Changing the Subject, Psychology, Social Regulation and Subjectivity, London, Routledge.

Ussher, J. (1991) Women's Madness: Misogyny or Mental Illness?, London, Harvester Wheatsheaf.

Ussher, J. (1997) Body Talk; the Material and Discursive Regulation of Sexuality, Madness and Reproduction, London, Routledge.

Ussher, J. and Nicholson, P. (1992) *Gender Issues in Clinical Psychology*, London, Routledge.

Wagner-Martin, L. (1987) *Sylvia Plath, a Biography*, New York, St Martin's Press.

Waites, M. (2003) 'Homosexuality, Heterosexuality and the Age of Consent in the United Kingdom', in Sociology, Vol. 37, No. 4, pp. 637–55.

Walby, S. (1990) *Theorising Patriarchy*, Oxford, Blackwell.

Walker, L. E. (1984) *Women and Mental Health Policy*, Beverley Hills, Calif., Sage.

Walker, Z. and Seifert, R. (1994) 'Violent Incidents in a Psychiatric Intensive Care Unit', British Journal of Psychiatry, 164, pp. 826–8.

Wallblinger, W. (1830) 'Friedrich Hölderlin's Life, Poetry, and Madness', trans. Scott J. Thompson, Walter Benjamin Research Syndicate, www.wbenjamin.org/holderlin. html accessed October 2002.

Wallcraft, J. (1996) 'Becoming Fully Ourselves', in Read, J. and Reynolds, J. eds *Speaking Our Minds*, Basingstoke, Macmillan and Open University Press.

Wallcraft, J. and Michaelson, J. (2001) 'Developing a Survivor Discourse to Replace the "Psychopathology" of Breakdown and Crisis', pp. 177–89 in Newnes, C., Holmes, G. and Dunn, C. eds *This is Madness Too, Critical Perspectives on Mental Health Services*, Ross on Wye, PCCS Books.

Ward, M. and Applin, C. (1998) *The Unlearned Lesson, the Role of Alcohol and Drug Misuse in Homicides Perpetrated by People with Mental Health Problems*, London, Wynne Howard Books.

Ward, N. (1999) 'Twelve of the Fifty-One Shocks of Antonin Artaud', New Theatre Quarterly, Vol. 15, No. 58, May, pp. 123–30.

Warner, R. (1985/1994) *Recovery from Schizophrenia: Psychiatry and Political Economy*, London, Routledge and Kegan Paul.

Warner, S. (1996) 'Special Women, Special Places: Women and High Security Mental Hospitals', pp. 96–113 in Burman, E. *et al.* eds *Psychology, Discourse, Practice: From Regulation to Resistance*, London, Taylor and Francis.

Warner, W. B. (1986) *Chance and the Text of Experience*, Ithaca, NY, Cornell University Press.

Warren, M. (1988) *Nietzsche and Political Thought*, Cambridge, Mass., The MIT Press.

Weedon, C. (1997) *Feminist Practice and Poststructuralist Theory*, 2nd edition, Oxford, Blackwell.

Weedon, C. (1999) *Feminism, Theory, and the Politics of Difference*, Oxford, Blackwell.

Weeks, J. (1985) *Sexuality and its Discontents: Meanings, Myths, and Modern Sexualities*, London, Routledge.

Weinberg, G. (1973) *Society and the Healthy Homosexual*, New York, Anchor.

Westwood, S. (1994) 'Racism, Mental Illness and The Politics of Identity', pp. 247–65 in Rattansi, A. and Westwood, S. eds *Racism, Modernity, and Identity*, Cambridge, Polity Press.

Wetherell, M. and Edley, N. (1999) 'Negotiating Hegemonic Masculinity: Imaginary Positions and Psycho-Discursive Practices', Feminism and Psychology, Vol. 9, No. 3, pp. 335–56.

Whiffen, V. and Clark, S. (1997) 'Does Victimisation Account for Sex Differences in Depressive Symptoms?', British Journal of Psychology, 36, pp. 185–93.

White, A. (1990) *Within Nietzsche's Labyrinth*, New York, Routledge.

White, M. and Epston, D. (1990) *Narrative Means to Therapeutic Ends*, Adelaide, Dulwich Centre.

Whitehead, S. (2002) *Men and Masculinities*, Cambridge, Polity.

Whitehead, S. and Barrett, F. eds (2001) *The Masculinities Reader*, Cambridge, Polity Press.

Whitmer, B. (1997) *The Violence Mythos*, Albany, State University of New York Press.

Whitmont, E. (1982/1997) *Return of the Goddess*, New York, Continuum.

Wild, J. ed. (1999) *Working with Men for Change*, London, UCL Press.

Wilkinson, S. (1994) 'Women and Madness: a Reappraisal', Feminism and Psychology, Vol. 4, No. 2, pp. 261–305.

Williams, R. (1965) *The Long Revolution*, London, Penguin.

Williams, R. (1980) *Problems in Materialism and Culture*, London, Verso.

Wilson, A. (1991) *Understanding Black Adolescent Violence: Its Remediation and Prevention*, New York, Afrikan World Infosystems.

Wilson, A. and Beresford, P. (2002) *Madness, Distress and Postmodernity: Putting the Record Straight*, pp. 143–58 in Corker, M. and Shakespeare, T. eds *Disability/Postmodernity – Embodying Disability Theory*, London, Continuum.

Wilson, D. (2005) *Death at the Hands of the State*, London, Howard League for Penal Reform.

Witz, A. (1992) *Professions and Patriarchy*, London, Routledge.

Young, I. M. (1990) *Justice and the Politics of Difference*, Princeton, NY, Princeton University Press.

Yovel, Y. (1994) 'Nietzsche, the Jews, and Ressentiment', pp. 214–36 in Schacht, R. ed. *Nietzsche, Genealogy, Morality*, Berkeley, University of California Press.

Zaitchik, M. and Mosher, D. (1993) 'Criminal Justice Implications of the Macho Personality Constellation', Criminal Justice and Behaviour, Vol. 20, No. 3, September, pp. 227–39.

Zeitlin, I. (1994) *Nietzsche, a Re-examination*, Cambridge, Polity Press.

Index

aggression 18, 181; and suicide 179;
    therapeutic 168
Ahmed, S. 63, 129
Alcoff, L. 141
Allison, D. 22, 56, 61, 215n, 217n
ally 7, 204
Althusser, Louis 225n, 228n, 229n
Apollo 75, 76
Artaud, Antonin 8, 46, 47–8, 79, 96,151;
    adopts mother's maiden name 92;
    asylum experience 90, 92; authentic
    madman 94, 96; electroshock 93;
    failure of *The Cenci* 95–6; and
    Nietzsche 80–2; Theatre of Cruelty
    82–3; 95–6; *To Have Done with the
    Judgement of God* 86; unpower 84
Ascheim, S. 56–7, 59–60
attention deficit hyperactivity disorder
    (ADHD) 11
authentic self 138
authenticity 145–7
autism, high functioning 10
autobiographical writing 4–5, 141, 142,
    203; critical 5–8, 49
aversion therapy 152

Bauman, Z. 31, 32, 35, 36–7, 166
Bell, C. 150
Bennett, David 243n
Bentham, J. 29, 31
Beresford, P. 169, 171, 235n
Best, S. 47, 213n
Bhabha, H. 187–8
Binswanger, Ludwig 119
bio-behavioural research 172, 243n
biography 46, 64, 101, 202; critical 46,
    48–9, 50–1, 52, 78, 115; Foucault and
    100, 102; narrative therapy and 201

biological foundationalism 123–4
biomedical psychiatry 146, 152
black and ethnic minorities men 12;
    medicalisation 173, 175, 176; seen as
    dangerous 12, 162, 174–5; and
    schizophrenia 152–3
black rage 174–5, 176
Black Skins, White Masks (Fanon) 175,
    187
Bloch, D. 128
Bly, R. 14, 19, 20
'Body without Organs' 135, 221n
Boyne, R. 223n
boys 20; attention deficit hyperactivity
    disorder 11; bio-behavioural research
    172, 243n
Bracken, P. 27, 34, 190–1
Brah, A. 33, 176
breakthrough 38
Breggin, P. 245n
Brown, W. 143–4, 145–6, 172–3, 198–9
Busfield, J. 11, 150
Butler, J. 107, 126; performativity of
    gender 124, 125

Callinicos, A. 51, 56
Campbell, P. 168–9, 206, 210n
Canetto, S. 178
Chadwick, P. 156–7
Chamberlin, J. 140, 143
Chesler, P. 14–15, 18, 156
Church, K. 5, 6, 142
Clare, A. 177, 179, 217n
Clifford, J. 27
clinical discourse 87–91, 190–2
Clunis, Christopher 175–6
Cobbs, P. 174
Coleman, R. 157, 161, 169